I have had the distinct pleasure of seeing John Vonhof work with endurance athletes before, during, and after some of the world's toughest foot races, and I can say with great confidence that no one knows feet better than John. Based on years of research and experience, he has compiled *the* ultimate guide on foot care for athletes. *Fixing Your Feet* contains practical treatments of foot problems and reveals tried-and-true secrets about how to prevent them. Whether you are a recreational hiker, an adventure racer, or an elite ultramarathon runner, this book has the answers you've been looking for.

—Lisa Bliss, MD, Medical Director of
the "World's Toughest Foot Race," the Badwater Ultramarathon

John Vonhof has more practical experience fixing feet than anyone I know. At the Badwater Ultramarathon he helps participants by working on blister prevention and repairing feet, enabling them to endure exposure to heat, friction, and moisture (the main causes of blisters). John is the expert, has the experience, and is the go-to guy for feet. *Fixing Your Feet* is comprehensive and complete; it is a must-read for foot care.

—Marshall Ulrich
adventure racer and seven summiter who has crossed
Death Valley 22 times; author of Running on Empty

If you are an extreme athlete, you need this book. It's confession time. As a veteran of more than 80 marathons as well as ultramarathons up to 100 miles, and being a podiatrist for 18 years, I thought I knew it all. John's comprehensive approach of asking the so-called medical experts as well as the real experts out in the trenches for their tried-and-true advice will bring you more value for your endurance event than a podiatry degree ever will.

—Bill Johncock, DPM
Fellow, American Academy of Sports Medicine
Board Certified, American Board of Podiatric Surgery

Just about everything I have learned and passed on about working on endurance athletes' and soldiers' feet I have learned from watching John completely and patiently repair blistered feet that I would have considered candidates for amputation. I am truly in awe of what John does with bad feet. The shame is that his reservoir of knowledge is so comprehensive that had his patients listened to him ahead of time on prevention, they would likely not have needed his services. There is no one alive today, in my experience, who has the knowledge and experience on how to prevent and—if you didn't listen the first time—fix endurance athlete foot problems than John. I cheerfully and humbly doff my hat to him.

—Anthony C. "Woofie" Humpage, CSCS, FMS
USA Triathlon Certified Coach
Badwater Ultramarathon medical team
Developer of SELECTED! a program for U.S. Army Special Forces

I consider *Fixing Your Feet* a must-have for every sports podiatrist! It is an invaluable resource.

—**Rob Conenello, DPM**
Global Clinical Advisor, Special Olympics
Honorary Police Surgeon, New York Police Department
Vice President, American Academy of Podiatric Sports Medicine

When a foot problem arises, this book's clear, concise explanations and fixes are wonderful. The book is comprehensive; every relevant topic is addressed. If you run ultras and you have at least one foot, you should have *Fixing Your Feet*.

—**Karl King**
president of SUCCEED Sportsdrink, LLC,
and inventor of S! Caps

Fixing Your Feet is the go-to foot care reference for the endurance athlete, period. Don't prepare for your next event without it.

—**Tim Jantz, DPM**
podiatrist and ultrarunner; www.foot-doc.net

If there's one thing that can turn an ultrarun or adventure race into a nightmare experience, it is sore and injured feet. Blistering and other foot ailments are not a "luck," or lack thereof, situation. Prerace care and conditioning, maintenance during a race, and the knowledge of how to deal with issues as they arise are crucial. Vonhof is *the* undisputed foot guru. His advice is sound and simple, and it comes as much from his own experience as his time spent at hundreds of races, working with thousands of athletes. *Fixing Your Feet* guides you through caring for and maintaining your feet. Although he teaches you how to patch blisters and deal with a variety of foot ailments, his objective is to have you running pain free from start to finish. He promotes prevention. And the recipe is easy. Read *Fixing Your Feet*. Do. Run.

—**Lisa de Speville, adventure racer,**
ultrarunner, and editor of www.ar.co.za,
South Africa's adventure racing website

I began using John's techniques from a photocopied handout at my very first expedition race and it was a godsend. As soon as I got home, I ordered the book and it became my bible. John and I became friends when we met at Primal Quest and I consider him my mentor. I highly recommend *Fixing Your Feet* to anyone who puts their feet through adverse conditions. You will wonder how you ever raced without it!

—**Maddalena Acconci, also known as M. A.**
Emergency Medical Responder/Advanced Wilderness First Responder
Medical Coordinator, Frontier Adventure Racing, Canada

In preparing for the 2009 four-day, 120-mile Nijmegen March in Holland, I had issues with shoe fit, blisters, toenail problems, and much more. While searching for answers, I found *Fixing Your Feet* and even e-mailed John. I was put on the right path, corrected all the errors in my training, and learned foot care—enabling me to cross the finish line and win my medal.

—William Hunter
93rd Nijmegen Marches, Medal reward #1, 50 x 4 kilometers
www.trainingforthenijmegenmarch.com

I have always had issues with blisters, particularly on long mountain runs. Since reading *Fixing Your Feet* and implementing John's techniques, I have not had any blister issues. This includes long runs in the mountains and pacing at Badwater for four years, including one double crossing and one starting at Las Vegas. For those with foot issues, this book is the solution to your foot problems.

—Scott Morgan
ultrarunner, endurance athlete, climber, and coach for www.sealfit.com

---

Thank you for your amazing ability to give the runners such superb foot care and to educate while doing it. Your vast and incomparable knowledge of foot care for athletes in *Fixing Your Feet* is, without a doubt, the *best* in the entire world! I marvel always when I get the chance to work with you, as each time I come away learning more yet craving more. With your medical background and amazing focus and memory, each runner gets the unique opportunity to learn about his individual needs while you expertly patch and care for those sore feet.

—Denise Jones, Badwater Blister Queen

I can't praise *Fixing Your Feet* enough. It's written for us, the walkers and hikers and runners who need advice on what to do before and after we stress our feet.

—Wendy Bumgardner
About.com Guide to Walking, walking.about.com

This is it—the best book ever written on foot care. Everyone who has been bothered by foot problems or wants to prevent them should own this book.

—Bill Trolan, MD, author of the Blister Fighter Guide
and medical consultant to adventure racing teams

I reference *Fixing Your Feet* often when consulting with customers about their foot troubles. There simply is no replacement for the amount of relevant content introduced in *Fixing Your Feet*. The product recommendations are unbiased and based on experience with real athletes. *Fixing Your Feet* is a must-read for serious runners, hikers, and team sports athletes.

—Jason Pawelsky, Tamarack Habilitation Technologies,
ENGO Patches; www.goengo.com

Last week I successfully completed the Racing the Planet: Australia 2010, 250K race. It is the first time that I have completed a race of this distance, and having read your book really helped make the race a truly enjoyable experience. Of the 185 starting competitors, only 118 completed the race, and most competitors had a lot of problems with blisters from the first day. I truly believe that if I had not read *Fixing Your Feet* three months prior to the event, I would have been exactly in the same position. Instead I managed to complete the week with feet in great condition—and not a single blister.

—Nathan Wilson, ultrarunner, Australia

As a walker, runner, hiker, and podiatrist, I have found *Fixing Your Feet* full of essential information for athletes at all levels. Anyone with a foot problem would benefit from this book. An absolute must for runners, adventure racers, and ultrarunners!

—Christine Dobrowolski, podiatrist and author of Those Aching Feet

Fixing Your Feet is the encyclopedia of foot care! Whether you're looking for daily foot health tips or ways to survive prolonged and severe foot floggings in ultra-endurance sports, this is your one-stop source of foot info. John has done his homework and presents it in an organized and easy read. You've saved my feet!

—Terri Schneider, ultrarunner, adventure racer, and triathlete; www.terrischneider.net

Fixing Your Feet is the most comprehensive, easy to read, organized foot care guide on the market. Originally I purchased it for personal use; now I carry it with me during my travels, often using it as a conversation stimulator. Everyone likes to talk about their feet, and John does a great job helping me help others.

—Tammy Hanna, ENGO Patches; www.goengo.com

Through our experience as ultrarunners, we've noticed that our foot care needs continue to change, due to different environments, changes in training and racing, and even changes in our feet. We keep coming back to *Fixing Your Feet* for the most useful and comprehensive foot advice, and we always find the answers we're looking for. This new edition keeps us up to date with the latest products and trends. We couldn't ask for anything more!

—Gillian Robinson and Don Lundell ultrarunners and founders of www.zombierunner.com

Fixing Your Feet is the most comprehensive book that I have ever seen on foot care. As a person who has been running for more than 31 years and has run more than 100,000 miles, I know just how important it is to maintain proper care of your feet. I appreciate John's statement that there is no one method to treat each problem. What works for one runner may or may not work for another runner. I encourage every runner to use this book as a valuable resource.

—David Horton, ultrarunner and Pacific Crest Trail speed record holder; www.extremeultrarunning.com

FIXING YOUR
Feet
prevention and treatments
for athletes

John Vonhof

Fifth Edition

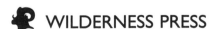 WILDERNESS PRESS

Fixing Your Feet: Prevention and Treatments for Athletes

1st Edition 1997
2nd Edition 2000
3rd Edition 2004
4th Edition 2006
5th Edition 2011
   3rd printing 2013

Manufactured in the United States of America

Published by: **Wilderness Press**
              c/o Keen Communications
              P.O. Box 43673
              Birmingham, AL 35243
              (800) 443-7227; FAX (205) 326-1012
              info@wildernesspress.com
              www.wildernesspress.com
Visit our website for a complete listing of our books and for ordering information.

Distributed by Publishers Group West

Many of the designations used by manufacturers and sellers to distinguish their products are claimed as trademarks. Where those designations appear in this book and the author is aware of a trademark claim, they are identified by initial capital letters. These products are listed in alphabetical order for the sake of simplicity. The order does not imply one product is more helpful or less helpful than another.

SAFETY NOTICE: Although Wilderness Press and the author have made every attempt to ensure that the information in this book is accurate at press time, they are not responsible for any loss, damage, injury, or inconvenience that may occur as a result of using this book. The information contained here is no substitute for professional advice or training. Readers are encouraged to seek medical help whenever possible.

Library of Congress Cataloging-in-Publication Data

Vonhof, John.
   Fixing your feet : prevention and treatments for athletes / John Vonhof. -- 5th ed.
      p. cm.
   ISBN-13: 978-0-89997-638-9
   ISBN-10: 0-89997-638-7
   1. Foot—Care and hygiene. 2. Running injuries—Prevention.3. Hiking injuries—Prevention.
   I. Title.
   RD563.V63 2011
   617.5'85—dc22
                              2010037007

Dedication

This fifth edition of *Fixing Your Feet* is dedicated to Denise Jones, the Badwater Blister Queen. Denise is my sounding board as we talk about foot care and how to fine-tune our taping, patching, and product ideas. She is a special, caring person who loves to help others with her foot care expertise. I value her friendship immensely—she walks the talk. Thanks, Denise.

Acknowledgments

Thank you to the thousands of athletes who, over the life of this book, have shared their experiences, asked for foot care help, and given me encouragement to keep writing about *Fixing Your Feet*.

Special thanks go to my wife, Kathie, for her continued patience through yet another rewrite and research process, and my son, Scott, who, after one of my 12-hour track runs in 1996, gave me the original idea for this book.

Thanks to the staff of Wilderness Press for believing in the ongoing potential for this fifth edition of *Fixing Your Feet*. Again, they continue to take it to a high level of professionalism.

My Motivation

Run with perseverance the race marked out for you. —*Hebrews 12:1*

Foreword

Whether participating in a 5K or 150K race, all athletes need to train appropriately to avoid injury. Train correctly and you can experience the wonders of the outdoors and the thrill of competition. Train incorrectly and you may sustain a significant injury that will not allow you to compete, nor reach your goal. In extreme situations, where athletes are out in the wilderness, injuries can have deadly consequences. Good athletes train appropriately and prepare for whatever obstacles might come their way.

Spending years competing as an endurance athlete, including adventure racing and triathlons, has taught me the importance of preparation and prevention. I can remember finishing 24-hour races having crossed several riverbeds, hiking over mountain passes and through slot canyons, thankful that my feet, though sore, were fine. Unlike the poor soul I passed at a checkpoint tending to a horrific blister requiring him to drop out of a race, I've learned the importance of taking care of one of the most important parts of my body—my feet. Our feet connect us to the surrounding terrain, propelling us toward our next destination. *Take care of your feet and the world is yours to enjoy. Ignore your feet and life can be a miserable experience.*

I've witnessed the impact of injuries to the feet as Medical Director for Racing the Planet (**www.racingtheplanet.com**). These ultraendurance running events challenge athletes to cross more than 150 miles over seven days through some of the harshest terrains around the world. My research has shown that for the majority of athletes who experience some sort of race injury, it's an injury related to their feet. Yet almost 25% of these athletes will not need medical care. How can that be? The answer lies in training and prevention. The majority of foot injuries are blisters, which can be managed appropriately if identified early. In fact, our medical team spends a good amount of time reminding athletes to protect their feet. Strategies include using lubricants, changing socks, checking skin for hot spots, and staying well hydrated and well nourished. However, mismanage blisters or other lower-extremity injuries, and athletes can experience serious illnesses, including skin infections, that cause them to drop out of the race.

That is why *Fixing Your Feet* is such an important resource. This comprehensive book provides some of the most detailed information regarding your feet and how to prevent or treat injuries, from one of the experts in the field. Looking through the pages, you'll learn about the basics of footwear, including new information regarding minimalist and barefoot running versus shod or traditional footwear. Preventive strategies focus on the role of clothing, compounds, taping, and the impact of various extreme conditions on your feet. Treatment recommendations will help you manage typical foot injuries relating to skin, muscles, and ligaments. Throughout, practical tips abound. It's why I typically recommend the book as a resource for any medical personnel helping with an ultraendurance running event or a wilderness expedition. Whether you are an athlete competing in a race or part of the medical team taking care of athletes, I recommend you keep *Fixing Your Feet* nearby.

—Brian J. Krabak, MD, MBA
Medical Director, Racing the Planet 4 Desert Series
Sports Medicine Physician, University of Washington
and Seattle Children's Hospital
Rehabilitation, Orthopedics, and Sports Medicine

Contents

Foreword   viii

Introduction   1

Getting the Most out of *Fixing Your Feet*   4

The Best of 15 Years of Foot Care   6

Part One: Foot Basics   **19**
  1. Seeking Medical Treatment 21
  2. You Can Have Healthy & Happy Feet 24
     Think "Feet" 24
     A Daily Ritual 24
     Talk to Your Doctor 25
     Summer Foot Care Basics 25
     Winter Foot Care Basics 26
     Aging Feet 26
  3. Sports & Your Feet 28
     Sport Similarities 29
     Differences in Terrain 30
     Conditioning 32
     Biomechanics 34

Part Two: Footwear Basics   **41**
  4. The Magic of Fit 43
     Buying Footwear 45
     Know Your Feet 47
     Components of a Good Fit 50
     Tips for a Good Fit 52
     Customizing Your Footwear 53
  5. Footwear & Insoles 55
     Brand Loyalty in Footwear 57
     The Anatomy of Footwear 58
     Running Shoes 59
     Sports Shoes 62
     Hiking Boots 64
     Choosing Lightweight Footwear 68
     Custom Shoes 69
     Sandals 70
     Insoles 72
  6. Barefoot & Minimalist Footwear 76
     Shoes vs. Minimalist Footwear 77
     The Value of "Going Bare" 78
     The Science on Barefoot Running 79
     Function & Form 80

Barefoot Precautions 81
Minimalist Footwear Choices 85

7. Socks... 94
Sock Fibers & Construction.. 96
Buying Socks... 99
Specialty Socks 100
Going Sockless.. 105

Part Three: Prevention   107
8. Making Prevention Work............................. 109
Components of Prevention... 112
Finding the Right Combination 115
9. Compounds for the Feet 117
Powders.. 117
Lubricants 119
Skin Toughening Agents & Tape Adherents................ 121
Antiperspirants for the Feet 124
10. Taping for Blisters 129
Tapes 130
Working the Tape 133
Three Taping Techniques... 135
Taping the Feet 137
11. Orthotics 143
Custom-made Orthotics 145
Over-the-counter Orthotics.. 147
Using Your Orthotics 147
12. Gaiters 150
Making Your Own Gaiters 151
Repairing Gaiter Straps 152
13. Lacing Options.. 156
Lacing Tips... 157
Lacing Methods... 157
14. Self Care for Your Feet 162
Skin Care 162
Pedicures 165
Foot Massage 167
Hydration, Dehydration, & Sodium........................... 169
Changing Your Shoes & Socks 171
Keeping Your Shoes Fresh 173
15. Extreme Conditions & Multiday Events 174
Cold & Wet 176
Trench Foot 180
Frostbite... 181
Snow & Ice 182
Heat... 185
Sand 187
Jungle Rot.. 189
Foot Care in Multiday Events..................................... 191
Aching Feet 195

16. Teamwork & Crew Support **197**
    Teamwork 197
    Planning for Foot Care 198
    Team Responsibilities 199
    Crew Support 199
17. Providing Foot Care for Athletes **201**
    Being Part of a Foot Care Team 201
    Setting Up Your Station 202
    Tips on Managing Blisters 202
    Advising about Post-event Care 204
    Your Tools 204
18. 12 Mega-distance Athletes Talk about Foot Care **205**
19. Preventing Blisters **218**
    Things You Can Do for Your Feet 219
    Things You Apply to Your Feet 219
    Things You Put Around Your Feet 220
    Things You Do in Combination 221
    Things You Do in General 221

Part Four: Treatments   223

20. Treating Your Feet **225**
21. Blisters **228**
    Hot Spots 229
    Beyond Hot Spots: Blisters 230
    Types of Blisters 235
    General Blister Care 236
    Advanced Blister Patching 241
    Extreme Blister Prevention & Patching 245
    Beyond Blisters 254
    Fixing Blisters, Their Way or Yours 255
    Post-event Blister Care 256
22. Strains & Sprains, Fractures & Dislocations **257**
    Strains & Sprains 257
    Strengthening Exercises 264
    Fractures 268
    Stress Fractures 269
    Dislocations 271
23. Tendon & Ligament Injuries **273**
    Treating Tendon Injuries 274
    Achilles Tendinitis 278
    Ankle Tendons 282
    Bursitis 284
    Plantar Fasciitis 284
24. Heel Problems **294**
    Heel-pain Syndrome 294
    Heel Spurs 294
    Haglund's Deformity 296
25. Toe Problems **299**
    Strengthening Your Toes 299

The Basics: Toenail Trimming 299
Black Toenails 300
Big Toe Problems.. 304
Hammertoes, Claw Toes, & Mallet Toes 305
Ingrown Toenails 307
Morton's Toe... 308
Overlapping Toes 309
Stubbed Toes 309
Toenail Fungus 310
Turf Toe 313

26. Forefoot Problems **315**
Bunions 315
Metatarsalgia... 317
Morton's Neuroma 318
Sesamoiditis 320

27. Numb Toes & Feet **322**
Transient Paresthesia 322
Peripheral Neuropathy 323
Raynaud's Syndrome.. 324

28. Skin Disorders **326**
Athlete's Foot 326
Calluses... 327
Corns 331
Fissures.. 332
Plantar Warts.. 332
Rashes... 334

29. Cold & Heat Therapy............................. **336**
Cold Therapy 336
Heat Therapy 337
Combination Cold & Heat Therapy................................. 338

30. Foot Care Kits **340**
Basic Self-care Kit for Home Use 342
Fanny-pack Kit.. 342
Event Kit 343

Part Five: Sources & Resources   **345**

Appendix A: Product Sources.......................... **347**

Appendix B: Shoe & Gear Reviews **349**

Appendix C: Medical & Footwear Specialists **350**

Appendix D: Feet-related Websites **351**

Notes **352**

Glossary **355**

Bibliography **359**

About the Author....................................... **361**

Index   **362**

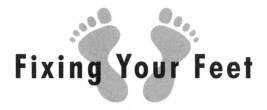

Fixing Your Feet

Introduction

"One thing is for sure: when one's feet hurt …
it definitely gets one's attention."

—Denise Jones, the Badwater Blister Queen

For years, I have signed copies of *Fixing Your Feet* with the following inscription: best wishes for happy and healthy feet. That and helping people have been my motivations for more than 15 years of learning as much as possible about foot care. I love to see athletes able to finish their races without foot problems.

Those reading this fifth edition of *Fixing Your Feet* are, by their very nature, active people. They love the outdoors. They love challenges, often pushing their bodies beyond the norm. Oftentimes this is done in less than ideal conditions—rain, cold, snow, sand, and on feet that hurt. And more often than not, on blistered feet. If there is one injury that has plagued the majority of athletes, it's blisters.

Mark Swanson, an ultrarunner, sent an e-mail to a listserv in response to a comment about blister prevention. He wrote: "Let's remember the lesson John keeps emphasizing—what works for you may not work for the next person and what works for you now may not work for you next time. But what works for you will help some people and may work for you for a long time!"

There is a lot of value in these two sentences. A common saying is, "We are each an experiment of one." That applies to foot care, and especially blister prevention. Ever since I wrote the first edition of *Fixing Your Feet,* I have tried to get people to learn about how to prevent blisters with a variety of techniques and products.

Yes, blisters are the number one issue, the number one question that athletes ask about. I wish I could tell you the one answer that would solve all your blister problems. But there's not one solution. In this book are hundreds of tips to help prevent blisters and, if you get them anyway, products to fix them. You need to find which ones work for you. By doing your homework, you'll be closer to solving your foot problems. This goes for other foot problems too.

Fixing Your Feet is filled with information to help you keep your feet happy and healthy. Rather than looking only for a quick solution to your problem or injury, I encourage you to learn as much as you can about what caused the problem or injury. It is important to eliminate the cause to achieve a long-term solution. Start with the new chapter on "Getting the Most Out of *Fixing Your Feet*."

In the publishing world, not many books make it to a fifth edition. *Fixing Your Feet* has done so because it continues to offer solutions.

In each edition, the foreword has presented a perspective that emphasized a unique point:

■ Our feet are our primary mode of transportation and require our attention and preparation. **—Billy Trolan, MD, first edition**

■ Most of our foot problems could have been avoided with proper care. **—David Hannaford, DPM, second edition**

■ Our feet will take us to new challenges and adventures if we make the conscious choice to care for them. **—Dan Barger, the Primal Quest Expedition Race founder, third edition**

■ If your feet are happy, you're happy. If your feet are miserable and want to quit, you are miserable and want to quit. **—Demetri "Coup" Coupounas, fourth edition**

■ Our feet connect us to the surrounding terrain, propelling us toward our next destination. Take care of your feet and the world is yours to enjoy. Ignore your feet and life can be a miserable experience. **—Brian J. Krabak, MD, fifth edition**

This edition includes two new chapters. The first, "Barefoot & Minimalist Footwear," was prompted by the changing footwear marketplace. The second, "Providing Foot Care for Athletes," is aimed at those who work at events to provide foot care to runners, walkers, and adventure racers—anyone needing help. I have a special place in my heart for those trying hard to repair feet so the athlete can continue. The fifth edition has updates and changes throughout, including coverage of new products and new techniques, particularly in the "Taping for Blisters" and "Blisters" chapters.

Fixing Your Feet is for you— solutions for your feet. I would love to hear from you. Send me an e-mail at john@fixingyourfeet.com and let me know your story about your feet.

Foot Fetish

My feet are runner's feet;
a little rough around the edges,
with black nails on the toes where I have nails at all
Lovingly decorated with bright colors.

My toes are warriors, of a sort.
They carry the entire continent of my body on adventures
and rise to challenges that could crush them.
Some days they are worn and calloused,
but they are strong and fierce adversaries for the
rocks they overtake.

My arches are the springboard of my soul.
They give me lift with every step I take
and cushion all my landings.
They are always ready
when I want to jump for joy.

My heels respond when the shepherd
of my spirit nips at them to run.
They strike again and again,
to thwart frustration,
to redeem the day.

My feet are runner's feet;
a little rough around the edges,
but they are strong
and they are willing
and oh, I love them.

—Lisa Butler, ultrarunner

Getting the Most Out of
Fixing Your Feet

In the 15 years since *Fixing Your Feet* first came out, I have answered many questions about foot care. I have patched thousands of feet at ultramarathons, multiday stage races, adventure races, marathons, and walking events. If there is one thing I have learned, it is this: the majority of athletes wait until they have problems to learn how to care for their feet.

When problems develop, everything becomes reactive—working to solve an existing problem. Preventing foot problems is being proactive—working to solve problems before they develop. Being proactive takes time up front. Being reactive takes time and resources often when they are not available or when using them may jeopardize the outcome of the event. I prefer proactive.

So here you are, holding this book in your hands. Maybe it's the first time you've seen it or maybe you had one of the earlier editions. The question is how can you get the most value out of it?

I would start by skimming the contents, the foreword, and the introduction. That will give you a feel for the depth of information inside. Then, read the chapters that catch your attention—maybe because you are dealing with those particular issues.

If you are new to learning about foot care, set aside some time to read through "Part One: Foot Basics" and "Part Two: Footwear Basics." They are the starting point for everything else in the book. Then skim through "Part Three: Prevention," and highlight the material that catches your attention. When you have time, go back and read the chapters that apply to your situation. Pay close attention to the chapter on taping.

Part Four: Treatments is important to cover when you can take in all the information. If you arc experiencing specific problems with your feet, read those chapters first. Then skim the others. Be sure to read and study the chapter on blisters.

Anytime you see products that sound interesting, check them out on the listed websites. Not all of the products are right for you, but I guarantee that many are.

Nathan's story, opposite, is a perfect example of how to get the most out of *Fixing Your Feet*.

Nathan's Story

As I was finishing the material for this fifth edition, I received an e-mail from Nathan Wilson, who lives in the Kimberley region of northwest Australia. The week before, he had finished the seven-day, 250K stage race known as Racing the Planet: Australia. Previously Nathan had finished some marathons and ultramarathons, the longest one being 100K. Of the 185 starting competitors in Racing the Planet: Australia, only 118 completed the race, and most competitors had problems with blisters from the first day.

Three months before the race, Nathan bought *Fixing Your Feet.* He read it and learned a great deal about what he needed to do in preparation for this grueling event. Importantly, he learned how to deal with the problems he had experienced in earlier races. He learned how to pretape his feet and had the right tapes. In fact he taped his feet three times during the race. He carried seven pairs of Injinji toe socks and Teko merino wool blend socks to wear over the toe socks. He used Hydropel ointment at the start of each day. He used Sorbothane insoles for added shock absorption. For river crossings, he took off his shoes and socks and, once on the other side, cleaned his feet and reapplied Hydropel. Each evening he cleaned his shoes and insoles. When he got into camp each day, he dried his feet and coated them with iodine and, in one instance, benzoin, to dry them further. He watched his electrolytes to avoid swelling of his feet and hands. For him, the race was an enjoyable experience.

Nathan was proactive from the beginning. Contrast that to others, who did not have adequate protection for the wet conditions, did not know how to use the contents of their "required" foot care kit, did not pretape, used the wrong tape, had not conditioned their feet and bodies for the weight of their packs, and were reactive to problems.

Nathan wrote, "I realized that the part of the book that focused on working on your feet prior to a large event really had an impact on me. After reading people's stories of soaking their feet, removing calluses, and filing their toenails, I was motivated to do the same on a near-daily basis. It also motivated me to work on my ankle strength and my calves to help my feet. I suppose if I had not done this prep work, all of the taping, Hydropel, toe socks, and so on would have helped some, but it might not have made such a difference. A lot of people have asked about the race and the blisters 'I must have had.' I just laugh and tell them that I didn't get a single one."

Nathan thanked me for getting him through Racing the Planet: Australia, a very tough event. I commend Nathan for doing things right. I hold Nathan up as an example of how to use the material in this book. I could not have found a better example of being proactive. I challenge you to do likewise.

The Best of 15 Years of Foot Care

In 1996 I spent a year writing the first edition of *Fixing Your Feet*. In the 15 years since then, I have learned a lot that is worth repeating. This chapter comes from my experiences, learned in the field and shared in my blog. You may find some of this repeated elsewhere in the book and there is a reason for that. This is important stuff. It includes answers to questions and comments I also hear over and over. Allow me to share a bit of what I have learned. I also encourage you to check out and subscribe to my *Fixing Your Feet* blog by going to **www.fixingyourfeet.com**.

Five Tidbits of Wisdom

1. Taking care of your feet is your job. Do not count on someone else to take care of your feet.

2. Fit is key. Shoes that are too short or that are wrong for the event will make your feet hurt and lead to problems.

3. Your feet must be conditioned to endure the rigors and stresses of your chosen sport or sports. Train in race conditions in the shoes and socks you will wear on race day. Work up to distances that you will tackle in your event.

4. A little toenail care goes a long way in preventing blisters and black toenails. Properly trimmed and filed nails will not catch on socks and will be less likely to lead to toe blisters.

5. Calluses can and usually do lead to problems with blisters or with the thickened and hardened skin folding up on itself when it becomes macerated from being wet. They will become painful.

The Golden Rule for Your Feet

The signature line on Mike's e-mail caught my eye: "Treat your feet as you would have yourself be treated." As a runner, he had e-mailed me about one of my blog posts, and his mention of "running's golden rule" caught my attention.

Because feet have always interested me, I asked him to tell me more. Mike says, "I think it means the same as the Golden Rule: take care of your feet and they will take care of you; treat your feet with respect and kindness and they'll support you in tough times; be your best friend to your feet and they'll be your best friend when you need one most."

I like that. Too often we relegate our feet to the end of the line. Sure, we buy good footwear and socks, but that's it—we forget about the feet themselves. We forget quality toenail care and then wonder why we get black toenails. We forget about callus control and then wonder why we have to deal with blisters underneath them. We fail to deal with corns, athlete's foot, and other problems common to feet. We get blisters but don't take time to figure out why we get them or learn measures to prevent and treat them.

We forget the golden rule: "Treat your feet as you would have yourself be treated." Actually, it is pretty easy. A few minutes a day is all it takes.

Basic Foot Care—It's Your Job

In January 2006 I had the opportunity to serve on the medical team at The Coastal Challenge, a seven-day, 150-mile stage race in Costa Rica. There's no better way to see a country than on foot. Some 51 athletes from around the world were there to experience the trails, roads, beaches, and rain forests of a beautiful country. The people were warm and very friendly. The food was great. The scenery was fantastic; the wildlife, colorful and exotic; and the weather, hot and humid. We had great fun.

Of course I was there to patch feet—so that's what I did. I made some observations over the course of seven days. What I want to share here is pretty basic—but what many forget.

When you are starting an adventure, whether a backpack, a 50-mile run, a fast pack, a walking vacation, or an adventure race, you are responsible for your feet. Not me. Not the medical crew, if there is one. It's your job. Let me explain.

You need to come to an event prepared to manage whatever your feet toss at you. That means having a foot care kit appropriate for the length (both in miles and days) and type of event. Having a foot care kit means that you also know how to pretape to prevent hot spots and blisters, repair any blisters you get, apply any patches you have, care for your toenails, and manage calluses or any other unique features of your feet.

The medical staff doing foot care at the Costa Rica race had lineups every evening. Three of us were patching feet. We had a lot of materials but quickly went through much of it. It is difficult to patch feet in the evening and then be expected to patch feet at the aid stations the next day, and then again that evening. We would have run out of materials in a few days. Fortunately, some of the runners had their own materials and patched their own feet. I commend them. They really helped us.

You also need to come into an event with feet that are properly prepared. That means reducing your calluses. I know, I know, you really like your calluses. Then at least reduce them so they aren't as thick. The little calluses on the bottom of your toes can quickly become bothersome. Those on your heels can ruin your whole event. Work on your toenails so they won't create toe blisters and black toenails. See the "Toe Problems" chapter for more on toenails. Put miles on your feet to condition them for the rigors of the event you will be doing. Running 20 miles a week will not prepare you effectively for doing a 150-mile, seven-day event. Also, prepare your feet by having quality shoes and socks—not ones that are worn down.

So what's the bottom line? It's your job to be prepared. It is not the job of the medical staff to patch you up every night and every morning, and at every aid station during the event—especially when your feet are not prepared coming into the event. Many times we can work small miracles, but please work with us. Then watch us as we work and take the time to learn so the next time you can help us out.

Lisa Bliss, MD, who helps at the Badwater Ultramarathon, supports my comments. "If runners think we are there for blister care, then they will not take the time or effort to learn about it themselves and train appropriately in advance of the race," she says. "It's not that I don't mind helping; I just don't want runners to be helpless about prevention and treatment."

Self-Education

Podiatrist Rob Conenello, who managed feet at the seven-day Sahara Race in Egypt, said, "I would go daily to the athletes' tents to help them prevent injury. The key is to educate the participants on how to tape themselves and care for small problems."

Self-education takes many forms. It's getting your feet in the best shape and condition possible for the events you do. It's getting inside your footwear. Literally. Buy a pair of shoes or boots and you'll get the stock, standard insole. Depending on the manufacturer, it may be good, or it may be a basic, nonsupporting piece of heavy cardboard. Take it out and see if it is worth keeping. Fortunately, footwear makers are learning that their buyers want overall quality—and that includes insoles. Check for bad seams and stitching in the shoe. Know your foot type and research reviews to find the best shoes. Know what makes for a well-fitting shoe.

Find what works best for your feet. As Gordon Wright, Media Director of Primal Quest, said, "I don't have anything to add from my seven years of adventure racing but one word: Injinji socks. I was always prone to blisters between my toes, and literally have not had one—in many, many miles—since I started wearing them."

Learn how your skin reacts to powders and lubricants to reduce friction. Learn how to tape your feet and patch a blister—in five different ways with different products. Learn how to trim your toenails. Learn how to strengthen your feet and ankles. Learn what words such as *proprioception* and *onychocryptosis* mean and how they affect your feet.

Are Your Feet Prepared?

When I talk to runners preparing for a race, some seem to be well prepared. They know about blisters and what kind of socks to wear. They either have experience with foot issues or want to learn more. Others seem unconcerned or unprepared.

The main question I ask is, "Are your feet prepared?" I give them a half page of tips, which are reproduced below. The tips can easily apply to anyone running or walking a marathon, or doing any similar event. Are they magic? No. But many people, even athletes, seem to forget the commonsense tips that can make their event a better experience.

Preparing Your Feet for a Race

BEFORE THE RACE

- Toenails too long catch on socks: trim them short.
- File toenails smooth.
- Use a callus file to smooth calluses.
- Clean out lint and junk from inside shoes.
- Check your shoelaces and replace if frayed.

MORNING OF THE RACE

- Apply a layer of your favorite lubricant or powder.
- Smooth your socks around your feet.
- Avoid tying laces too tightly.

DURING THE RACE

- If you feel a hot spot, apply a pad, a bit of tape, a dab of lubricant, or even an energy gel wrapper between your sock and shoe.
- Loosen shoelaces if you have pain on the top of your foot.

AFTER THE RACE

- If you have blisters, soak your feet in Epsom salts and warm water three times a day.
- Drain blisters only if they are in a pressure area.
- Trim edges of loose skin around blisters.
- If feet are swollen, elevate and ice.

With Footwear, Try Then Adjust

A triathlete recently said after running a marathon, "My left instep is still quite bruised. It took a pounding from the stretchy triathlon shoelaces that I used and —whoops!—never adjusted quite properly. Lesson learned: too loose is better than too snug."

In other words, she put the laces in her shoes and ran in them without adjusting them to fit her feet. This is an easily made and common mistake. When you make changes to your footwear, learn to try . . . and then adjust as necessary. You can apply this same failure to other parts of your footwear.

A few don'ts when it comes to footwear:

■ Wear new shoes for a walk, race, or hike without trying them first—it's easy to miss a bad fit, a rough inside seam, or a wrong fitting arch. Walk around the house in them for a few hours.

■ Wear new socks in an event without first trying them inside your shoes—the socks may be thicker or thinner than your previous socks, making the fit different.

■ Replace insoles without checking if they are thinner or thicker than the old ones, which can change the space for your feet inside your shoes.

Don't Give Up on Footwear

Maggie was having tremendous problems getting a good fit with her footwear. She wrote, "This is by far the most frustrating thing I have experienced in my quest to find my personal 'very best way.' Occasionally I have come up with a combination that has had very acceptable results, only to have the same strategy fail miserably on the next outing."

Many more people have the same problem. Some have had only a few minor problems while others have had lots. I like to hear from those who never have foot problems. They may be doing everything right, be genetically blessed with good feet, and likely have put lots of miles on their feet in order to have the right conditioning. Others, such as Maggie, have tried every idea under the sun—without success. These are the ones I love to talk to. They are dedicated to finding what works and will give up at nothing.

Maggie and others are on a quest to find the best fit, as well as the best shoe and sock combination possible. They love their sports. They love being outdoors, running, hiking, or walking. It is a part of who they are. But they want to do it with happy feet.

Maggie described her feet to an online hiking forum and told us what she had tried, and what had worked (not much) and what hadn't worked (lots). Many fellow hikers responded with ideas. Many were very good. In the end, I printed out about ten pages of back and forth e-mails, read them to grasp what had been suggested and tried, and then made my own recommendations. What a learning experience!

You may be frustrated as Maggie was. My advice? Don't give up. There is a solution. There are shoes out there that will fit. With the search you'll learn about fit, socks, insoles, orthotics, lacing techniques, heel counters, forefoot width, pronation, supination, shoe lasts, narrow feet, wide feet, Morton's toe, bunions, and much more. Read shoe reviews in magazines. Do Web searches on different shoes with the word *reviews* in the search box. Quiz your shoe store salesperson. Ask questions. Try different pairs by different manufacturers. Don't leave the store with a shoe that doesn't feel right. Don't settle for second best. Your feet deserve the very best.

Preventing Blisters

If there is one thing I have come to know, it's this: the very best way to prevent blisters today may not work tomorrow.

I wrote the above in response to a hiker who said he knew the secret to preventing blisters. He wrote, "The very best way to prevent blisters is to wear sock liners under your socks. Nothing works better to prevent blisters."

I wrote back to him, "There is not *one* 'very best way' for everyone to prevent blisters. I've patched thousands of feet over the past eight years and have seen it all and heard it all. I feel there is a very best way for each of us. It may mean using powder, lubricant, liner socks, double layer socks, toe socks, pretaping, toughening your skin, keeping your skin as soft as a baby's bottom, and a host of other ideas. It may also be a combination of ways. Just as long as you understand that the very best way today may fail tomorrow. It's important to know your options."

Many others have learned this the hard way. They love their calluses, only to get deep blisters underneath. They wear the wrong socks. They fail to get the best fit possible. They don't trim toenails and then blister on the tips of their toes. They find that yesterday's solution is now today's blister. It can happen to anyone—and it usually does.

I appreciate the solutions that people find. I've found them too. I've heard the comments, "Wow! My blisters are gone. I found the best socks." That's great. I'm happy. But be careful. Take a bit of time and know your options. Socks are good but learn how to tape. Learn about insoles, fit, lacing options, and more.

You know your own feet better than anyone else so you have to experiment to find what works best for you. That's why one of the chapters in this book is "Preventing Blisters."

Let Your Feet Breathe

Are your feet comfortable? I mean, do they get to relax like the rest of you? If you are like most people, you get home from work and change into something comfortable. You know, loose-fitting clothes that are soft.

So what do you put on your feet? Socks and comfortable shoes? Thongs or sandals? Or maybe you even choose to go barefoot? What's the right choice?

In the same way that your body needs something comfortable, your feet do too. After a day cooped up in socks and shoes, or nylons and heels, give your feet a break. Let them out for some air. They need to breathe too. Wiggle your toes. Rub your feet. According to the American Podiatric Medical Association, our feet have approximately 250,000 sweat glands and produce as much as a pint of moisture per day. Your feet need their space and they need to be let out for air at least once a day. Be nice to your feet and let them breathe.

Size Matters

We all have heard the old adage that "size matters." Here I am talking about shoe size. A common problem when buying shoes and boots is that people will tell the salesperson, "I wear a size 9½." Well that may or may not be true. Over time, our feet change—typically getting larger. The fat pads on the bottom of our feet become thinner as we get older. We may get bunions or our calluses may thicken and affect fit. You may have been a 9½, but now you may be a 10. You might even be a 9.

It's wise to get your feet sized each time you purchase a new pair of shoes. The Brannock Device is the tool that stores use to measure your feet to determine shoe size. Be sure to measure each foot. Measure sitting and standing—although standing is the most important measurement. Many of us have one foot a bit larger than the other foot, so always buy shoes to fit the larger foot.

This easy measurement is important to get the best fit possible. Remember, though, after measuring your feet and trying on a pair of shoes, the shoes still may not feel right. Shoes can vary in construction and one company's shoes may run smaller or larger than those of another company. Once on your feet, the shoes need to feel comfortable. If not, move up or down a half size and see if that helps. Because after all, size matters and that's the first place to start in your search for new shoes.

What Changed?

Let's begin with a story from an unnamed runner: "I'll start by saying that I've never had problems with blisters in the past, except for one little problem four years ago. So this last weekend I start the AT100, and by mile 16 I've got hot spots going on the sides of both heels. Got out the duct tape and did my thing, but by mile 32 both heels have blisters going, and I've got hot spots on the balls of both feet as well. I retape, moleskin, etc., but to no avail. By mile 48 the blister on the heel of my right foot has broken; the hot spots on the balls of my feet have turned into half-dollar-size blisters. Retape and go. At mile 57, I retape again; the side of the heel of my right foot is bleeding. Coming back into an aid station the blister on the ball of my right foot has popped and I rather painfully 'squish' with every step. By this point I've had it, and at mile 67 I drop. I did nothing different than I've ever done—same shoes, same socks, and the same lubricant. Everything was identical to my other 30 races where I've had no problems whatsoever. So what happened here?"

Blisters can be puzzling because they seem to develop on different parts of the foot at different times and for different reasons. If this happens to you, a question is in order. A friend asked for advice after working hard to rid his feet of calluses. His feet were fine for a long time afterward and then, one day, they got trashed during an ultra. He asked for help. I asked in both cases, "What changed?"

The answer is sometimes simple and easy. Other times, it's complex. People tell me they never blistered before today, or they blistered in a new area, or had problems with their toes, or something else. Or they tell me they worked hard to rid their feet of calluses and now something happened and their feet are trashed. Some tell of bad blisters deep underneath calluses. Or bad toe blisters.

Never mind the problem. The question is always the same, "What changed?" Another angle on the question is, "What felt different?" Even if you used the same shoes, socks, and lubricant as before, other factors could be different. Perhaps there was a change in hydration, temperature, and humidity. Maybe your training changed, and you didn't put in the necessary miles before the event. Trail factors include slope, dust and grit, rocks, mud, and water. Perhaps water went down your legs while you were sponging off, or you didn't wear gaiters, or the mesh upper of the shoes allowed dust and grit inside that caused the hot spot. The insoles could be old and should be replaced if any of their fabric is folding down, or if a rough edge is exposed. The shoe's heel counter could be too rigid, or the heel counter fabric frayed, or the juncture of the insole and heel counter bothersome—all factors that could cause blisters. It could even be how tight you tied your shoes to secure your heel in place and the amount of heel ups and downs. Socks often bunch up and cause problems. Maybe you changed to a new sock. Or worse yet, wore non-moisture-wicking socks or never changed socks. How quickly after a hot spot developed and how well you taped the hot spots and blisters could also be a factor. Many times we blister more easily in certain places when walking as opposed to running, and that could also have been a factor. The lubricant you put on your feet could have worn off and was not replaced, or the lubricant softened the skin and led to blisters. Maybe your toenails were not trimmed and caught on your socks, causing toe blisters. The toe box could have also been too short or too low. Your feet could have been wet too long and the skin macerated into blisters. You could have slightly turned an ankle and thus changed your gait, causing pressure and blisters in never-before problem areas. And the list goes on.

Chances are that *something* changed. You need to figure out what it was. It could be something simple or complex or even a combination of changes.

Many athletes find that they have been fine and blister free for years and then an event comes along and their feet are trashed. Sometimes it is just one of those days. No two events are the same; few of us can do events time after time and not experience problems with legs, stomach, mind, or feet. So if your feet had been good and healthy and they blistered or had other problems, ask yourself, "What changed?"

Trimming Toenails

How hard can it be to trim your toenails? I guess for a lot of folks, it's a huge deal and something they never do. In all the years I have been patching feet, I have observed that untrimmed toenails are the number one cause of problems leading to toe blisters and black nails. Socks will catch on nails that are too long or that have rough edges. This puts pressure on the nail bed, leading to blisters under the toenails, blisterrs at the tips of the toes, or painful toenails as they are pushed back into the cuticle. Nails that are too long are also prone to pressure from a toe box that is too short or too low.

So what are some tips to keeping your toenails under control? Toenails should be trimmed straight across the nail—never rounded at the corners. Leave an extra bit of nail on the outside corner of the big toe to avoid an ingrown toenail. After trimming toenails, use a nail file to smooth the top of the nail down toward the front of the toe and remove any rough edges. If you draw your finger from the skin in front of the toe up across the nail and can feel a rough edge, the nail can be filed smoother or trimmed a bit shorter.

You can use an emery board from your drugstore, a cheap "use it a few times and toss it" file. Better yet, invest a few bucks in a nice metal file that will last a long time and serve you well. To trim your nails, there are regular nail clippers, nippers, and scissors made exclusively for thicker toenails. If your local drugstore or pharmacy doesn't stock them, check out **www.footsmart.com** for a great selection.

A little bit of care in toenail trimming goes a long way in preventing toe blisters and black toenails, as well as making your socks last longer.

The Little Toe Triangle

We each have two. Little toes, that is. The number of problems with these little appendages has impressed me. "What problems?" you ask. It's all about that little triangle of skin where most problems occur.

If you look at your little toes, your toes may be well rounded and soft. Or they may have the often-typical triangle look where the skin on the bottom of the triangle is hard and callused. The skin on the bottom of the toe forms the point of the triangle. The problem is that on many of our little toes, this bottom point is hard and callused skin. The hard skin is prone to blisters forming underneath as pressure from the toe box creates friction. Often this hardened skin is partially under the skin of the next toe, another pressure area. The outside of the foot, the little toe area, is often more wet and damp than the inside of the shoes, leading to macerated skin. Once softened, this skin can easily blister underneath, or worse yet, the skin can separate, leading to major skin problems.

One of the last runners whose feet I patched at Primal Quest had struggled for the whole event with macerated skin on his feet. When he came into a transition area, the skin had stripped off the bottom point of this triangle—of both feet. I'm sure it was painful and very uncomfortable. Once patched, he continued on as best he could.

The little toe is so small that it is hard to patch well. The use of Micropore or Kinesio tape is a good choice. Even better, in my opinion, is reducing the hard callused skin. Injinji toe socks can also be helpful. Good shoes are vital too. Shoes with a good toe box that allows the toes room to wiggle are best. Once the skin has blistered, 2nd Skin is good to use as a patch. Cut it to fit the blister. Too much and it becomes bulky and rubs on the neighboring toe.

During a race or hike, be watchful of your little toes. This small but potentially troublesome triangle of skin deserves special care.

Time on Your Feet

Over the years I have seen many people complete marathons and ultramarathons. Most do well, suffering the usual malady of blisters, toenail issues, and an occasional ankle sprain. There are some, however, who finish their events with feet that they can hardly walk on. Complaints range from, "My foot feels like one big blister" to "I can't walk!"

These athletes usually have one thing in common. They have stressed their feet beyond what their feet are comfortable doing. There are several typical scenarios. The most common is that they have simply done too much too soon. The second most common is that they have encountered conditions beyond what they were prepared for. Because all of us, even non-athletes, can learn from these experiences, allow me to explain.

Sudden increases in mileage put undue pressure on the bones, tendons, ligaments, and muscles of the feet. If you typically walk 3 miles a day and then suddenly walk 10 miles, you can expect your feet to feel sore, hot, and painful. Increasing your running miles from a 10K (6.2 miles) to a half-marathon (13.1 miles) will result in similar complaints. The rule of thumb for runners has always been to increase weekly miles by no more than 10% a week. This is good advice for all of us.

Whenever we go for a walk or run, we might run into the unexpected. We step off a curb or roll our foot on a rock and turn an ankle. We hike on a trail and are not used to uphills and downhills, the tree roots and rocks, and the uneven terrain, and our legs, ankles, and feet become sore. It's hot and we sweat more than normal, and this moisture leads to hot spots and blisters. We wear a new pair of socks, thinner than normal, and our feet move around inside the shoes, creating blisters. We wear a new pair of socks, thicker than normal, and the pressure inside the toe box leads to painful toenails.

Whatever our activity, we need to do the time. We must put the time on our feet to get them ready and in shape to handle the stresses we will ask them to endure. If you have a vacation or a marathon coming up, count backward on your calendar and block off time to get yourself ready—including your feet. Putting in the time on your feet will lead to happy feet.

Touching Feet

During two weeks in 2004, I touched more bad feet than ever: first at the 100-mile Western States Endurance Run and then at the Atacama Crossing, a seven-day, 150-mile stage race in Chile.

In each event, I treated many athletes who had not properly trimmed their toenails. This, coupled with shoes that were too short or with a too-small toe box, led to the expected toenail problems. Several runners had nails lifting off the nail bed or had black toenails, which required relieving the pressure under the nail.

I learned that many athletes had done their homework and found a good combination of shoes and socks that worked for their feet. Quite a few used Injinji toe socks, usually as a liner, and then another heavier sock over the top. Many used SmartWool socks, again often two pairs on each foot. A number of the top runners, who had no foot problems, talked of how they worked hard at getting rid of calluses—and how that helped them. Charlie Engle, who finished second in the Atacama Crossing, told how it took him a year to get to smooth skin. Many pretaped as a preventive measure.

Even though I knew it, it was again confirmed that there is only so much that can be fixed. We cannot make a patch for those athletes who enter events injured and then come to us for help. We cannot take away a problem that an athlete has ignored. Calluses, poorly fitting shoes, overuse injuries, untrimmed toenails, nails thickened with fungus, and fissures or cracks in the skin—to mention a few—can be treated, but there is still usually some degree of discomfort, yet several athletes came to us expecting miracles.

Informed Athletes

I am always happy to see informed runners and racers. They know, for the most part, what their feet need. The athletes with the fewest foot problems share the following characteristics:

- Many pretape their feet to protect against hot spots and blisters.

- Most use moisture-wicking socks.

- Most change socks and shoes when necessary and before problems set in.

- Most know about their feet's problems, knowing when they have Morton's foot, bunions, calluses, bad toenails, or anything else out of the ordinary.

- Many have tried to rid their feet of calluses, knowing that a blister under a callus is the worst kind to get.

- Many use powder to keep their feet dry.

- Many use a good state-of-the-art lubricant to avoid friction.

- Most know the importance of shoes that fit well.

- Many file down their toenails.

- Many carry different tapes and blister patches.

Still Learning

What disturbs me is that there are still large numbers of athletes who seem to give little thought to their feet. The athletes with the most foot problems share the following characteristics:

- They shove feet into shoes without straightening their socks.

- They wear the wrong socks and do not look inside their socks for seams that cause toe blisters.

- They have sacrificed fit and buy a shoe because a friend recommended it and not because it was the best shoe for their feet.

- They try to fix blisters with Band-Aids.

- They fail to change their socks often enough when their feet are wet.

- They fail to trim their toenails and wonder why they get black toenails and toe blisters.

- They fail to put in the miles that their feet need to be toughened for the rigors of racing.

- They speed through checkpoints feeding their faces but not tending to their feet.

As Billy Trolan, MD, said in the foreword for the first edition of *Fixing Your Feet*, "The one factor that continues to amaze me is that individuals and teams will spend vast amounts of money, time, and thought on training, equipment, and travel, but little or no preparation on their feet. Too often the result has been that within a few hours to a few days, all that work has been ruined. Ruined because the primary mode of transportation has broken down with blisters." That was written in 1997 and is still true today.

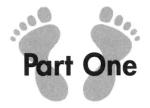

Part One

Foot Basics

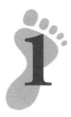

Seeking Medical Treatment

The information and advice given in this book is provided to athletes to use in their efforts to resolve foot problems. Not all foot problems or injuries will be resolved successfully by following the tips or using the products mentioned in this book. There are times when it is important to seek professional medical help.

Never ignore an injury. Pushing through an injury or returning to your sport too soon after being injured can lead to additional injuries. You do not want to turn a temporary injury into a permanent disability. Too often athletes rely on self-diagnosis rather than consulting with a medical specialist. If during or after running or hiking you have persistent foot problems or recurring pain that you cannot resolve, you are advised to seek medical treatment from a medical specialist who can provide his or her medical expertise for your problem. Consider yourself fortunate if you can learn firsthand from a medical specialist.

Primary Medical Specialists for Feet

ORTHOPEDISTS are orthopedic surgeons, experts of the joints, muscles, and bones. This includes upper and lower extremities and the spine. Look for an orthopedist that specializes in the foot and ankle. The American Academy of Orthopaedic Surgeons and the American Orthopaedic Foot and Ankle Society can provide referrals.

PODIATRISTS are doctors of podiatric medicine (DPM) that work on the feet up to and including the ankles. They specialize in medical and surgical problems including foot diseases, deformities, and injuries, such as nail, skin, bone, tendon, and diabetic disorders. Podiatrists treat such disorders with surgery, custom-made orthotics (shoe inserts), physical therapy, injections, casting and braces, prescription medication, and medicated creams and ointments. The American Podiatric Medical Association and the American Academy of Podiatric Sports Medicine can provide referrals.

If you have chronic foot problems, or you are uncertain what your feet are trying to tell you through their pain, consider consulting a podiatrist or orthopedic surgeon. Listen to your whole body and especially your feet. Be attentive to when the pain begins and what makes it hurt more or less. Then be prepared to tell the specialist about the problem, its history, what you have done to correct it, and whether it worked or got worse.

There is a wide range of skill overlap between orthopedists and podiatrists. Each can treat most of the same foot problems. When searching for a medical specialist for your feet, talk to doctors about their training, experience, and whether they have a specialty field. Each of the two specialist fields has doctors who specialize in sports medicine, and these would be my first choice. Weigh this information when making a decision about who to turn to for help. Additionally, a variety of other specialists can provide assistance in strengthening, alignment, rehabilitation, and footwear design and fit.

Foot Specialists

PEDORTHISTS work with the design, manufacture, fit, and modification of shoes, boots, and other footwear. Pedorthists are board certified (C.Ped) to provide prescription footwear and related devices. They will evaluate, fit, and modify all types of footwear. A C. Ped. can help find a shoe built on a last (the form over which a shoe is constructed) that best matches a person's feet, and then construct a custom orthotic that meets his or her particular biomechanical needs and interfaces with the shoe in a way that improves its fit and performance. The American Orthotics and Prosthetics Association and the Pedorthic Footwear Association can provide information and referrals.

SPORTS MEDICINE DOCTORS specialize in sports-related injuries. They are typically doctors of internal medicine with additional training in sports medicine. When treating athletes with lower-extremity injuries that do not improve with their initial treatment, they may refer the athlete to a podiatrist or orthopedist. Most are members of the American College of Sports Medicine (which does not provide referral services).

PHYSICAL THERAPISTS are licensed to help with restoring function after illness and injury. Most work closely with medical specialists. Physical therapists use a variety of rehabilitation methods to restore function and relieve pain: massage, cold and heat therapy, ultrasound and electrical stimulation, and stretching and strengthening exercises. The American Physical Therapy Association can provide referrals.

ATHLETIC TRAINERS are licensed to work specifically on sports-related injuries. Rehabilitation methods may be similar to physical therapy but can additionally focus on maintaining cardiovascular fitness while injuries heal. The National Athletic Trainers' Association can provide referrals.

MASSAGE THERAPISTS work with athletes in reducing pain and tightness in muscles, tendons, and ligaments—the body's soft tissues. The American Massage Therapy Association can provide referrals.

CHIROPRACTORS are doctors of chiropractic medicine who specialize in the alignment of the body's musculoskeletal system. Pelvis, back, and neck pain and muscle imbalances are often treated by a chiropractor. Some may specialize in sports injuries. Two organizations, the American Chiropractors Association and the International Chiropractic Association, can provide referrals.

When the time comes to seek medical attention, ask others in your sport for referrals, look in the Yellow Pages, or search online. If you have a choice, choose a sports medicine specialist over a general doctor. For contact information for the professional organizations mentioned above, check "Medical and Footwear Specialists" on page 350.

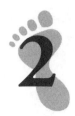

You Can Have Healthy & Happy Feet

This chapter was suggested by a reader who commented, "Many people don't have a clue about their own feet, about how things work and why, or about regular and preventive maintenance." As athletes, feet should be one of our most important concerns. They get us where we are going and back again. We toss on a fanny pack or backpack and trot off without a thought to what that means to our feet. We shove them into shoes and boots without taking time to look at them. We add miles too fast, stress them with uneven terrain, let them become too dry or too wet, and then wonder why our feet hurt.

Think "Feet"

As Coup wrote in the fourth edition foreword, "It's about your FEET." The only way to have feet that are healthy and happy is to be proactive in foot care, to stay on top of minor problems before they become major problems. That means you buy high-quality shoes and socks, take care of your skin and toenails through self care, condition your feet with the miles you need for the sports you will participate in, don't stress them beyond what they can do, and rest them when they need rest. Many foot problems happen because we forget to think about our feet.

A Daily Ritual

Each morning before putting on socks, take a few seconds to run your hands over your feet to check for anything out of the ordinary. If you find something, refer to the index to find the corresponding section in the book. Ask yourself some questions:

- Do I see any redness?

- Are there any cracks or cuts in the skin?

- Do my nails need trimming?

- Is there redness or tender areas at the nail beds?

- Do I see any scaly skin?

- Does anything itch?

- Do I have any old blisters that need attention?

- Is there pain anywhere?

- Do I have any callus buildup that needs attention?

- Do I see any corns or plantar warts?

- Does anything feel funny?

Talk to Your Doctor

Your doctor can do a foot check whenever you have a physical. He or she can help catch problems before they become medical emergencies. Ask what you should watch for. Typically watch for sores that don't heal, ingrown toenails, swelling, cold feet, numbness, a burning or tingling feeling, or unresolved or abnormal pain—even melanomas. Problems with our feet can develop into long-term health issues, which can rob us of our mobility and independence. The American Orthopaedic Foot and Ankle Society says that many of the more than 4.8 million visits to doctors made each year for foot and ankle problems are problems that could have been prevented with better footwear and foot care.

Summer Foot Care Basics

Summers are fun. We get outdoors and explore. We walk more, hike, run, and participate in sports. Many of these activities, however, put added stressors on our feet. This section discusses what we should do to prepare our feet for summer.

Many of us go barefoot in the summer. If you are outside, be watchful for cuts and abrasions to your skin. Use an antibiotic ointment if necessary. Going barefoot will cause the skin on the bottom of your feet to harden and turn into calluses. Calluses are always a good topic of discussion because while many people like them, many more don't. Some feel that the callus protects the area from blistering. The problem occurs when a blister develops under a callus. If you like calluses, try to keep them under control and not too thick. Use the Heel Smoother Pro, a pumice stone, or callus file to keep them manageable. Also watch for cracks in the heels. These cracks are called fissures and can be several layers of skin deep. Once cracked, the skin has to heal from the inside out. The use of a skin moisturizer in the morning and evening can do wonders to keep your feet in shape. When applying a moisturizer or callus remover cream in the evening, occasionally wrap your feet in a plastic bag or plastic wrap to hold the cream on the foot.

When you wear flip-flops and sandals, be aware that the same rules apply here as going barefoot. You can also develop a very thick and hard "corner" of skin at the edges of the heel. Be attentive to the condition of the skin on the bottom of your feet and care for it as described above.

Keeping skin soft can help the toes. Many of us develop a hardened layer of skin at the bottom of our toes, especially the baby toes. This can easily develop into calluses and then blister. A file and skin moisturizer can help.

Toenails need to be kept trimmed and filed smooth. Trim them straight across to avoid an ingrown nail. File the nail smooth so when you draw your finger across the tip of the nail, you can't feel rough edges. Nails that are too long or have rough edges can catch on socks and push the nail back into the nail bed. They also hit the front of the inside of the toe box, putting pressure on the nail, which can cause black nails. If the nail comes loose, be sure to keep it covered with a Band-Aid so it won't come off when pulling socks on or off.

This is a good time to drag all your shoes out of the closet and give them a once-over. Check for worn-out uppers, worn-down soles that could change your gait and cause problems, and compressed midsoles that offer no cushioning and support. Put these shoes aside and save them for gardening and chores. If the shoes are OK, check for worn-out paper-thin insoles. Replace them to give the shoes more life.

Strong ankles make walking, hiking, and running easier. Use a wobble board or ankle exercises to strengthen these important joints. A good exercise is to stand on one foot, or even on a soft pillow, with arms outstretched; when you master this, close your eyes. Ankle exercises help to promote better balance, ankle strength, and the ability to respond in mid-stride to changes in the terrain.

Winter Foot Care Basics

In the winter you still need to work on your skin and toenails, and keep calluses in check. Because you're not barefoot or in sandals as much, you may forget to check your feet as often as you do in the summer. In addition, be watchful for dry skin. The cold, snow, and ice make it important to wear good socks and keep your feet warm. The thick socks can make your feet sweat more so be watchful for athlete's foot. The use of antifungal foot powder can help prevent problems. Winter is a good time to go through your sock drawer and toss old and worn socks. Do the same with shoes, replacing old insoles, laces, and, if necessary, tossing the shoes too.

Aging Feet

Being aware of how your feet change as you age can help you prepare and make good choices. At a meeting of the American Academy of Orthopaedic Surgeons in Orlando, experts with the Foot and Ankle Society described the variety of foot problems that emerge with age and how to tell which ones can probably not be blamed on normal aging.

Cherise M. Dyal, MD, the chief of the Foot and Ankle Division of Orthopaedic Surgery at the Montessori Medical Centre in New York explained, "There are five things that occur naturally with aging. The size increases as your feet get longer and wider; you lose some of the padding on the bottom of your foot, so you thin out your fat pad and tend to lose some of the spring in your step; your foot tends to become a little stiffer, so you lose some of the range of motion in your foot and ankle; you tend to have some problems with balance; and there is a very mild settling of the arch that's seen as a flattening of the foot. Those are the natural changes."

It has been well documented that foot problems increase with age. A good resource as we get older is the book *Great Feet for Life: Footcare and Footwear for Healthy Aging* by Paul Langer, DPM. According to Paul, the most common foot complaints by older adults are toenail and skin problems, calluses or corns, swelling, bunions, and arthritis.

Here are some tips to deal with aging feet.

■ Make sure to have your feet sized each time you buy shoes.

■ Choose shoes with additional cushioning and support.

■ Switch to insoles with more cushioning in the heel and support in the arch. Sorbothane and Spenco insoles with gel are good choices.

■ Pay close attention to your toenails. They often thicken as you age so be sure to keep them trimmed and filed properly.

Ten Easy Steps to Happy Feet

Here are my top ten foot care tips to keep your feet healthy and happy. Each of these tips is explained in depth in this book.

1. Make sure your footwear fits.

2. Buy high-quality footwear.

3. Wear moisture-wicking socks.

4. Practice self care of your feet.

5. Manage your toenails.

6. Strengthen your feet and ankles.

7. Rest your feet.

8. Condition your feet for your sport.

9. Learn how to prevent blisters.

10. Carry a small foot care kit.

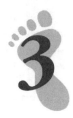

Sports & Your Feet

Running, hiking, and adventure racing place extreme demands on our feet. Soccer, football, and court sports stress the feet and ankles with their quick changes in direction and sudden stops. Skiing and snowshoeing encase our feet in unforgiving hard boots that also stress our ankles. The surfaces we play and compete on vary from dirt, rock, grass, asphalt, and concrete to wooden courts, tracks, snow, and ice. Every sport offers wide ranges of difficulty. We challenge ourselves with ultramarathons on trails or roads. We test our limits in adventure races under extreme conditions. We tackle the multisport fun of duathlons and triathlons. Whatever our sport, our feet take a beating.

A run may be a relatively short road 10K or a grueling ultrarunning event of 100 miles with more than 40,000 feet of mountainous ascents and descents. It may be in a short- or medium-length duathlon or triathlon, or a longer Ironman or Ultraman Triathlon. There are also further extremes: 24-, 48-, and 72-hour runs, six-day runs, and 1000-mile races. The terrain may be paved roads, tracks, fire roads, trails, cross-country, or any combination. You may run without any gear, with a single water bottle, or with a fanny pack or lightweight backpack loaded with extra socks, food, and water bottles.

A hike may be a day trip with a day pack, an overnighter with a mid-weight 40-pound backpack, or a ten-day high-Sierra trip with a pack that tips the scales at 65 pounds. You may be a traditional backpacker with a full-size pack that carries all the comforts of home, a fast packer with a 30-pound pack, or an ultralight backpacker with a 16-pound pack. Typical backpackers may cover 6–10 miles in a day, ultralight backpackers can easily cover 30 miles, while fast packers may cover 40 or more miles. The hike duration may be a night in your local hills, a week in the desert, three weeks in the Sierra, or several months on the Appalachian Trail or the Pacific Crest Trail.

Many athletes are choosing multiday running and walking events. The event that started the rage is Racing the Planet's seven-day stage races, where each participant carries all his or her own gear, including food, as they navigate 150 miles in places such as China, the Sahara, Chile, and more (**www.racingtheplanet.com**). RTP's events, the newer six-day Gore-Tex TransRockies Run, and other similar events are geared for people looking for adventure and challenges, in a doable event. Of course, this multiday format also brings with it lots of foot problems.

Adventure racing includes events with names such as Primal Quest, Eco Challenge, the Raid Gauloises, and the Beast of the East. These are typically competitive team races with up to five participants who must all finish together. Combining sports disciplines such as trail or cross-country running, mountain biking, rappelling, climbing, kayaking, canoeing, horseback riding, swimming, glacier climbing, and others, these races pose challenges along an often unknown course with constantly changing terrain. Many are multiday events over distances up to 450 miles. In these team events, the whole team is only as fast as the feet of its slowest member. Robert Nagel, one of the world's best adventure racers, recalls his experiences in the 1996 Extreme Games: "Our team had a strong and growing lead when my feet caused us to grind to a crawl. We continued, barely, losing more than 12 hours in the process, but still managed to take third place." He remembers that ESPN continued to show tapes of his feet 16 months after the event! After that experience, he worked hard to perfect a foot care regimen that would prevent such a disaster from happening again.

Most sports require considerable use of the feet, and participation in these sports requires an athlete to keep his or her feet happy and healthy. Many of these athletes have learned the finer points of keeping their feet in shape. They rely on the many sources of conventional wisdom about foot care, but while much of this wisdom is good, the best advice often comes from athletes who, through trial and error, have found unique solutions for the prevention and treatment of their foot problems. Ronald Moak, an Appalachian Trail thru-hiker (1977) and Pacific Crest Trail thru-hiker (2000), sums it up best: "I would like to think that after 30 years of backpacking, I'd have solved the little dilemma of my feet. But, alas, I'm not that naive." Ronald has the right idea—it's good to listen to all forms of advice and then try different things. Don't be afraid to go against conventional wisdom. Just because it didn't work for others, that doesn't mean it won't work for you.

Sport Similarities

What do the sports discussed above have in common? Foot-stressing sports have many similarities. They pound the feet, stress the joints, and strain the muscles, often to unnatural extremes. They may take place over a day, yet often are done over several days, or even a week or more. While athletes participate in these sports, their feet become highly susceptible to hot spots, blisters, and problems with toenails, stubbed toes, bruises, sprains, strains, heel spurs, plantar fasciitis, and Achilles tendinitis. All of these sports can be more enjoyable by solving these common foot problems.

Runners put considerable weight on their feet with each step. Though hikers move slower than runners, they often find their feet stressed by the weight of a fully loaded fanny pack, lumbar pack, or backpack. Adventure racers may stress the feet faster in shorter events or longer over multiday events in which they compete in multiple sports and carry the special equipment they require. The longer multiday adventure races often tax the feet more than we can imagine with the regular exposure to water, constantly changing adverse conditions, and lack of time to do proper foot care.

In Roland Mueser's book *Long-Distance Hiking: Lessons from the Appalachian Trail,* he describes what he found when he surveyed hikers:

> Problems with feet were endemic. Half of the hikers experienced blisters at the start; many of these were attributed to thrusting tender feet into stiff, heavy boots. During his first few days in Georgia, one hiker was forced into a hospital for an entire week with so many serious blisters that his trip was terminated. And even later when hikers' feet became toughened, the combination of rain, heavy boots, and wet socks meant trouble for one out of five on the trail. One foot-troubled backpacker reported having seven blisters at one time. And more than one hiker, squirming out of boots, was horrified to see socks soaked with blood.[1]

Studies have shown that "carrying heavy external loads (i.e., a heavy backpack) during locomotion appears to increase the likelihood of foot blisters."[2] In addition, the type of physical activity performed is a factor in the probability of blister development. As we intensify our activity and as the duration of the activity increases, frictional forces are increased. Heavy loads, high-intensity activities, and long-duration activities are what we do as runners, hikers, and adventure racers. In our events, most of us experience at least two of these three stressors. Ultrarunner Suzie Lister typically experiences few problems with her feet while running ultras. However, when she participated in the 1995 Eco Challenge, the added weight of a pack on her back and the multiday stresses of adventure racing caused many problems with her feet: blisters on top of blisters and swollen feet.

The similar stresses among sports make the preventive maintenance and treatments for blisters and other foot problems necessary for all sports. This book approaches the different disciplines—running, duathlons and triathlons, hiking and backpacking, and adventure racing—as one and the same when dealing with one's feet. Proper foot care is the most important variable for a successful outing.

Differences in Terrain

The terrain is an important part of your running, hiking, and playing environment. While a flat, smooth, and resilient surface may seem ideal, it is not. Most runners spend the majority of their running miles on roads and trails, while most hikers spend their time on trails. The ideal surface is one that keeps changing the stresses on our body. This will help prevent injury and make you stronger. Changing surfaces develops muscles and reflexes. Don't always choose the same surface. Mix it up.

Variations from our normal running or hiking surface can produce problems as we compensate for uphills, downhills, concave surfaces, or irregularities of the surface. Be aware of compensations in your stride or gait due to changes in the surface.

Dirt & Trails

Dirt and trails provide a soft running and hiking surface. Trails or fire roads can open new vistas to the adventuresome athlete. Some trails are well groomed, while others are barely maintained. Soft dirt trails provide excellent shock absorption and can be a good surface to use if recovering from an injury.

Whether running or hiking, pay close attention to trail hazards such as rocks, roots, wet leaves, mud, and other potential hazards, any of which can cause a turned ankle or a fall. On rainy days, slippery mud and grasses can present problems with footing. Watch for uneven terrain, roots, and holes on grassy sections of trail. Trail dust, dirt, pebbles, and rocks can be kicked up into the sock or between the sock and the shoe. These irritants can cause hot spots, blisters, or cuts. Gaiters worn over the shoe or boot tops can help prevent this problem (see "Gaiters," page 150).

Hiking on trails while wearing a backpack presents the added problem of maintaining one's balance with a top-heavy load while negotiating rocks, roots, and uneven trail. Attention to your footing can help prevent a turned ankle. Striding uphill stretches the Achilles tendons and the calf muscles, and makes the pelvis tilt forward. Going downhill increases the shock impact to the heels when landing and tilts the body backward. Constantly going up- and downhill may also cause problems with toes, toenails, heel pain, plantar fasciitis, and more.

Grass

Grass is a forgiving surface and a great choice if you are prone to road-impact injuries. Be careful of uneven grassy areas, holes from burrowing animals, the slipperiness of wet grass, and the occasional rock.

Roads

Road running is the mainstay of most runners. The asphalt surface of most roads provides a softer surface than concrete sidewalks. However, roads have slanted, concave surfaces curving down toward the sides. The concave surface puts more stress on the downward side of your shoes and your body. The foot of the higher leg rotates inward, while the foot of the lower leg rotates outward. Spend a few minutes on your favorite roads to check the angle of their curve and be aware of it. Avoid prolonged running on slanted surfaces or at least spend equal time on both road shoulders. Keep your eyes open for potholes and manhole covers. Of course, the biggest hazard to road runners is vehicles. Where possible, run opposite the flow of traffic and safely to one side of the road, and choose roads with wide shoulders.

Concrete & Sidewalks

Concrete is approximately ten times harder than asphalt. While the surface is usually smooth, your bones, muscles, and connective tissue get hammered. This surface can cause foot, leg, or back pain through the jarring of the joints. Shin splints, stress fractures, and compartment syndrome are common injuries from running on concrete. Care must be taken to watch your footing on sidewalks to avoid the tapered edges of driveways and drop-offs at curbs. The use of good, cushioned shoes and gel insoles can make concrete bearable—but try at all costs to avoid running on concrete.

Courts

Court play is usually on either asphalt or wood. Tennis courts may be indoors or outdoors. Basketball, racquetball, and other indoor sports are usually on wood. While an asphalt or wood court surface is hard and unforgiving, the main foot stresses for athletes playing on them are caused by sudden, quick movements and sudden starts and stops. Cushioned or motion-control shoes, depending on your feet, will protect your ankles. A good shoe fit, coupled with moisture-wicking socks and insoles, will prevent hot spots and blisters.

Sand

Walking or running on sand is hard work. Though sand is soft, its surface is not typically flat. Your heels may sink in more than the forefoot and the uneven sand may cause a turned ankle. If you have access to a beach, try to stay near the water on the wet and fairly hard sand.

Snow & Ice

Walking or running in the snow or on ice can be challenging. There may be snow on top of a layer of ice. Your shoes cannot make good traction unless they have been modified with small screws or special traction gear. Falling is a hazard and muscle pulls can be common as you slip or slide.

Tracks

Most of us at some time run on tracks. True, they can be boring. Running in circles, actually in ovals, lap after lap after lap after lap may not be your idea of a good run, but there may be a time for it in your running schedule. A track allows us to calculate with accuracy how fast we are running. I have used a track for occasional speed workouts. Prior to my first 24-hour track run, I spent three hours running at a local high-school track to get a feel for the repetitiveness of track running.

The continuous running in one direction stresses the outer leg, so change direction every now and then. Dirt tracks should always be checked for ruts and uneven surfaces that could cause you to trip. Running in the outer lanes is less stressful when rounding the curves.

Conditioning

Conditioning means more than getting your body in condition. It also means getting your feet into the best shape possible for your sport. Your feet will respond to training in the same way your legs respond. Increasing your running or hiking time by increments will allow your feet time to adapt to the added stresses of the additional mileage. Doubling your mileage too quickly will likely lead to potential problems. If you are working up to a marathon, an ultra, or a multiday hike, do back-to-back training days to work your feet into their best possible condition. Toned and strengthened feet can reduce the occurrence of injuries, as well as sore and tired feet.

" I *personal experience*

n 1991, I walked through immigration in the old Stapleton International Airport in Denver, wide-eyed and fresh from Australia and sporting some nice, neat, size 9 wing tips, comfortably encasing my soft corporate toes. Years later I am outgrowing my somewhat less than nimble size 11 trail shoes, with nary a hope of ever squeezing back into my old wing tips. This rather dramatic change in foot size is due entirely to conditioning. In 1984, when I started adventure racing in Australia, I had a size 8 shoe, but the intervening 22 years spent running and hiking around for prolonged periods with a pack on my back has resulted in a physiologic adaptation.

"This is really just conditioning. The same effect can be seen in farmer's hands, which grow to quite unusual sizes over decades of manipulating heavy machinery and tools. It is not uncommon to walk into a bar in the Midwest and see the little old farmer, neatly shrunk inside his once tight-fitting Wrangler jeans, with absolutely enormous gnarled hands nursing a beer.

"So, to get these nice big, abuse-proof peds, spend some time on them. Lots of time. So much time that they hurt really bad. I don't usually say this, but in the case of feet, no pain, no gain. Don't go out and get bloody blisters, but do go out for those really long hikes, with a pack stuffed with baguettes, Camembert, bottles of red wine, and the kitchen sink and really abuse your lower leg structures. Work the crossword every day and you will get good at it; wield a hammer all day and you will get calluses on your hands; hike with a heavy pack for hours and you'll get bigger, tougher feet!"

—Ian Adamson, adventure racer

Brick Robbins was an adequately trained runner when he started his thru-hike of Pacific Crest Trail, but he quickly found that running had not conditioned his feet. The extra weight of a backpack caused additional stress to his feet. After 100 miles his feet were sore and bruised. By the time he reached Idyllwild—another 70 miles down the trail—he had killer blisters that took another 270 miles to heal. Although his feet were in good shape from running, they needed additional conditioning for the weight of a pack. There are no shortcuts to conditioning your feet. Your feet will become conditioned to longer distances by gradually increasing your mileage.

When Karen Borski thru-hiked the Appalachian Trail in 1998, she had very few foot problems. A year before the thru-hike, however, her feet were so out of shape that after an 8-mile day hike they would be riddled with huge blisters on the sides of the heels. Wearing a pack, she found that after only a few miles, blisters would begin to develop on the soles of her feet, usually the balls of the feet where the main pressure is felt. Karen recalls that she was "so frightened and worried about these blisters that I was afraid I would not be able to thru-hike." To fix the problem, she first bought new boots that were slightly too large so that during the course of a hike, as her feet naturally swelled, they wouldn't become too tight and rub. Then she started hiking with a pack every weekend. After hobbling around for most of the following week nursing these awful blisters, she would go out and do it again. When calluses finally began to develop, she took up running on the weeknights, both to get her body in shape and to help toughen her feet.

So, what is the best way to condition your feet? Your feet must be conditioned to endure the rigors and stresses of your chosen sport or sports. Train in race conditions in the shoes and socks you will wear on race day. Do short hikes with a pack on your back before taking off to tackle a multiday hike. Use a wobble board to strengthen your ankles. Toughen your feet with barefoot walking. Work up to distances that you will tackle in your event. Work out the kinks; find the best shoes and socks for what you will be doing. Learn how to trim your toenails and reduce calluses. Discover the proper insoles that provide support to relieve your plantar fasciitis or heel pain. Strengthen your toes and ankles. In short, do your homework before you head out to tackle the big one. Your feet will thank you.

If you are training for a race or event, at least 60% of your training should be done while wearing your pack with about the same amount of weight as you plan to carry during your race. This works your upper and lower body and trains the muscles, tendons, and ligaments of your ankles and feet to handle the extra weight. You must also train on somewhat the same terrain you'll face during a race—rocks, sand, up and down hills, even with wet feet. Knowing in advance how your feet respond to these conditions will help you anticipate problems. Finally, you must train for the same distances as the race itself. One or two long runs a week is much better than five or six short runs. To the under-trained, the multiple days of pounding on your feet can take a cumulative toll and make every step painful.

Biomechanics

Many athletes who have participated in extreme sports have learned firsthand how one minor problem can be magnified over time and eventually have major consequences. Typically this happens when a blister affects the gait, a backpack's weight throws off balance and stance, or stressed or weakened muscles cause an imbalance in the body's mechanics. Every athlete has different strengths and weaknesses, different degrees of flexibility, and different muscle skills and body types. These factors affect the way we walk, run, and move. Add on a fanny pack or backpack, or put a flashlight in one hand and a water bottle in the other hand, and your biomechanics change. Each time your foot lands, it absorbs about two-and-a-half times your body weight. For every mile you travel, your feet hit the ground around 800 times each.

The Importance of Alignment

You all know the foot bone is connected to the ankle bone, and the ankle bone is connected to the leg bone. True, correct alignment of all those bones at the joints keeps you moving relatively pain free now, and prevents many degenerative changes down the road. Total body alignment is essential to the success of any athletic activity.

Even more important to the healthy functioning of the feet and their ability to carry you through life is the spine—the very specific focus of chiropractors. The spinal cord carries sensory and motor information from your feet (and everywhere else for that matter) to your brain and back again. If one of the vertebral bones is even slightly misaligned or fixated, it can affect the communication lines and your feet and brain can be broadcasting misinformation. The joints of your feet and particularly your ankles contain nerves called proprioceptors that send messages about the changes in terrain that you are walking, standing, or running on. The brain then interprets and makes the miniscule changes in every joint in your body, from the tilt of your skull to the tuck of your tailbone, to keep you upright.

Chiropractors come in many styles. I recommend one who specializes in sports chiropractic and who adjusts extremities as well as the spine. Those chiropractors are certified in orthopedics and can design a rehab program of strengthening and stretching. Always get referrals from other runners and make sure the chiropractor is a good fit for you.

—Pam Adams, chiropractor

Maryna, a holistic practitioner who was part of the medical team at the Canadian Eco Challenge, emphasizes how your whole leg and, indeed, your whole body needs to function in a unified, integrated way. She saw a lot of blisters caused by legs being out of alignment in various places from hips to knees to ankles. Misalignment causes radical changes in all phases of your footfall from strike to break over to push off. Problems can work from the legs down or from the feet up. An understanding of biomechanics will help us visualize the cause and effect.

Understanding Biomechanics

Biomechanics is the study of the mechanics of a living body, especially the forces exerted by muscles and gravity on the skeletal structure. The foot, which includes everything below the ankle, is a complicated but amazing engineering marvel. With an intricate biomechanical composition of 26 bones each, together the foot bones account for almost one-quarter the total number of bones in the entire

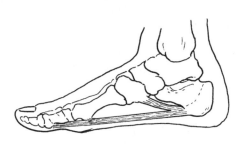

Side view of the bones of the foot

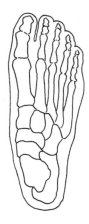

Top view of the bones of the foot

body. Thirty-three joints make each foot flexible. About 20 muscles manage control of the foot's movements. Tendons stretch like rubber bands between the bones and muscles so that when a muscle contracts, the tendon pulls the bone. Each foot contains 109 ligaments that connect bone to bone and cartilage to bone and hold the whole structure together. Nerve endings make the feet sensitive. With each step you walk or run, your feet are subjected to a force of two to three times your body weight, which makes the feet prone to injury.

The big toe, commonly called the great toe, helps to maintain balance while the little toes function like a springboard. The three inner metatarsal bones provide rigid support while the two outer metatarsal bones, one on each side of the foot, move to adapt to uneven surfaces.

Your feet are each supported by three arches. The transverse arch runs from side-to-side just back from the ball of the foot. This is the major weight-bearing arch of the foot. The medial longitudinal arch runs the length of the instep, flattening while standing or running, giving spring to the gait, and shortening when you sit or lie down. The lateral longitudinal arch runs on the outside of the foot. Both longitudinal arches function in absorbing shock loads and balancing the body. These three arches of the foot are referred to singularly as the foot's arch.

Our feet have four ranges of motion. Upward motion is called dorsiflexion and downward is plantar flexion. Inward motion is known as inversion while outward motion is eversion.

With a basic understanding of the foot's construction, it becomes increasingly important to be aware of how we affect our body's biomechanics. At some point in training for an event, we need to try to mimic the event itself. Wear the same shoes and socks that you plan on wearing during the event. Wear the same clothes. Carry the same weight in a fanny pack or backpack. Even get out in the same weather. Although we may not realize it, these factors can change our stride, work different muscles, and put pressure on different body parts—including the feet.

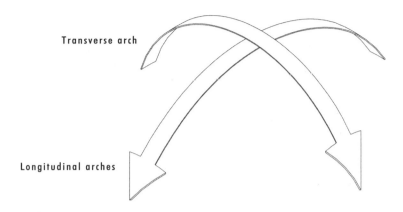

Transverse arch

Longitudinal arches

Avoiding Biomechanical Problems

The body lines up over the foot. When the foot goes out of alignment, the ankle, knee, pelvis, and back may all follow. Analyzing the way we stand, walk, and run helps a podiatrist or orthopedist determine whether we have a mechanical misalignment and how it can be corrected. He or she will also want to see your running shoes to analyze the wear patterns on the soles.

An example of biomechanics is the functioning of the foot's arch. A low arch, or flat foot, typically occurs when the foot is excessively pronated, turning it inward. A high arch supinates the foot, rolling it outward. Both of these structural variations can cause knee, hip, and back pain. When one arch flattens more than the other arch, that inner ankle moves closer to the ground. That hip then rotates downward and backward causing a shortening of that leg during walking and running. The pelvis and back both tilt lower on the shortened leg side and the back bends sideways. The opposite leg, which is now longer, is moved outward toward the side that puts added stress on its ankle, knee, and hip. The shoulder on that side then drops toward the dropped hip. All of these are compensations as the body adapts. Muscles, tendons, ligaments, and joints are stretched to their limit. The body is out of alignment. Pam Adams, a chiropractor, gives her perspective on how this all works on page 35.

The stresses on our bodies can result in inflammation, often the cause of foot pain. Running on unbalanced and uneven feet may result in fatigue. Fatigue gives way to spasms that may cause a shift in the shape of our feet. Corns, calluses, bunions, spurs, and neuromas may develop when joints are out of alignment.

Do not fall into the trap of drawing erroneous conclusions about your injuries or the type of shoes or equipment that you need for your running style. A podiatrist or orthopedist should check pain associated with running. Heel pain that we try to resolve with a heel pad may not be caused by a heel problem but by arch problems. This in turn may throw off the biomechanics of the body's alignment. If you begin a run and right away experience knee pain, you most likely have a problem with the knee. If the pain comes after running for a while, it is most likely not a knee problem but a biomechanical problem. Likewise, you may think that because you are a heavy runner, you need a shoe with lots of cushioning. Based on that decision, you buy a cushioned shoe, the most cushioning insoles, and wear thickly cushioned socks. But, in reality, what you may need is a stability control shoe. This is where the help and expertise of medical specialists comes in. They are trained to determine biomechanical problems.

In 1991 Craig Smith and his brother set out to hike 300 miles of the Continental Divide Trail. With training and planning done, they started with heavy packs that tipped the scale at almost 58 pounds each. Two days and 22 miles later, Craig had developed severe pain in both knees. Forced to abort the trip, they cached as much gear as possible before starting back. With Craig's knees wrapped with torn T-shirt strips, it took them four days to backtrack the 22 miles. It took several weeks of conditioning therapy before he could finally walk without a limp. Craig now packs lighter, does exercises that focus on strengthening the knees, and uses a walking stick on downhills. He could have easily been a victim of biomechanical problems that centered in his knees.

Remember that most athletes have foot problems or become injured by doing too much, too soon, and too fast. To avoid biomechanical problems, use proper footwear, pace yourself, do strength training, and train in the gear you will use in your event.

CONDITIONING PRODUCTS

The **DYNA-DISC** is made of the same material as a gym ball and is inflatable with just a standard ball needle and pump. It comes in 14- or 24-inch diameters. The Dyna-Disc has both smooth and knobbed sides. Perfect for balance training, lower back, pelvic stabilization, and weight-shift exercises. Lifestyle Sports also offers balance and wobble boards. **www.lifestylesport.com**

OPTP (ORTHOPEDIC PHYSICAL THERAPY PRODUCTS) has a wide range of devices for balance/proprioception, massage, stretching strength training, and more. **www.optp.com**

POLES can be used to hike farther and more comfortably, absorb shock, keep your knees healthy, and help maintain balance. Walkers, hikers, backpackers, and adventure racers have discovered the benefits of poles. Made of either aluminum or carbon fiber, many models offer antishock support and carbon tips. Poles are made by Black Diamond, Komperdell, Leki, MSR, and REI. Typically called hiking or trekking poles, they can be found in sporting goods and camping stores. Some people use two, but others are comfortable using one. Check your local outdoors store for lightweight models.

WOBBLE AND ROCKER BOARDS can be used to improve balance and strength, retrain injured muscles, improve muscle memory, and build core strength. Fitter First has the most comprehensive line of boards, as well as training charts and programs. **www.fitter1.com**

Form & Health

As long as you have good form, whether walking, running, hiking, paddling, or biking—any activity where you are using your feet for movement—you stand a better than average chance of not injuring yourself due to a biomechanical problem. But if a pack rides wrong on your back making you lean to the side, or if weak abs make you lean forward, or tired arms cause your shoulders to drop, or spent quads cramp up, your body is tossed out of alignment. This will ultimately work its way down to your feet. As they compensate for your biomechanical problems, your gait and stride change, and your feet develop their own problems.

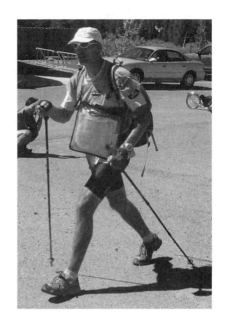

Use hiking poles for support and to help the knees.

So what is gait? We'll take our definitions from Wikipedia, the free encyclopedia. Its definition is "the way locomotion is achieved using human limbs."

Wikipedia also says, "Walking is the most common human gait. It is characterized by alternating steps of left and right lower limbs. It generally provides useful speeds of progression for daily activities with near-optimal energy efficiency. . . . Running is nearly identical to walking except that the person is actually airborne once each beat. This is the chief high-speed gait of humans. The beats happen faster and the distance traveled per beat is also much higher. Running requires much more energy than walking. . . . Jogging is a sub-gait of run where the pace is much less and the legs nearly never go out of the body's center line."

Thus gait can be best described as your own particular style of walking or running, which determines the distribution of stress to various parts of your legs and feet. While there is no single proper gait that suits everyone, if you experience pain or discomfort (particularly back, hip, or knee pain) while walking or running, a gait analysis from a podiatrist or physical therapist may be in order.

Dr. Stephen M. Pribut, in an article "Gait Biomechanics" on his website **www. drpribut.com,** explains a gait analysis: "In the gait examination, we will observe for symmetry. We will look for clues regarding leg length inequality. Arm swing asymmetry, uneven head bounce, unilateral pelvic drop, and uneven stride length are all indicators that there is a leg length inequality. Other factors to note are the heel contact point, an apparent bouncy gait, excessive pronation of the foot, early heel off, and the angle of gait."

Your best bet is to maintain good form by thinking smart and training wisely, whatever the discipline. Make sure your shoes are not worn down—replace them before they lose their support and cushion. Wear good insoles to balance the foot and provide good heel and arch support and alignment. Strengthen the ankles and knees with specific exercises. Do upper body exercises to strengthen your abs, back, and shoulders for carrying your pack. Work your arms so they can help maintain balance and proper form. Learn how to tape a sprained ankle or turned knee. Condition yourself in incremental stages without huge jumps in mileage or extremes. Train with the gear you will use in an actual race—building up to appropriate weights rather than carrying everything all at once. Use hiking poles for support and to help the knees. Learn your body's weak links and find exercises to strengthen those muscles and joints.

Every one of us, at one time or another, can fall victim to biomechanical problems as we race to extremes. Train smart and race smart, and you can stay healthy, starting with your feet.

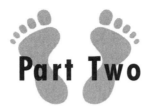

Part Two

Footwear Basics

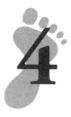

The Magic of Fit

The website **www.foot.com** gives the following statistic: "The average person will walk more than 115,000 miles in a lifetime, which is enough to walk the circumference of the earth four times over. Additionally, the average person does not wear a properly fitting or comfortable shoe." I agree.

Fit is key. Again, repeat after me: "*Fit is key.*" Without properly fitting shoes or boots, your feet will encounter many problems that can initiate many others. If your footwear is too loose, your feet will slide around, creating friction. If your footwear is too tight in certain areas, your feet will experience excessive pressure. Wearing too loose or too tight footwear will change the biomechanics of your foot strike, which in turn will affect your gait and throw off your whole stride and balance. This will stress your tendons and ligaments. When your feet and toes are pinched in too-tight shoes with socks that make the fit even tighter, the blood circulation is reduced. To top it all off, you will endure aches and or pain, and will be more tired from dealing with all of the above. Sounds like fun, right? Unfortunately many athletes have resigned themselves to this type of process. They go out strong for as long as their feet last—which in many cases is not as long as they had hoped and often is well before the finish line or the end of their journey. Does it have to happen this way? You decide.

Fit starts with properly fitting shoes with a quality insole. No matter how good your socks are or how well you apply tape or how good any other component is, if the shoes fit incorrectly, you will have problems.

In *Advanced Backpacking*, Karen Berger makes a good comment on the fit of boots—and the same advice applies to any sport shoe. "Like most marriages, the mesh between boot and foot is not always a good match. If you look at the feet of several people, you'll undoubtedly see a range of bumps and bunions, arches, and anklebones—all of which are encased in the same hard leather cage. It takes a bit of time, accommodation, and softening for boots and feet to settle into a comfortable routine."[3] Because our feet are so different, many factors go into achieving a good fit.

Rich Schick, a physician's assistant and ultrarunner, believes the key to getting the proper size shoe is the insert: "If the foot does not fit the insert, then the shoe will have to stretch to accommodate the difference or there may be excessive room in the shoe, which can lead to blisters and other foot problems." He thinks there is too much confusion about straight lasts, curved lasts, semicurved lasts, and so on:

> You don't need to know any of this if you use the insert to fit your shoes. The same holds true for the proper width of shoe. Simply remove the insert from the shoe and place your heel in the depression made for the heel [in the insert]. There should be an inch to an inch and a half from the tip of your longest toe to the tip of the insert. None of your toes or any part of the foot should lap over the sides of the insert. If they do, is it because the insert is too narrow or is it because of a curved foot and straight insert or vice versa? The foot should not be more than about a quarter inch from the edges of the insert either. This includes the area around the heel, or the shoe may be too loose. Check to see if the arch of the insert fits in the arch of your foot. Finally, if all the above criteria are met, then try on the shoe. The only remaining pitfalls are tight toe boxes and seams or uppers that rub.

Many shoe and boot companies suggest specific models that are best for certain types of activities and sports, and for certain types of feet. They do this because many shoes are made for a specific type of foot—and many people have feet that will work better with one type of shoe than another. Look for the buyer's guides in the magazines of your sport. Runners can find shoe reviews in *Runner's World, Trail Runner, Running Times*, and *UltraRunning*. Backpackers and hikers can check out *Backpacker* magazine's boot reviews, and *Outside* magazine's Buyer's Guide for helpful information.[4] For information on shoe reviews and gear review sources, see page 349 in the appendix. Other sport-specific magazines may offer similar reviews. Many websites are now posting reviews, and some offer reader comments or reviews.

Be Careful Out There

The newspaper and mail often bring us ads from discount sports and department stores. They typically advertise shoes with names that are unknown to the well-read athlete. Who has heard of these shoes? Many major shoe companies make shoes aimed at these stores. They may be good shoes, but I wouldn't buy them for serious walking or running.

While most athletes are careful and know enough to buy running shoes at a running store, many more people are not. Pity the beginning walker or runner who buys shoes without the quality help from a qualified salesperson. They'll get no help with fit—important things such as foot type, toe box space, arch support, and heel counter grip, to say nothing of shoe type, such as motion control, cushioning, and so on. They'll get no help finding the right shoes for whatever they plan to run and no information about the shoe's life expectancy.

They take their shoes home, lace them up, and start running. A small percentage of them will still be going a year later. But many more will have quit because their feet hurt, or after wearing the shoes down—and not knowing when to get new ones—they got injured and quit.

If you know someone who is starting to run or even walk seriously, take a moment and share a bit of your experience on buying good footwear. Many shoe companies make mid-range or even cheap shoes, and I don't want these substandard shoes to have a negative influence on people wanting to get out and exercise. We all have to be careful out there.

Can there be more than one shoe that is right for your feet? Are there perfect shoes? Christopher Willett went through four pairs of shoes on his 2003 Pacific Crest Trail thru-hike (2,600-plus miles) and bought them as he went. Wearing size 15 running shoes, he didn't really have the option of buying from an outfitter along the trail. He would call or use the Internet from various towns along the way and have new shoes and socks sent up trail. He started in Brooks Adrenaline GTS and liked them in the hot 563-mile Southern California section. He wished the next shoe, the Asics Eagle Trail, had a more protective sole but liked the tread. While the New Balance 806s were structurally good, he felt they had a poor tread design; it is the only shoe that he would not wear again. He finished the last 670 miles in the Asics Gel Trabuco V and liked their durability and tread. Would one of the shoes have worked for his whole thru-hike? If they had been the NB 806s, the answer would be no. Probably any of the other three would have worked the whole way, but Chris might have had problems sticking with one shoe given the varying weather and terrain of the trail. Even the most perfect shoe can have small issues: breathability, tread design, cushioning, sole protection, and so on. Each of these issues can make them perfect for one set of conditions and wrong for another.

Buying Footwear

Buying shoes has evolved to a level of complexity never before seen. Buyers have to study the latest issue of their favorite running, ultrarunning, adventure racing, triathlete, or outdoors magazine or website, or try to read through the materials posted on manufacturers' websites to comprehend the language they're speaking. Does Impact Quotient Technology really matter to you or me? Does IGS really guide my foot "from heel to toe in a much more natural, comfortable stride"? I know what a truss is, so is a Trusstic System something similar?

We're not buying a car, just a pair of shoes. But the complexity of the selection process recently was turned up several notches. If you want to find the best shoes, you now have to read the fine print—and understand what the fine print means. Many of the acronyms and terms above are puzzling unless you read further. Some of the shoe company's websites are very helpful, offering images and understandable explanations of what these things mean. But some are downright useless.

The bottom line: We need to find a shoe that fits well, lasts more than a few miles, and doesn't rub us the wrong way. And after we buy the shoes and find that we love them, we hope they don't discontinue them in six months when the new models are released. There is something to be said for brand loyalty. I have it and I suspect many of you also do—especially when you've found a pair that fits well.

In today's marketplace, we are in a shoe buyer's heaven. Everywhere we turn, there's a shoe store, and in almost every magazine and on every website, there are ads galore for new shoes and boots. But are all things equal? Here is where I chime in with a big resounding NO.

First, we are faced with the typical mall store, usually a chain shoe store that employs people without any degree of knowledge of how to fit shoes. Many times, they also sell shoes that one would never find elsewhere. For example, New Balance, a great shoe company, sells shoes to these stores that are not found in running stores and running magazines. They are different, not as well made, yet perfect for the typical mall shopper.

Specialty outdoor stores, such as running, backpacking, and camping stores, carry shoes that are well made and well known. This is important because we can find reviews of these shoes online and in sport-specific magazines. This allows us to shop with a high degree of knowledge that the shoes we buy are made for our sport and will perform well. These stores also have salespeople who can fit shoes and help you choose between several pairs.

There are running shoes (and this means road shoes and trail shoes), walking shoes, cross trainers, and other sport-specific shoes. I can walk in running shoes but would not run in walking shoes. I can run and walk in most cross trainers, but you would be wise to not use walking and running shoes for a serious game of basketball or other court sport. I can run on trails in most road shoes, although I may sacrifice traction and support. While I can also run on roads in trail shoes, they are often clunky, heavier, and not as flexible.

My preference is to use shoes for what they are intended. I have road and trail shoes and I use them for their intended purpose. Your choice in footwear is important. When shopping for shoes, look for those made for your sport. When participating in sports, use shoes designed for that specific sport.

Personally, I would never buy shoes from any source without trying them on, and walking in them, running a short bit, or using them on an incline board. I prefer to frequent my local running stores, walking stores, and hiking or outdoor stores. I avoid, like the plague, the chain stores that often have shoes that I have never heard of—even if they are from major well-known companies. I get mail-order catalogues from companies that sell all types of shoes and related gear, and I often check out Internet sites where shoes are also sold. If I recognize a particular shoe and know that it fits my foot, I might buy from one of these sites, but with rare exceptions, I buy from my local stores. I value the service, the help with fit, and their look at my gait as I try out the new shoe. They will look at my old shoes (so yes, take your old shoes along), ask what I will be using the shoes for, ask about my foot type, ask about any injury history, and maybe which shoes I have worn in the past. When they bring out the shoes, they will often point out the shoe's features. They'll have me try on the shoes, and they will check for correct spacing in the toe box (both length and height). They will ask me to walk in the shoes and maybe even to go outside and run to get a feel for the shoes. My bottom line: I want a shoe that works on my foot, a shoe that fits as well as possible, and a shoe that's right for whatever sport I throw at it—and that requires the help of a good salesperson.

Buy your shoes wherever you want, but remember, fit is one of the most important elements of using your shoes and boots without problems. Your local shoe store is dedicated to providing you with high-quality choices in shoes and service you can't get through mail order. There is more than one pair of shoes for your feet. There may be a half-dozen models that will fit well. The experts at your local store will help you select several brands and models to come up with a good final choice.

Know Your Feet

With knowledge of biomechanics and your specific foot type, you can make a better choice than shopping blindly. When shopping for shoes or boots, try on several different pairs from several different companies. This will help you identify those that initially feel good versus those that just don't feel quite right. Knowing how different shoes and boots fit your feet will help in the final selection.

A biomechanically efficient athlete lands on the back outside of the heel and rolls inward (pronation) to absorb shock. The foot flattens as the motion moves forward, rolls through the ball of the foot, and rotates outward (supination) to the push off. Overpronation is the inward roll of the foot as you roll off the heel.

There are two main schools of advice for preparing to purchase shoes. One school suggests asking a friend to watch or even to videotape your feet as you walk or run to determine how they land and your general form. This information and the wear patterns on your old shoes can help you decide whether you should look for shoes that compensate for underpronation, overpronation, or severe overpronation, or whether you can get by with shoes for neutral pronators. Use this information to select shoes from one of four categories: flexibility trainers for underpronators, stability trainers for overpronators, motion-control trainers for severe overpronators, and neutral trainers for neutral pronators.[5]

| Under-
pronation | Neutral | Over-
pronation | Severe
overpronation |

Another school suggests that you first consider your running and biomechanical needs, including your most common running surface, and then select one of five categories that best matches your needs: motion-control, stability, cushioned, light-weight training, or trails. Secondly, determine whether your foot type is normal, flat, or high-arched (discussed below). Use this information to select shoes from within that category.[6]

Take your old shoes with you when you shop for new shoes. The wear patterns on the soles can help you or the salesperson determine how you run and the best shoes for your running style. Normal wear is on the outer heel and across the ball of the foot. Pronators show wear both on the outer heel and the inner forward side of the shoe. Supinators typically show wear on the heel to the forefoot along the outer edge of the shoe.

The key to a good fit in running shoes is to know your foot type. To determine this, walk on a hard surface with wet, bare feet to see your imprint.

The Three Arch Types

FLAT-ARCHED FEET leave an imprint that is almost completely without an inward curve at the arch. Looking down their leg, these athletes will typically see their feet turned outward like a duck's feet. They will typically do best in a semi-curved or straight last shoe that offers good stability and/or motion control. They are often overpronators. The use of an arch support is usually helpful.

NORMAL-ARCHED FEET leave an imprint that shows the forefoot and heel connected, but with an inward curve at the arch. Standing and looking down their leg, these athletes will see their ankles and feet follow the vertical line down their lower leg. These athletes will typically do best in a semicurved last shoe because they are generally efficient in their gait. They might benefit from a cushioned or stability shoe with moderate control features.

HIGH-ARCHED FEET leave an imprint that shows the forefoot and heel connected by a very narrow curve at the arch. If your feet are turned inward, you will typically do best in a curved last shoe with good cushioning. Athletes with high arches are typically underpronators and should avoid motion-control shoes.

A common problem when buying shoes and boots is that people will tell the salesperson, "I wear a size 9.5." Well that may or may not be true. Over time, our feet change, typically getting larger. The fat pads on the bottom of our feet become thinner as we get older. We may get bunions or our calluses may thicken and affect fit. You may have been a 9.5, but now you may be a 10. You might even be a 9.

It's very important to get your feet sized each time you purchase a new pair of shoes. The Brannock Device is the tool that stores use to measure your feet to determine shoe size. Be sure to measure each foot. Measure sitting and standing—although standing is the most important measurement. Many of us have one foot a bit larger than the other foot and you should always buy shoes to fit the larger foot.

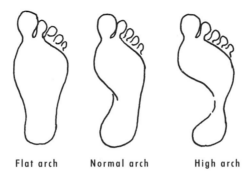

Flat arch   Normal arch   High arch

This easy measurement is important to get the best fit possible. Remember, though, after measuring your feet and trying on a pair of shoes, they still may not feel right. Shoes can vary in construction and one company's shoes may run smaller or larger than those of another company. Once on your feet, the shoes need to feel comfortable. If not, move up or down a half size and see if that helps.

Shop around until you find running shoes that feel right on your feet. A correct fit will help in blister prevention. Valerie Doyle remembers her fight to beat blisters. When she learned how to buy shoes that fit properly, she found they solved her blister problem. The same applies to fitting boots. Studies have found that tight footwear can increase the forces exerted by the shoe or boot on the foot, increasing blister probability, while loose-fitting footwear increases the movement of the foot inside the shoe or boot, causing increased friction forces on the foot, which in turn increases blister probability.[7]

Walk in the shoes or boots for a while to be sure they are comfortable and do not have any pressure points. Some shoes and boots will be higher at the ankle and may put pressure on your foot. Others will not bend at the same forefoot and toe point, making an uncomfortable heel to toe transition or pinching the toes. There may also be a seam inside the shoe or boot that rubs your foot and creates pressure and a potential blister. Pay close attention to the overall fit.

Fitting shoes means more than simply handing you a size 9 shoe and pushing down on the toe and saying, "Yup, it has enough room." When trying on shoes, the toe box (the front part of the shoe that covers the toes) is one of the most important parts of your shoe, and a good salesperson will make sure to emphasize this factor. Those little (or large) toes at the end of your feet need room, both height and width. The right toe box can save your toes. The wrong toe box can cost you your toenails.

In shoes with the right toe box, your toes will feel comfortable and have room to wiggle and breathe. Shoes with the wrong toe box will squeeze your toes—giving them no room to wiggle and breath. This squeezing may happen from the sides and/ or the top. The side squeeze will push your toes together and maybe even underneath each other. A squeeze from the top will put pressure on your toenails. When going downhill, this pressure often results in subungual hematomas or black toenails. If your nails are not trimmed properly and are too long, jamming the toes into the front of the shoe will put additional pressure on the nails and cause nail bed problems.

One rule of thumb is that when standing in your shoes, you need a thumb's width of space between the end of your longest toe and the front inside of the shoe. Generally this works. You may want more space when you are going to be involved in a multiday race, hike, or event. In that case, consider buying shoes a size or two larger than normal. You'll note I said "space between the end of your longest toe." For the majority of us, that means your big toe. But for about 15% of the population, it means the toe next to the big toe. This is a condition called Morton's foot or Morton's toe. This condition, usually hereditary, requires shoes to be fit to that toe.

You may find shoes that fit well with one exception. The toes may pinch or you may have corns or bunions that create pressure in specific areas. Some runners will cut slits into the side or the toe boxes of shoes to provide a better fit. Other runners will actually cut out a portion of the shoe over the problem area. If you do this, be careful not to sacrifice the integrity of the shoe. Be aware of an additional problem this may cause: Dirt and small rocks can easily get into the shoe and lead to hot spots and blisters.

If you have narrow or wide feet, consider shopping for shoes or boots that offer variable lacing capabilities. These shoes and boots will have lace eyelets that are not lined up in an up-and-down row but spaced horizontally farther apart. See "Lacing Options" (page 156) for information on how to lace for different types of feet.

The American Academy of Orthopaedic Surgeons gives suggestions for buying shoes. Foremost, they remind us that shoes should always conform to the shape of your feet; your feet should never be forced to conform to the shape of a pair of shoes. Their suggestions apply equally well to buying boots.

Components of a Good Fit

Fit can be achieved with simply a little common sense and a bit of luck. Out of all the shoes and boot to choose from, there is more than one brand and style that will fit your feet well. When you find them, buy several pairs. Rotate them, but save the best pair for the race or event you are training for.

Apply common sense when trying on the shoes or boots.

Commonsense Tips for Trying on Shoes

- Try on and fully lace both shoes.

- The shoes should feel comfortable. You should feel no discomfort in any part of the shoe's fit.

- Feel around the inside of the shoe for rough spots where the parts of the uppers are stitched together.

- Your feet should have some room to breathe and swell.

- Your toes should have plenty of room to move and wiggle, and the toe box should not be too short in height or length. Aim for at least 0.5–1 inch of space between your longest toe and the front interior of the shoe.

- The tops of feet shouldn't be pinched when the shoes are laced properly.

- Your little toe should not be pinched by the shape of the front of the shoe. Likewise, your big toe joint should fit at the widest point of the shoe.

- Be sure the shoe's counter (the part that wraps around your ankle and heel) does not rub your foot wrong. Your heels should be snug in the heel counter of the shoe and should have little up and down movement. There should be a firm grip of the shoe to your heel, but not too firm.

- The arch of each foot should be supported, but the shoe arch should not be too high, or too far backward or forward, for your foot type.

- The shoes' shape (last) should be comfortable and not overly curved or straight for your foot type.

- The shoes should fit well with the same type of socks you will be wearing in your training and/or race event.

- The shoes should flex well for the type of terrain you will encounter and at the right point of your foot. This will help provide support to your ankles and prevent uncomfortable heel to toe transition or pinching of the toes.

- The shoes should provide adequate protection for the bottom of your feet from rocks and uneven terrain.

- The fit of the shoe should come from the shoes themselves, not from tying the laces.

- The laces should stay tied the way you like them without coming undone.

- The shoes should have outsoles for the type of event or race you will be doing. They should help keep your feet in place inside the shoes.

- If the insoles that come in the shoe are weak and flimsy, replace them when you are buying the shoes—get a pair that provides support and cushioning.

- If you will be using orthotics or special insoles, make sure that they fit in the shoes without pushing your feet too high in the shoes' uppers or too far forward.

Tips for a Good Fit

Whether buying shoes for running, hiking, court sports, soccer, or golf, it is important to get a good fit. When you purchase footwear, consider the whole picture, not just the shoe or boot you hold in your hand. Your footwear must work with your choice of socks, insoles, and orthotics (if your wear them), and also with the activity you will be using them for. Hiking boots that feel OK when you walk around the store may feel different when you get home and try them when carrying a 30- to 40-pound pack on your back.

Here are some suggestions for getting the best possible fit.

- Use shoe buying guides as just that—do not eliminate a shoe from your consideration until you have tried it on.

- Try shoes in a range of prices—don't save a buck at the expense of your feet. The differences between several pairs of shoes can be amazing.

- Judge a shoe by how it fits on your foot, not by the marked size.

- When going to try on or buy shoes, take a pair of your socks along rather than rely on the store's basket of socks that have been on who knows how many feet.

- Do not buy a pair assuming that they will fit better later, unless they are leather boots. In most cases, today's shoes and boots require no breaking-in period.

- Have your feet sized each time you buy new footwear. Measure both sitting and standing to determine your elongation factor.

- Fit new shoes to your larger foot and your longest toe.

- Try on shoes at the end of the day, preferably after running or walking, because your feet normally swell and become larger after you have been standing and sitting all day.

Footwear purchasers frequently forget to allow enough toe space when buying shoes and boots. When your foot is in the shoe, the arch naturally flattens. Since your heel is held in place by the shoe's counter, your foot can only move forward. If the shoe does not have this bit of extra space in the toe box, the toes become cramped. Toenail problems, blisters, and calluses may develop.

Our Aging Feet

As we age, our feet change. Make no mistake, that fat pad on the bottom of your foot is getting thinner as you get older. Our feet spread out, getting longer and wider, so we may move up a size or more in footwear. Additionally, we usually become a bit stiffer in the joints. Your arch may also flatten more than normal. Just because we are aging doesn't mean that our feet have to hurt or that we have to stop walking, running, or whatever our activity is. As long as we remember how our feet change as we age and buy footwear that fits, we can stay physically active. So the natural question is, "What should we do?" Here are three steps to keep your aging feet happy.

1. Have your feet measured each time you buy shoes.

2. Buy shoes that fit the shape of your foot and have a wide and long enough toe box.

3. Invest in a good pair of insoles that provide cushioning and support. Sorbothane and Spenco insoles with gel are good choices.

Customizing Your Footwear

When you shop for shoes or boots, run your fingers around the inside to determine whether there are any rough spots, overlapping or raised seams, or other potential pressure points that could cause hot spots or blisters. These may be able to be rubbed flat or softened. Ask the store for another pair to determine if the spots are common to that style or just one particular shoe or boot. If these spots are common to that particular shoe or boot, your choice is to have the shoe modified by a pedorthist or a shoe repair shop, or find another style that fits correctly.

The contour around your heel and ankle has to be smooth from the base of your foot all the way up to your ankle or the top of your heel. If a shoe or boot has any ledges, ridges, or extrusions around the ankle or heel, they will rub into your feet and potentially cause a problem. These extrusions may be there due to stitches, due to extra foam, or by design. Hiker Buck Jones has had two such bad experiences with heel and ankle rubbing. In the first, he was an hour into a short hike in his new pair of trail running shoes when he discovered that the ledge in one had made a hole in his sock and was working on his ankle. He recalls, "I applied duct tape and moleskin to my foot and also patched the shoe with duct tape and moleskin so that the ledge was minimal." He was able to finish his hike with little more wear on his foot. His second experience was with a friend who was a beginner hiker. Shortly after starting the hike, she was bothered by a hot spot. The boot had a stitch around the heel and it was causing a blister. He applied duct tape and moleskin on the foot and under the void of the stitch. By mending both the foot and the shoe, they were able to prevent further skin damage. Now before Buck buys a pair of shoes, he checks for a bad design around the heel and ankle area.

If you have difficulty finding quality shoes that fit your particular type of foot, consider searching for a certified pedorthist (C. Ped). Kirk Apt, C. Ped, describes the work of a pedorthist:

Even those with no medical conditions, but with common discomfort and general foot fatigue, can find relief by utilizing the expertise of a C. Ped. Specifically, pedorthics is the design, fit, manufacture, and modification of footwear and orthotics to help alleviate problems due to congenital deformity, injury, disease, or overuse. C. Peds function as part of allied health care teams, where a person can go to a medical doctor (family doctor, orthopedist, podiatrist, and so on) and get a diagnosis and a prescription for a conservative, nonsurgical remedy. The patient may then be referred to a C. Ped, who can fill the prescription for therapeutic shoes and/or custom orthotics. Shoes are built around 3-D foot-shaped models called lasts, which are identical mirror images of feet of a given size. Unfortunately, real feet are seldom mirror images of each other. A C. Ped. can help find a shoe built on a last that best matches a person's feet, and then construct a custom orthotic that meets their particular biomechanical needs and interfaces with the shoe in a way that improves its fit and performance. In this way, athletes, active people, and those who work long hours on their feet can be accommodated with footwear designed specifically for their unique feet. In my practice, I work with both patients who have a doctor's prescription, and with others who want their footwear to fit and perform better. I often work with a physical therapist. Together, we do a pedorthic assessment where we determine the condition of the feet and analyze the gait of a person. Using this information, I can recommend a specific shoe or design and construct a custom orthotic.

Look in the telephone book or ask your orthopedist or podiatrist for references. Information on the Pedorthic Footwear Association can be found under "Medical & Footwear Specialists" in the appendix (see page 350).

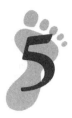

Footwear & Insoles

Many people consider footwear as simple basic equipment that takes little thought. Yet the war against foot problems can be lost over ill-fitting shoes, boots, or socks that cause blisters or insoles that are not right for your activity. Choose your footwear based on which sport you will be doing, the terrain expected, and your level of experience. Find the right shoes or boots and the right socks based on what feels right and fits correctly—not by price. Tom McGinnis, who thru-hiked the Appalachian Trail in 1979, makes a good observation: "Good boots and bad socks can be miserable. Cheap boots and good socks can be a dreamland." This chapter focuses on types of running shoes, sport shoes, hiking boots, custom shoes, sandals, and insoles. Minimalist footwear, such as Vibram FiveFingers, are discussed in the next chapter. Socks play such a large role in preventing problems that they are discussed at length in their own chapter.

Our feet are unique. Yours may look similar to mine, yet they are as different as our fingerprints. Although our feet may fit into the same size and shape of shoe or boot, our feet actually mold into the footwear differently. Corns, bunions, susceptibility to blisters, toe length, the type of arches, and the shape of our feet are just a few of the factors that affect the fit of our footwear. Even how we react to and recover from the stresses of running and hiking is important in choosing shoes and boots.

Only you can determine what type of footwear you need to wear. Certainly runners wear running shoes, but there are many types of running shoes. Hikers and adventure racers have many choices in hiking boots, but many make the choice to wear trail running shoes instead of boots. Many of the top adventure racers wear trail running shoes for their whole event, even on snow and ice and while wearing crampons. Just remember the ifs. If you are used to hiking in trail running shoes, if your ankles are strong, and if the shoes provide the necessary support while wearing a pack, then trail running shoes may be right for you.

Regarding trail shoes, Cathy Corning makes a good point:

> Trail shoes are constructed a bit differently than road shoes. Pronation is an important consideration for road shoes but not for trails. Think about

it. On the road, it's the exact same movement over and over and over, and pronation is a big deal. On the trail, every footfall is completely different will all sorts of soft, hard, and twisted surfaces, and your foot lands differently every time. Pronation is really not a consideration. Trail shoes are far more focused on stability, with your foot sitting lower in the shoe and closer to the ground to help stabilize your foot on uneven surfaces. Even the base of the trail shoe is slightly wider than a road shoe for more stability.

An important consideration in choosing footwear is shoe construction and ventilation. Footwear constructed with Gore-Tex fabric is good at keeping moisture out—but also tends to hold in sweat. In extreme cold, shoes that drain may be a better choice. Footwear made with mesh is lightweight—but the mesh allows grit and dust to get inside the shoe. Your shoes may be lighter and cooler, but the grit can increase friction. Gaiters can help control what gets in your shoes.

Several years ago I spent a trail-running weekend with friends in the Northern California High Sierra. In between the fast hiking and running, while watching my step, I kept an eye on what others had on their feet. Most had good footwear—either trail running shoes or larger heavier boots. There were some, however, who wore the wrong footwear. They wore running shoes made for roads, or court shoes. These shoes provided no traction on the slippery rocks and no protection from the sharp rocks, and they did not give their feet and ankles the needed support. One friend wore her road shoes and ended the first day with three blisters and very sore feet. I saw several hikers with court shoes and a pack—a very poor combination. Trouble occurs when you end the day with blisters, damaged or black toenails, a turned ankle, or simply very sore feet. You may associate the discomfort and pain with the activity. Instead, the right footwear would have made the hike much more enjoyable. Whether walking, hiking, running, trail running, playing court sports, adventure racing, climbing, or biking, the right footwear can make all the difference.

When shopping for shoes or boots, try on several different pairs from several different companies. This will help you identify those that initially feel good versus those that just don't feel quite right. Knowing how different shoes and boots fit your feet will help in the final selection. When going to buy new shoes, you may have a preferred shoe, sometimes based on magazine ads or on the recommendations of others, but buy only those that fit best. Whichever type of shoe you wear, be sure to train in them. Never wear a new pair in a race. Always wear them before the race to make sure they fit well and there are no problems.

Kevin wrote that he wears a size 7 shoe and has found that the mid- and outsoles are the exact thickness in all shoes regardless of the shoe size—not proportionally thinner. "While shopping, if you pick up a large shoe of a particular model and try bending it, then pick up the smaller size of the same model and try bending that one, you quickly notice how much more rigidity a small foot has to work against. Try repeating that ten times, and you see your arms get tired, not to mention bending it 25,000 times or more over a long day hike! It's not the shoe getting stressed; it's your feet and ankles trying to overcome the rigidity that a smaller, shorter foot has to work harder to overcome. When I am buying new shoes, I pick up each model and bend their size 7 and compare stiffness. I find quite a difference between models, so it helps me in the selection."

John Schumacher, in the *Sacramento Bee* newspaper, wrote about Stacy Dragila, a 2000 gold medalist in the pole vault. She had gone to Athens for the Olympic Trials in 2004 with high expectations—but came home devastated. And yes, it was the shoes. Dragila had provided input for a new shoe design for Nike. When Nike rolled it out before the U.S. Olympic Trials in Sacramento, Dragila decided to make the switch. Her old jumping shoes were a little loose in the heel. The new pair, reinforced to last longer, felt nice and snug at first. As she wore them in the trials, she felt a little Achilles flare-up. "I just attributed it to stress, being at the trials, not sleeping as well as I probably should," said Dragila. "I never thought it was the shoe." By the U.S. Olympic training camp, both Achilles tendons were bothering her. She couldn't do her normal workouts, and during qualifying discovered she couldn't make a full approach on the runway. She tried heights she had easily done before but couldn't make them. "I just knew I was doomed," she says. Doomed, she admits, by her own hand. Or shoe. "When you're a fine-tuned athlete or sports car, you don't change the wheels," she said. "I wish somebody had told me. I don't blame anybody but myself. I shouldn't have tried to break in something new in a crucial time of training. In hindsight, looking back, stay with what you've got."

Socks vary in thickness, and changing socks can change the way your feet fit inside your shoes. When trying on shoes, wear the same socks when trying on shoes that you wear during races. When buying new socks, be sure they will not alter the fit of your shoes. If your new socks make your shoes fit tighter, you may be able to fix this with new slightly thinner insoles.

TIP: Best Friend to Worst Enemy

Whatever sports shoes you wear, remember to inspect them regularly for problems. Frank Sutman was on the second day of a six-day 80-mile backpack trip when one boot's outsole split from the midsole to the ball of the foot. He suffered through four days of flapping sole, picking up pebbles, rocks, and sticks and even being tripped up. The moral of his story: Check your boots and shoes before major activities and periodically to keep small problems from becoming major inconveniences. Split outsoles, ripped or torn fabric that lets dirt and rocks into the shoe, cracked heel counters that create folds in the inner heel material, or broken laces retied into a bothersome knot over the top of the foot are all preventable.

Brand Loyalty in Footwear

When athletes talk about footwear, you often hear, "Be loyal and don't jump from brand to brand or style to style." How true is that statement? Let's look at a few different perspectives on the subject.

From the manufacturer's perspective, it makes perfect sense. If buyers are loyal and stay with the manufacturer's shoes, life is perfect. They have an ongoing market that remains faithful and so their shoes will always sell.

From the shoe store's perspective, it makes life easier. They'll keep ordering the same shoes from the same manufacturers. Sure, they'll take chances on new shoes, but if buyers remain loyal to the old shoes, they'll have a harder time convincing athletes to switch brands.

So, that leaves our perspective: the customer. Why would athletes remain loyal to one brand? Let's identify some reasons, keeping in mind that the inverse is true too—when one of the reasons fails, the athlete is often open to a change in shoes.

■ The shoes work well for my sport.

■ The shoes fit.

■ They've never caused problems.

■ I hate taking a chance on a new shoe.

Certainly, shoe companies would like us to be loyal. One obvious problem is that companies often seem to disregard the people who buy and wear their shoes. They will change or discontinue shoe styles with no warning. If you've found shoes that work, every spring and fall is tense as you wait to see if your favorite shoes are still being made. I know athletes who buy several pairs of shoes once they find a pair that works for their feet. They don't want to take a chance on the shoe companies not honoring their loyalty. I don't blame them.

The Anatomy of Footwear

By understanding the parts of a shoe or boot, you can make informed choices about which running shoe, cross-trainer, or boot is best for your sport—and for your feet. The parts of a shoe are fairly common, regardless of what kind of footwear you are looking for.

Parts of a Shoe

The shoe's **COUNTER** is the part that wraps around the heel of the foot.

The **EYELETS** are the holes the shoelaces run through.

The **COLLAR** is the part at the top that wraps around your ankle.

The **HEEL TAB** is the notch that surrounds the Achilles tendon.

The **HEEL** is the back bottom of the shoe.

The **INSOLE** or **SOCK LINER** is the inner insert on which your foot rests. These are typically interchangeable.

The **MIDSOLE** sits between the shoe's upper and outsole.

The **OUTSOLE** is the shoe's bottom layer.

The shoe's **SHANK** is the part of the sole between the heel and the ball of the foot.

The **TOE BOX** is the tip of the shoe that shapes and protects the toes.

The **UPPER** is the top of the shoe that surrounds the foot.

Tossing Shoes & Boots

There comes a time when shoes and boots need to be thrown out. You may feel a difference in the cushioning of the shoe—they may feel flat or lack the spring they once had. You may experience foot, ankle, or knee pain. The footwear may simply be trashed. Some athletes, especially runners, log the miles they run in each pair of shoes, and then move the worn ones to garden duty. There is no hard-and-fast rule, but many suggest 500–600 miles as the maximum from a pair. How long your shoes will last depends on your technique, running surface, mileage, weight—and the shoe itself. The newer technologies in some shoes can extend their life beyond other shoes. Here are a few tips and reminders to keep in mind when evaluating your shoes:

- Write the purchase date in the tongue of the shoe or on your calendar.

- Exposure to heat and water will shorten the life of shoes.

- Never put your shoes in the dryer—air-dry them.

- Heavier runners should replace shoes more often.

- Buy a second pair, or even three pairs, and rotate shoes in your workouts. This can give you a better feel for worn shoes.

Kevin shared this tip: "I wear New Balance 833s. They wear out fast, before the uppers are even dirty. I couldn't take the idea of tossing them out and ended up with nearly a dozen used pairs. When my knees start to ache, it tells me the shoes are going. I tried this company, Resole America (**www.resole.com**), and have been satisfied with the result. The resoled shoes don't last as long as the originals, but for me it's better than tossing them out. Plus because I have five pairs now, I can rotate to make them last longer. When these wear out, I'll send more in to be resoled. The company sends prepaid mailers for the old shoes. Prices are fair and they do all types of shoes, from street shoes, running shoes, hiking boots, work boots, and more."

If your old shoes still have some life in them, consider donating them to one of the companies that sends shoes to Third World countries. The U.S. site **www. soles4souls.com** and Canada-based **www.soleresponsibility.org** are two organizations that serve as collection points

Running Shoes

There are many sources of information about which shoes may be the best for you. The five main sources are the shoe companies, local running stores, magazines and catalogues, running friends, and the Internet. Recognize the difference in the quality of help available at some chain shoe stores in shopping malls versus stores that specialize in running shoes and equipment. A specialized footwear store usually has personnel who are athletes themselves and can watch you run, look at your old shoes, and recommend specific brands of shoes and styles based on what they see and your answers to their questions.

To understand running shoes, you need to be aware of their construction. The first construction component is the last, the form over which a shoe is constructed.

Running Shoe Last Patterns

BOARD lasts have the shoe's upper material glued to the shoe's board, which runs the length of the shoe. This generally produces a fairly rigid and stable shoe.

COMBINATION lasts have the shoe's upper material stitched to either the forefoot (slip-lasted) or the rear foot (board-lasted). This design offers additional stability at either the foot plant or the toe's push off.

SEMICURVED lasts are molded straight toward the rear foot while having some curve toward the forefoot. This mold provides stability and flexibility.

SEMISTRAIGHT lasts are built to curve slightly from the toe to the heel. This provides some flexibility and a high degree of stability.

SLIP last shoes are made with the upper material stitched directly to the midsole without a board. This offers maximum flexibility.

STRAIGHT lasts are built along the shoe's straight arch to provide maximum stability.

Basic Categories of Shoe Construction

NEUTRAL shoes are made for the runner who has good biomechanics and would be categorized as a neutral pronator. These shoes generally have a good blend of flexibility and stability.

FLEXIBILITY shoes are made for runners who are underpronators, who have foot motion toward the outside and need a shoe that offers more shock-absorbing pronation than their body can deliver.

STABILITY shoes offer high stability and cushioning. Midweight or normal-arched runners without motion problems who are looking for good cushioning typically use these shoes. These runners usually overpronate slightly beyond neutral and need a shoe with extra medial support. Most are built on a semicurved last.

MOTION-CONTROL shoes provide the most control, rigidity, and stability. Heavy runners, severe overpronators, flat-footed runners, and orthotic users often choose these shoes. They are typically quite durable shoes, but they are often heavier. Most are built on a straight last and offer the greatest level of medial support.

TRAIL RUNNING shoes usually offer increased toe protection, outsole traction, stability, and durability. Runners who run mainly on trails usually use these shoes.

CUSHIONED shoes are those with the best cushioning. These are typically used by those who do not need extra medial support and by high-arched runners. Most are built on a curved or semicurved last.

LIGHTWEIGHT shoes are typically made for fast training or racing. These come with varying degrees of stability and cushioning and can be worn by runners with few or no foot problems. Most are built on a curved or semicurved last.

Buying Running Shoes

Running shoes are changing rapidly. The major shoe companies roll out new designs twice a year. Shoes now offer midsole air, gel, and tube chambers; springs; recoil plates; Gore-Tex and other membrane fabrics; breathable liners and mesh outer fabrics; and better support and stability. More models have been released for trails as this market has grown many times over.

Before you buy a pair of shoes, run your hands over the inside to check for seams that could cause an irritation and lead to blisters. Look at the stitching and the seam that bonds the upper to the bottom of the shoe. Then pull out the insole and make sure everything is smooth. Once you buy a new pair of shoes, wear them around the house to be sure they fit well and are comfortable. If you sense problems, return the shoes for another style or type. Even the same shoe model that you have worn in the past can have minor design changes in a new release. Wear them for a while until you are sure they fit well.

Shoe designs are always changing. Often our favorite shoes disappear from the shelves and we find ourselves forced to make new choices. Do your homework, study the shoe reviews and the ads, talk to your running friends, and try on various styles. Good stores will let you run in them. Ultrarunner Orin Dahl once found that his favorite shoes were no longer offered. Instead of the old shoes, Nike offered a new type of air shoe. He bought the shoes and began running in them. The new shoes were not as flexible in the forefoot, causing his heel to pull up and out of the shoe. To his dismay, he developed blisters at the back of his heels. He recalls how he turned the shoes over to the Salvation Army and began a search for a different pair. He has no doubt that the shoes were good shoes, but they were just not right for his feet and running style. As you look for shoes, remember that not every pair of shoes is right for your feet.

"I *personal experience*

did ten 100-mile runs in 1999: Rocky Raccoon, Umstead, Massanutten, Old Dominion, Western States, Vermont, Leadville, Wasatch, Angeles Crest, and Arkansas.

"I really didn't have too much of a problem with my feet that year. The Rocky Raccoon (the first race) is where I had the most trouble. It was 80°F and very humid, and I wore last year's shoes, which were size 11 (my normal size). Because the shoes were a bit worn and [my feet had] some swelling due to the humidity, I had several blisters between my toes. After the run, I drained them with a pin and then pretty much forgot about them.

"I then bought some Asics 2040s and Montrail Vitesse shoes in size 12. I always wear double-layer, blister-free socks. The rest of the [year], I had very few blister problems. The only consistent blister problem was with the Montrails. If I didn't put duct tape on the balls of my feet, they would develop blisters. They also rubbed on the outside of my left big toe. I did not need any tape with the 2040s. Even at the hot and humid Vermont 100, I had little problem with blisters, [and what problems I did have were] mostly as a result of wearing the Montrails. On rare occasions, I would get a small blister on the inside of the big toe on my right foot.

"I never put anything on my feet. I do, however, use Succeed electrolyte caps. This has helped me with stomach distress (I only drink water or, late in the race, Pepsi). I am sure that [the caps] also help with the blistering. I think experience has a lot to do with blisters. The more races I run, the tougher my feet become."

— Jeff Washburn

Sports Shoes

By sports shoes I mean any shoes specific to your particular sport. These may be soccer, football, baseball, or climbing shoes, or even cross-trainers. Even military boots can be considered in this category—the requirements for getting a good fit are the same.

When shopping for these shoes, apply the same basic principles that you would for other athletic shoes. Try several different brands and styles. Try them on wearing the socks you will wear during the activity. Lace them up and be sure that they hold your heel, that your toes have wiggle room, and that they feel comfortable.

Many sport-specific shoes such as those for soccer have a simple thin insole with virtually no arch or heel support. These can lead to arch problems, metatarsal pain, blisters, and more. The first thing I do when I find a shoe that fits well is to replace the standard flimsy insoles with a good supporting insole—but do this when buying the shoes to make sure they are big enough to accommodate the insoles.

Climbing shoes are meant to fit close to the skin. These are often worn without socks, so be sure there are no irritating seams that can cause blisters. If you will wear thin socks with the shoes, take them along when shopping for shoes. One problem area in climbing shoes is the tight toe box. If you have Morton's toe, hammertoes, bunions, corns, or other toe problems, be aware of how the tight fit will affect that condition. Understanding any preexisting foot problem will help you make an informed choice of shoes. Each of these conditions is discussed later in this book.

Military boots may not offer much in the way of selection, but you need to be aware of many of the fit issues discussed in the next section about hiking boots. Irritating seams, poor heel fit, thin insoles, toe boxes that are too narrow and too short, and boots that are not correct for the shape of your feet can lead to long-term problems. If given a choice in boots, try on several to get the best fit possible. Again, as with most other shoes, replace the insoles. Then choose a good moisture-wicking sock.

"O *personal experience*

n my feet, I wore a liner sock, SmartWool socks, and Wellco jungle boots with an enhanced cushioned midsole and Vibram-type sole. I coated my feet with BodyGlide. This combination had worked very well for me in training, with no blisters, and so I anticipated no problems. During the competition, however, I developed hot spots fairly early on the bottom of my feet. By mile 5, I was pretty sure that some of the hot spots had turned into full-on blisters; my suspicion quickly proved right. At about the 5¾-mile mark, I picked up a trot as the course came off a dike. As I did so, I felt an excruciating pain on the bottom of both heels. I realized two things: my feet were going to hurt a lot, and quitting just wasn't an option. . . . Somehow I did manage to qualify for the new unit.

"As an experienced triathlete, I made some right choices. However, with the combination of a heavier 45-pound pack, gravel roads, liner socks that were too tight, and unseasonable warm and humid weather, my feet were doomed from the start.

"I don't know that anybody teaches foot care to subjects in basic training. A lot of information is passed along through informal instruction in the ranger and infantry communities, but it may not be up-to-date and may not reflect lessons learned from people such as endurance athletes and adventure racers. The sad thing, however, is that if you showed up to a non-infantry (or non-special ops) unit on the morning that they'd decided to do a road march, you'd see some frightening equipment choices and personal preparation. There's very little foot care knowledge in many combat support units. It makes me shudder just to think about it."

—an Army Ranger, describing a 12-mile forced march that was part of the selection process for an elite special operations unit

Hiking Boots

Terry, a dedicated hiker, told me, "After a bazillion miles of backpacking and running, I should know everything about my feet. [Yet] when thinking about another thru-hike next year, I spend more time thinking about my feet than my backpack." We can learn from his insight.

My first pair of hiking boots was all leather, with thick Vibram soles. They laced all the way to my calf and seemed to weigh as much as my loaded backpack. Times have changed and so have hiking boots. They now fit better and are easier on your feet. Running-shoe technology has had a positive influence on hiking boots. Insoles, molding, padding, and midsole and outsole advances have made many as comfortable as lighter-weight boots. An ad by boot maker Sorel claimed, "Any boot can repel water. Ours will actually suck the sweat off your pinky toes." As technology advances, many boot makers such as Sorel will offer moisture-control systems to wick perspiration away from your feet. Gore-Tex fabrics are commonly built into boots for moisture transfer. Lacing systems are also changing for the better.

Kent Ryhorchuk has the right attitude about hiking footwear:

> When it comes to budget, I would not be stingy on anything related to your feet. Your feet will hurt badly enough without having to deal with blisters and chafing. Bad feet stopped or hobbled many people the year I hiked, mostly due to blisters—even some experienced Appalachian Trail hikers. The shoe-and-socks system I use for footwear is Montrail Vitesse shoes, flat Spenco green insoles, Birkenstock blue footbeds over the Spenco insoles (to control my metatarsal problems), SmartWool low-cut hiker socks, and Fox River X-Static liner socks. It took several years of hiking, trail running, and adventure racing to figure this out, but I went from getting blisters all the time to hardly ever getting blisters at all. The point is that I spent a lot of time on it, not that this system is necessarily right for anybody else. Everybody's feet are different.

Many hikers have been converted to using the newer lightweight boots. These are usually as flexible as running shoes and carry many of the running-shoe benefits of fit and comfort. Because of their flexibility and construction, many of these boots require very little or no break-in time. I completed an 8.5-day, 221-mile ultralight backpack of the John Muir Trail in regular running shoes. Unless you are used to hiking or running trails in running shoes while wearing a backpack, I do not recommend them for backpacking. Since I did the John Muir Trail in 1987, boots have changed. Today, I would consider a trail-running shoe or lightweight boot for the same hike. Newer lightweight boots tend to dry faster and drain better. The typical leather boot can soak up to a pound of water. That means you lift an additional 2,212 pounds to walk 1 mile.

Check out some of the features of new hiking boots at your local store. Many boots offer a combination of features: lighter weight, breathable uppers, high-traction and long-lasting outsoles, improved lacing systems, flexible footbeds, stable and cushioning midsoles, wider toe boxes, and Gore-Tex fabric incorporated into the uppers. Some boot companies have developed what they call their "hiking boot last," which is designed to be snug around the heel and arch, and with a roomy toe box. Both offer three different insoles for a better fit, and the use of different thicknesses of socks and the number of pairs worn can adjust the fit even more.

Boots falls into three basic categories: lightweight hiking (for trail hiking and light loads), midweight hiking (for on/off trail hiking and light backpacking), and heavyweight hiking (for on/off trail, heavy loads, and multiday trips).

Before you go shopping for boots, determine the type of hiking you will be doing and how much support and protection you will need for the weight you will carry. Then, look at the various features of different boots in each of the three categories. Finally, shop accordingly, but do not rule out a certain type of boot until you try them on your feet. A boot that pinches or rubs in the store will not feel better when you are out on the trail. Rob Langsdorf suggests taking time to really test a new boot before leaving the store:

> I usually wear mine around the store for an hour or more before deciding to take it. It takes time but consumes less time than having to return it or having to spend lots of time treating blisters. Then, break new boots in by wearing them around the house, to work, church, and so on, before going out on the trail. Begin with easy hikes before starting off on a long trip. Only when they feel good on a short hike are they ready for a longer one.
>
> I had a friend who bought a pair of boots but didn't break them in because she felt that wearing them around the house wasn't the feminine thing to do. She ended up with major blisters after 6–7 miles. By the end of our 15-mile weekend backpack, she was ready to throw the new boots away and swear off backpacking—all because she didn't want to look funny wearing her boots in town.

Switchback, a hiker, writes:

> Before you go on a hike, walk a few miles in your hiking footwear without socks. You will be amazed what your feet will tell you about potential hot spots, tight areas, and potential blisters. Listen to your feet when you do this experiment. Remember, each foot is different and will have different things to tell you. Socks not only protect our feet but can also mask problem areas. Then when you are out on your hike walking with your socks and shoes, you will know where potential problems might occur. This is

very valuable to you. Why find out about a foot problem after it has developed? Be proactive and not reactive.

Some boots will soften and become more flexible with forceful flexion of the soles and uppers, hand-working a waterproofing solution into the leather, or mechanical flexion of the uppers at a shoe shop. If your boots are too stiff, try one of these three methods.

Rod Dalitz shares a good tip for getting a good fit with hiking boots:

It's important to shape the heel to fit your foot. Find a heavy-gauge plastic bag and put the boot inside, with the heel immersed in a large pot of boiling water, for a few minutes. (It doesn't do the leather any good to be directly in boiling water!) Make sure the bag doesn't leak. When the boot is hot, the plastic cup in the heel can be molded by gentle hand pressure to a suitable shape.

Ed Acheson made several painful discoveries when he hiked the Pacific Crest Trail. Before he began his trip, he switched to a new pair on a salesperson's recommendation. The boots were too much boot for him and a half size too small—the salesperson told him they were sized larger than most. Ed remembers for the first 20 days having "more blisters than the number of days I had been out." To compensate for the blisters, he changed his gait, which in turn gave him knee problems. Before he could get new boots, he was forced to cross the Mojave in tennis shoes. He suffered for years from problems he attributes to the wrong boots.

And even after you have broken in your boots, be sure they still fit after not wearing them for a while. Wear them for at least one getting-reacquainted walk before going on a major hike. Your feet may have changed, and they may need to get readjusted to the boots before a long hike.

Airing Your Feet

If you are looking for a shoe to wear around camp, an alternative to sandals is lightweight closed-cell foam structure shoes. Sometimes called clogs, these shoes have a soft pliable feel and provide cushioning to your heels for all-day wear, all the while massaging the bottoms of your feet with their textured footbed to promote circulation. They're warm in winter and cool in summer, with a vented design and antibacterial material to reduce foot odors. They are an especially good way to air your feet after a long day on the trail.

One pair weighs less than 10 ounces! And because they are made from one piece of closed-cell foam, they won't come apart or break down. Choose from an open-back shoe or one with a heel strap. The colors are as wild or sedate as you want. All this for around $30. And they provide better cushioning and support than flip-flops.

I'd toss these on my pack for use as camp shoes without a second thought. They won't add much extra weight. They're easy relief after a day of hiking and wonderful to have waiting outside your tent to slip on when you venture outdoors. They're also great to wear in the communal shower on the road. They're dry in a minute, so you can throw them right into your gym bag.

The three most common lines are Crocs at **www.crocs.com**, Waldies at **www.waldies.net**, and Holey Soles at **www.holeys.com**. Vibram FiveFingers are a great lightweight alternative, with a glovelike appearance, stretchy upper, and a Vibram sole at **www.vibramfivefingers.com**.

Buying Hiking Boots

Before buying new boots, understand how they are changing. Boot designs are offering waterproof, breathable Gore-Tex liners; thinner leather for better hot-weather hiking; better lug soles for increased traction; lugs that extend up the rounded sides; better insoles; softer uppers for shorter break-in times; snug ankle collars to keep debris out; and more. Boots are being made better, but never buy a pair for their features alone. Buy them because they fit.

Before buying boots, check *Backpacker* and *Outside* magazines (and their web-sites) for their coverage on hiking boots. These articles evaluate most brands based on fixed standards while identifying their features and costs. Then check out your local backpacking supply store for the brands and styles they carry. Spend as much time as is necessary to get a good fit. Tell the salesperson what type of hiking you will be doing, for how long, and how much weight you plan on carrying. Try on several pairs of boots by different companies. Use your own socks. Walk in the boots. Squat in them. Look for a pair that fits right from the start and grips your heels. Take out the insoles and look at the boot's construction. Find the pair that fits and feels better than the others. Purchase a high-quality boot made for hiking rather than lighter-weight boots sold for general-purpose street wear. These fashion-statement boots will not hold up under the stresses of heavy trail use. Utilize the experience of the personnel of your local camping and backpacking stores to help you make a wise decision, but realize the final decision is yours based on how they feel on your feet.

Remember that the boots you select will each be picked up and put down many times each day. Hiking 12 miles each day would equate to about 25,000 steps[8], day after day. Feel the weight of your boot and think about each step. Heavier boots are not always the best. True, they may provide more ankle stabilization, but you could get more benefit from a lightweight boot and proper ankle and foot-strength conditioning before the hike. Ray Jardine, who has hiked the Pacific Crest Trail three times and the Appalachian and Continental Divide trails each once, estimates that each 3.5 ounces off a pair of boots could add about a mile to a day's hiking progress.[9] A review of one store's boot selection showed weights for a pair of boots ranging from 1 pound 9 ounces all the way to 3 pounds 9 ounces. Selecting boots that weigh 10.5 ounces less than another pair could mean an additional 3 miles hiked per day. An educated choice based on boot features, your personal needs, and the terrain ahead is necessary.

If you are planning a several-week hike or a several-month thru-hike on a multi-state trail, you will need to buy boots that are larger than normal to accommodate your feet as they become stronger and enlarge to their normal hiking size. Try on boots that are anywhere from one to two sizes larger than normal, which will allow your feet to fit into them properly. If you need to purchase new boots midway through a long trek, be aware of potential problems of breaking in new boots.

Mara Factor has experienced her feet changing:

> Be wary of buying multiple pairs before you start. Most people's feet change significantly as they hike. The shoes you wear day to day will adjust some-what and continue to fit your feet. New shoes, the same size as the ones you've been wearing for a while, often do not fit. Longer and/or wider sizes are often required after spending a few hundred miles on the trail. I used to be a woman's size 12 before I started long-distance hiking. Now I'm a men's 13 (I can't find women's 14s or 15s). I may be an extreme example, but most people do have some change along the way. It may be worthwhile to plan a side trip or two off the trail to go to an experienced outfitter who can remeasure your feet and make sure the next pair will fit properly.

When you do have problems with your feet, and you usually will at some point, you need to look at the boots and evaluate whether you need to replace them with another boot type and/or style. On long hikes, your feet do enlarge and change. Boots wear out. Over a couple of years your feet may also change. Be open to new styles and features in newer type boots and find the pair that best fits you.

If you are always having problems with your boots and a different set of boots does not help, consider trying a pair of running shoes, preferably trail running shoes. Be aware, however, of the differences. Running shoes do not provide the same degree of ankle support and overall foot protection. While some may prefer the increased ankle mobility of a low running shoe, this choice requires proper strength in the feet, ankles, and legs. My choice to wear running shoes when fast packing the 221 miles of the John Muir Trail was based on a trial overnight hike with a full backpack and years of running trails. I knew my feet and ankles could handle the stresses of the trail in running shoes, and I did not need heavier boots.

One week into hiking the John Muir Trail, Andrew Ferguson developed a hel-lacious deep blister on the back of his right foot, 1.5 inches in diameter. By nurs-ing the blister with Spenco 2nd Skin and tape, he hiked for three days in running shoes before reaching civilization and purchasing a new pair of boots. The red heel bothered him for two weeks and took six months to return to normal. Andrew is now a believer in running shoes for hiking. Many people prefer running shoes instead of boots for hiking.

Choosing Lightweight Footwear

Our feet need varying degrees of support. Whether you wear a fanny pack, carry a lightweight pack with 10 pounds, or carry a 35-pound pack, the correct footwear is important. If your ankles are weak, you'll benefit from a higher shoe. A good insole will provide support and cushioning, reducing the jarring of your feet. Good outsole tread will provide traction on rocks and on wet trails. Good spacing in the toe box will save your toenails. You can find all these things in a lightweight shoe. Reducing your pack and gear weight will allow you the option of lightweight shoes. Do not make the mistake of choosing lightweight shoes without also considering the weight of your gear and pack. A heavy pack and lightweight shoes can hurt your feet and lead to an uncomfortable outing.

For help in reducing your pack weight and saving your feet, the gurus of lightweight are Ryan Jordan and his team at **www.backpackinglight.com.** The book Ryan edited, *Lightweight Backpacking and Camping: A Field Guide to Wilderness Hiking Equipment, Technique, and Style* is a must if you are serious about going lightweight. Ryan emphasizes:

> Chapter 1 begins appropriately with the category of equipment that is arguably more important that any piece of gear or apparel a lightweight backpacker will use: footwear. Lee Van Horn's treatise on footwear includes a comprehensive discussion of lightweight backpacking shoes. Simply put, shoes have such a profound impact on the lightweight backpacking experience because (1) the type of footwear you are able to wear depends in large part on the weight of the pack, and (2) the type of footwear you choose governs the transfer of energy and shock to the rest of your lower torso and spinal joints. Since this book's manuscript was finalized, I've been diving into research about ultralight footwear and experimenting with shoes lighter than anything the market has previously seen. I've been strengthening my feet, hiking in shoes with less support that are more akin to slippers than hiking shoes, and have been making some dramatic discoveries. In particular, I've learned that with proper conditioning, the natural features of the feet (as long as the arch is supported and the heel pad retains its shape for shock absorption) are ideally suited for transferring energy to the rest of your body, and I'm finding that I can walk longer distances in less supportive footwear—with a light pack—than I've ever been able to do before.

Of course, lightening your footwear means you should lighten your load. Get a lighter fanny pack, hydration pack, or backpack. If carrying a pack, lighten its load. Go from a tent to a new ultralight tent or a tarp. Change to one of the lightweight stoves and take advantage of lighter walking or hiking poles. Eliminate gear that you never seem to use but just had to pack. Your feet will feel all these weight savings. A weight loss of a few pounds will feel like heaven. You'll travel farther and your feet will be more comfortable.

Custom Shoes

What happens when you can't find a shoe you like? Your options are limited. Shoe companies are not in the business of making custom shoes. If you have a narrow heel and a wide forefoot, overall narrow or large feet, or have typically struggled to find shoes that fit well, you have probably experienced shoe hell. Most shoes, because they don't fit your feet, lead to blisters, arch problems, tendinitis, squished toes, and more. Rather than find a shoe that fits your feet, your feet are forced to fit into shoes made for the masses.

An excellent choice is to check out the Hersey Custom Shoe Company. They offer ten shoe models for runners, walkers, race walkers, and hikers. The ten include trainers and lightweight trainers, high-mileage shoes, racing flats, walking and racewalking shoes, hiking shoes, trail runners, and a high-top for those who need ankle support. Their approach is very simple: "Tell us what you're looking for, and we'll let you know if we can help."

The Hersey staff will work with you to get the shoe you want, based on your unique foot needs. You will answer a set of questions about how often you run and race, what your usual race distance is, what shoes you have used in the past that have worked and that have not worked, and then a set of questions about your feet (pronate, supinate, abnormal wear, orthotics, shoe breakdown patterns, and so on). You will also send a tracing of your feet based on Hersey's specific instructions. Then choose your model and design options and the shoes will be made to fit your feet and your feet alone.

Do they cost more? Certainly. Are they worth it? If you have hard-to-fit feet, I'd bet they are. If you want a shoe that is solidly made and not an off-the-shelf made in who-knows-where shoe, I'd also bet they will appeal to you. The Hersey Custom Shoe Company can be found at **www.herseycustomshoe.com.**

Their custom shoes were named by *Runner's World* as the best in both men's and women's in 1985. This shocked the Hersey staff—but shocked the giant shoe companies even more. *Runner's World* and other publications were pressured to do away with independent judging of shoes.

Sandals

Sandals are a nice alternative to shoes and boots. They are becoming more popular as designs improve to provide better traction, foot control, and comfort. Changing from running shoes or hiking boots into an open pair of sandals can be refreshing. When your feet are tired, hot, or sore, sandals can feel like a small piece of heaven on earth.

Spencer Nelson recommends sandals for some uses:

> I have put in some quality training and raced in them to get a feel for their use. I always wear them with socks (usually SmartWool) and have worn them for flat 5-mile runs to 20 miles on trails to day two of the Tahoe Triple Marathon, which had 13 miles of downhill. They are good for my feet, and I will probably get another pair for the following positive reasons. They are very comfortable and better cushioned than they appear. I don't even notice that they are a sandal after four or five minutes; in other words the straps and open-air feel don't affect me. They are quick to dry on trail runs with water crossings. They keep my feet cool. They feel as good after around 200 miles as they did when I got them. Scree gets in and is easily kicked out . . . honestly! I have not had any problems with stubbing my toes or things of that nature.

Those who prefer the freedom of sandals over constricting shoes may find the Teva or Keen sandals to their liking. The Teva Wraptor was the first performance running sandal. Using a patent-pending strapping system and a fusion arch, the sandal offered adjustability, comfort, and control. The strapping system flexes to adjust to the runner's arch and assist in motion control. Both companies make sandals for cool, comfortable use, providing the cushioning, stability, toe protection, and support of a running shoe in a lightweight, airy sandal.

Wearing sandals while running or hiking takes practice. Small pebbles, gravel, leaves, or other debris can easily work their way underfoot. Shaking the foot or a light kick against a rock will usually knock these loose. Be especially careful of sticks on the trail that could inflict a puncture wound to your exposed feet.

If you wear sandals without socks, the skin of your feet will eventually toughen into calluses. Check the calluses regularly for cracks that can split through to uncalloused skin and bleed or become infected. If going without socks, a dab of sunscreen on the toes and tops of the foot will protect from bothersome sunburn. Both Keen and Teva sandals now come in half sizes. Consider wearing socks to protect your heel's protective fat pad and to avoid cracks and fissures in the skin. Some athletes have glued Spenco Hiker insoles onto the sandals, while others use Velcro to secure insoles or foot pads onto the sandal's footbed.

Switchback, a long distance hiker, recommends several things if you hike with sandals: "[use] a good insole glued into the sandal footbed, use hiking socks and a foot cream on your feet to keep them from chapping and drying out, and if your heels hurt, use a heel cup under or over the insole to provide a little extra cushion for the heels."

Tired of running shoes that fit him poorly, caused blisters and toenail problems, and seemed to collect dirt, Rob Grant bought a pair of sandals. He used his Tevas in a Sri Chinmoy 24-Hour Run. At 100K both small toes were swollen. The next day he ground down the ridge on the footbeds that fits under the toes. This corrected the problem. After putting 405 miles on the sandals, he reports no noticeable wear on the soles or the straps. Rob found that rubbing petroleum jelly on the inside of the straps helped to soften them. He feels that ankle support in sandals is comparable to that of running shoes.

S A N D A L   P R O D U C T S

KEEN FOOTWEAR makes sandals with the protection of a shoe and the comfort of a sandal. The sandals have a toe guard, traction outsole, a wide footbed, and a quick-release drawstring closure. **www.keenfootwear.com**

TEVA SANDALS are for walking, running, and water sports. The Wraptor 2 is made for running. It has a raised toe spring to protect from rocks, roots, and debris; a dual-density EVA midsole with a molded shank arch plate; a Heel Shoc Pad; a quick dry upper; and a heavily lugged traction rubber bottom sole. This sandal will work well on trails and roads. With a contour molded, waterproof suede footbed, the sandal would be comfortable in bare feet. **www.teva.com**

Insoles

Insoles are funny little things. Most of our boots and walking and running shoes come with removable insoles. Typically, we buy a pair of shoes and wear them until they wear out—without ever thinking about the insoles under our feet. You may think insoles are similar, but they differ quite a bit. They range from rigid to flexible, cushioned to hard, no arch to high arches, low to high heel cups, one material to multiple substances, and cheap to expensive, and they come in a multitude of coverings. Newer types can be heated in an oven and then after standing in them, you can mold them to the shape of your feet.

INSOLE PRODUCTS

The replacement insoles listed below are a sampling of what is available to the general public. New models and designs are constantly being introduced. Check your local running, hiking, and footwear stores or check the manufacturers' websites to see what is available. Many of the shoe and boot companies such as Montrail, Birkenstock, Merrell, and Vasque also make insoles. Many drug stores and pharmacies also stock insoles such as those made by Dr. Scholl's.

ENDURO-SOLE by Montrail ensures a custom fit via thermo-moldable CTX foam over a dynamic molded arch piece. Heat the insoles in an oven, put them into your shoes, and stand on them for two minutes to mold them to your feet. www.montrail.com

FOOTFIX INSOLES are made with a deep heel pocket for stability, a gel heel cushion for minimizing heel pain, and a built-in arch for underfoot support. www.footfix.com

HAPAD COMF-ORTHOTIC is a full-length or three-quarter–length insole. Many people have had considerable success with these. For more information, see "Orthotic Products" on pages 148–149.

ORTHOSOLE offers a Max Cushion insole that can be customized with your choice of three arch supports and two metatarsal pads for six combinations of support. www.orthosole.com

POWERSTEPS offer a Pinnacle insole with a semi-rigid shell, a deep heel cup, and a strong arch support. www.powersteps.com

SHOCKBLOCKERS INSOLES, by Oregon Aero, were originally created for the U.S. military. The two-layer insoles feature a highly shock absorbing Visco-Kinetic polymer layer and a high-wicking, low-friction fabric. Several insole models are offered. www.oregonaero.com

Take the ones out of your shoes. Are they flimsy? Do they easily bend in half? Are they lifeless with little structure to offer support? Are they flattened out? Do they look like squashed cardboard? If so, your shoes came from the "we-cut-corners-on-the-insole" shoe company. Toss them out and get a new pair. The old one may be contributing to foot problems including blisters and foot pain.

Insoles, sometimes called footbeds, are designed to provide extra support and/or cushioning during running and hiking. Some models are molded to cradle the heel, support the arch, and cushion the forefoot, while others have only an arch support or are flat. Replacement insoles are to be used in place of your shoe's standard insole. Many replacement insoles offer better heel support, shock absorption,

INSOLE PRODUCTS

RXSORBO makes an assortment of replacement insoles. Several designs use Sorbothane viscoelastic polymer inlays in the heel and forefoot for maximum foot-strike protection. Other designs use Sorbothane foam in the full insole. www.rxsorbo.com

SHOCK DOCTOR FOOTBEDS incorporate multiple shock absorbing, support, and comfort components to create a foot-hugging performance platform. www.shockdoctor.com

SOF SOLE offers an Airr insole made with a heel air chamber that extends under the arch. Made with a Coolmax top sheet to wick moisture. www.sofsole.com

SOLE CUSTOM FOOTBEDS use heat-to-fit technology as an excellent, inexpensive alternative to custom orthotics. The footbeds have Poron cushioning, a deep heel cup for stability, and an aggressive arch for support. When you heat the insoles in your oven, put them into your shoes, and stand on them, they mold to your feet. www.yoursole.com

SORBOTHANE PERFORMANCE INSOLES are made with their proprietary viscoelastic polymer, giving maximum shock absorption and energy return. Features a textured Poron foam top for moisture management. www.runlonger.com

SPENCO makes several lines of replacement insoles: Polysorb, Gel, Spenco RX, and Spenco for Her. The Greenline designs are made from closed-cell neoprene. Sold through stores. www.spenco.com

SUPERFEET footbeds are made in two systems: Trim-to-Fit and CustomFit. Their corrective shape and design offer a stabilizer cap that provides excellent support and stability to the bone structure of the foot, allowing the foot muscles to function more efficiently and the body to be correctly aligned. The Trim-to-Fit insoles come in nine color-coded designs for specific activities and footwear. The seven CustomFit designs are fitted at stores with staff trained in their fit system. www.superfeet.com

energy return, and reduction of friction than the insoles that come with the shoes. Some have a better arch support that will help with flat feet problems. The insoles listed below are typically found in running, camping, and sporting goods stores. Ask to see their product catalogs if their shelf stock is low or if you are looking for a particular type. Some stores offer custom-made insoles that may provide a better fit than a general insole.

There are basically two types of insoles available: foam and viscous polymer. Foam insoles are lightweight and inexpensive, and they retain heat. However, their impact absorption is not as good, and they lose their impact absorbing properties with use. In general, foam is more suited for runners because of the concern about weight. The viscous polymers, such as those offered by RXSorbo, are a great choice for athletes with sensitive feet or injuries that require protection to the foot's padding. Some insoles offer polymer at the heel and/or forefoot, and the rest is made of foam. This reduces the weight liability of all-polymer insoles.

Superfeet is a good example of an insole made to perform. Many insoles are made to provide shock absorption, support, or alignment. Superfeet are made to do all three. Their unique Encapsulating Stabilizer System provides the ideal biomechanical support. One of their eight models is worth trying before going to a more expensive orthotic.

If you have tried changing socks and other techniques to decrease your chance of blisters and still have problems, try changing insoles. You may find that a particular brand or type of insole may be better at reducing blisters on your feet. This is usually due to the fabric or components of the insole. Replacement insoles may be sized differently. Be sure to check the fit inside your shoes or boots. An insole that is narrow in the forefoot can create problems as the foot overlaps space between the narrow insole and the side of the shoe. Insoles may be different in other areas also. Some may have a higher arch that will put pressure on your foot, creating blisters. Others may have a narrow heel bed and cause friction where your foot rubs against the top edge of the heel cup. Finding and using the right insole can make a big difference in the overall fit and comfort of your footwear. But insoles are not made to last forever. Check them for breakdown and replace them when necessary. This will depend on how you run and hike, as well as your mileage.

Replacement insoles are not sold as corrective footbeds. If a particular brand or style of insole is uncomfortable or causes pain, try another type. One brand may fit your feet better than another brand. Some are quite rigid, while others are very cushioned. Try several until you find a pair that is comfortable for your activity. If you purchase insoles and they are too tight in certain areas of your feet, inquire with your local shoe repair shop or a pedorthist about thinning them with a belt sander.

Do not confuse these insoles with an orthotic. Always consult with a pedorthist, orthopedist, or podiatrist if you are having frequent foot problems. Repeated foot pain may be a sign of deeper foot problems that a general-use insole cannot correct. In that case, an orthotic may be necessary to correct an imbalance problem. See the "Orthotics" chapter for more information on the types available and what these can correct.

A study by the American Orthopaedic Foot and Ankle Society found that inexpensive off-the-shelf insoles are more likely to be effective than pricey, custom-made products. According to the society, many foot problems can benefit from the cushioning of a cheap insert more than the repositioning provided by a custom made insert. Many of these inserts are made from foam, silicone, plastic, wool, or combinations of different materials.

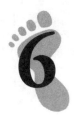

Barefoot & Minimalist Footwear

A few years ago, no one was talking about minimalist footwear. Then *Time* magazine named Vibram FiveFingers one of the best inventions of 2007. A few people got on the bandwagon. In 2009 Christopher McDougall wrote the book *Born to Run* and the issue exploded. McDougall set off to find out why his feet hurt and shared with readers the secrets of the Tarahumara Indians—and a better way to run. Barefoot running and running in minimalist footwear have become much more acceptable, and now the testimonials abound.

Mitch Kern shares his experience with barefoot running: "I've been running for years but my career has always been punctuated by injuries along the way. Like so many others I read McDougall's *Born to Run* and just had to buy a pair of Vibram FiveFingers. From there I transitioned into barefoot running and have been injury free ever since. I feel like I've learned just how to run for the first time. In the past, I was a heel striker/long strider, but now I take a very different approach—faster cadence and on the balls of the feet. I am convinced it is the way to go. People think I'm nuts, but man, oh man, what a difference."

Talk to a few people who are wearing Vibram FiveFingers or who run barefoot and you will discover a culture has developed. This unique line of footwear has five individual toes—for your toes—and with a Vibram outsole, it is akin to going barefoot. People who were previously unable to run now can. Those who had become accustomed to discomfort and pain from bunions, heel pain, and more have discovered relief. It is worth paying attention to.

Daniel Lieberman, a prominent researcher in the barefoot and minimalist movement, has written extensively on the subject. On his website he says, "We do not know how early humans ran, but our research indicates that humans were able to run comfortably and safely when barefoot or in minimal footwear by landing with a flat foot (mid-foot strike) or by landing on the ball of the foot before bringing down the heel (forefoot strike)."[10]

Running barefoot or in minimalist shoes is different than running in the usual running shoe. Most important, you land differently. Danny Abshire, the cofounder

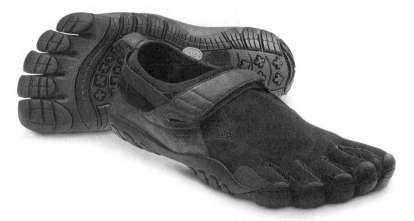

Vibram's FiveFinger KSO Trek for trails. Photo credit: Vibram

of Newton Running, says you acquire a connection with the ground as you run. You are more agile and run with finesse. Others in the barefoot and minimalist movement echo the same thought.

For purposes of this chapter, minimalist footwear is defined as any footwear that does not have the typical high cushioned heels, stiff soles, and arch support common in today's running shoes. The information and tips in this chapter, generally speaking, apply to someone wearing FiveFingers or other minimalist footwear, or those going barefoot. Many of those wearing minimalist footwear will also forego wearing socks.

And lest you think that going barefoot is only for walking and running, consider the group Barefoot Hikers. Barefoot Chris (his trail name), a member of Barefoot Hikers, recalls the reaction of hikers they encountered while on a weeklong barefoot backpacking trip on the Appalachian Trail. "They told stories of many other barefoot hikers, including at least two that had done the entire trail without shoes."

A quick online search for "barefoot running clubs" finds many cities with these running clubs. There are also clubs dedicated to walking and hiking barefoot.

Shoes vs. Minimalist Footwear

For years, everyone wore shoes, or if we were hikers, boots. We could choose between neutral, flexible, stable, motion-control, cushioned, lightweight, and trail shoes. We might stick to one design or try several. Many athletes went through pair after pair trying to find the perfect shoe for their feet, often in an effort to accommodate injuries. We had choices—as long as it was a shoe the shoe companies offered.

Yes, there were always a few runners who ran barefoot. Many times they received odd looks. Others looked for ultra lightweight shoes, which were few and far between. If you wanted to run, shoes were what you needed.

Kevin O'Neall shared his experience with wearing FiveFingers: "I was close to giving up running after 50-plus marathons and two dozen ultras because of chronic heel pain. My feet had developed golf-ball-size lumps where the Achilles tendons insert on the heel bone. After a year and a half wearing FiveFingers exclusively, the lumps are 90% gone. There is still heel pain, but it tends to fade while I'm running. At this point I prefer them to running shoes, even though they do make me a slower runner."

Of course, there are many arguments for and against barefoot running. Some claim that barefoot running is better for you. Others argue that barefoot running is dangerous and will lead to more injuries. And still others say that running shoes prevent injuries—or lead to injuries—depending on their point of view. Athletes will point to the few studies available to support their views—whatever they are.

The conspiracy theorists talk about the "big lie" from the shoe companies, which want you to buy their shoes. One ultrarunner, a proponent of the minimalist movement, wrote in an online forum, "They want you to buy heavy, stiff, supportive, motion-control shoes so that all the little muscles, tendons, and bones in your feet get weak, conforming to the brand you run in, so that they can upgrade you to the next model, which will invariably be heavier, stiffer, more supportive, more cushioned, more motion control, more expensive, and wear out faster." Personally, I don't believe that statement. I think there is room for regular shoes and minimalist shoes—and barefoot running. You have to make the choice and in my view, it should be an educated and informed choice.

Christian Griffith, an ultrarunner, made a valuable comment in an online forum about the barefoot and FiveFingers bandwagon that so many athletes are touting. He wrote, "It's a tool to help strengthen, lengthen, and improve flexibility in the leg muscles with the added benefit of forcing me to run what I view as 'correctly'—meaning upright, with a stable midline, mid-foot strike, and gently." Others in the forum agreed, emphasizing it as a way to learn and maintain good running form and to keep that form when moving back to shoes. While some athletes will stick to barefoot or minimalist footwear, many rotate between a combination of trail shoes, road shoes, barefoot, and minimalist footwear.

The Value of "Going Bare"

In the simplest of terms, going barefoot or using minimalist footwear makes your feet do more of the work they were intended to do. The bones, muscles, tendons, and ligaments all work together. You have a lighter gait. Instead of landing on your heels, you land more on the midsole and forefoot. With that comes a better connection between your feet and the ground. Barefoot Ted talks about this connection later in the chapter.

A 2004 study at the Sapporo International Half-Marathon in Japan captured foot strike positions of 283 runners; 75% of the runners landed on their heels,

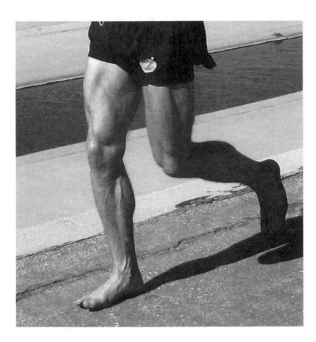

Running in bare feet
requires a mid-foot strike.
Photo credit: Barefoot Ted

24% landed mid-foot near the arch, and only 4% landed on their forefoot. The 4% were not the fastest.

When we wear shoes, most of us are heel strikers. Barefoot runners, as well as those in minimalist footwear, tend to strike the ground near or on the ball of the foot. I recently watched a 72-year-old woman—who, because of heel injuries as a child, had been unable to run—show me how she could now run. She was excited and had just finished her first 5K race. FiveFingers had allowed her to run again.

Our body adapts: muscles, tendons, and bones adjust to changes in footwear, our stride, and the way our foot strikes the ground. Many runners who have struggled with chronic injuries have switched to running barefoot or to minimalist footwear and have seen their injuries reduced or eliminated.

The Science on Barefoot Running

Articles in journals have talked about running shoes and barefoot running for some time. Here are a few examples.

- Barefoot running promotes front- and mid-strike, which allows the runner to take more advantage of elastic energy stored in both the Achilles tendon and the longitudinal arch of the foot. This develops more calf and foot muscle strength and avoids uncomfortable and potentially injurious impact.[11]

- A shoe with any heel height, trainers included, alters the entire body posture.[12]

- The sole and tips of our feet have 200,000 nerve endings connecting us to the world and helping us balance. The stimulation is a connection from foot to body and foot to brain. This sensory perception is often denied because of thick layered and inflexible shoes.

- When running barefoot, the runner compensates for lack of cushioning by adjusting the foot-landing angle to a more natural mid- to front-foot strike, giving it a softer landing.[13]

- Humans have engaged in endurance running for millions of years, but the modern running shoe was not invented until the 1970s. For most of human evolutionary history, runners were either barefoot or wore minimal footwear such as sandals or moccasins with smaller heels and little cushioning relative to modern running shoes.[14]

- The soft materials in modern running shoes allow a contact style [heel strike] that you would not use [if you were] barefoot. The foot no longer gets the proprioceptive cues that it should, and a midsole [foot strike] can impair the foot's ability to react to the ground. This can mute or alter feedback the body gets while running.[15]

Function & Form

The barefoot movement has taken the running community by storm. Athletes want to mimic the experience McDougall wrote about in *Born to Run*. Thousands have tried barefoot running, FiveFingers, and whatever new minimalist footwear that they have heard others talking about. They want the function and the feeling of venturing out with as little as possible on their feet. They are after the natural movement of going barefoot.

Unfortunately, this barefoot function requires a change in form that many do not consider. You cannot run barefoot, or in the new minimalist shoes, and land on your heels. You will become injured. This new style requires a mid-foot or forefoot strike. Newton Running calls it natural running, saying it will help you discover your optimal running form. Their website has videos and information describing this new form.

Think about how we move on our feet. When we walk, we naturally land on our heels first. When we sprint, we land on our toes. Ideally, we need a point in between.

When we run in normal shoes, we land on our heels and roll through to our forefoot and toes. Our heels strike first, in front of our center of gravity. This impact leads to a moment of deceleration, as the heel shock moves upward through the knees and spine. Then we push off with the muscular force of our toes.

When we run barefoot or in minimalist shoes, we naturally land on our mid-foot or forefoot. We lean slightly forward, with our center of gravity over where our forefoot strikes. Our stride is shorter with a quicker cadence. We land lightly and quickly lift our foot for the next foot strike. The body should be relaxed rather than tight or tense.

It takes time to unlearn old habits and learn the proper technique. Many become injured because they do too much too soon.

Barefoot Precautions

Whether you're going barefoot or wearing minimalist footwear, you need to start slowly. Your muscles need to get used to the new stresses on them. Tendons and ligaments need to be strengthened. Bones need to adapt to the new demands placed on them. Flexibility needs to be developed. None of this happens overnight. You need to ease your way into it. Doing too much too soon could cause damage to all those internal parts. Muscle tears, tendinitis, strained tendons, and stress fractures could result. Long-distance barefoot runner Tellman Knudson suggests starting with five minutes a day running barefoot, then putting your shoes on. After a week, add in another five minutes. Continue this for a few weeks and let your feet be your guide. If you experience swelling, internal pain, or a burning sensation, reduce the amount of time spent barefoot. You could also do this at the end of your run.

You are also changing from a heel striker to a forefoot striker. Landing on the balls of your feet adds new stresses on your Achilles tendon and calf muscles. Many of those starting out complain of Achilles and calf pain. Starting slowly will give these muscles time to strengthen. Landing on your forefoot or mid-foot doesn't mean that your heels don't come down; it just means that they don't touch first. You'll land more in the middle of the foot first and then your foot continues down until the

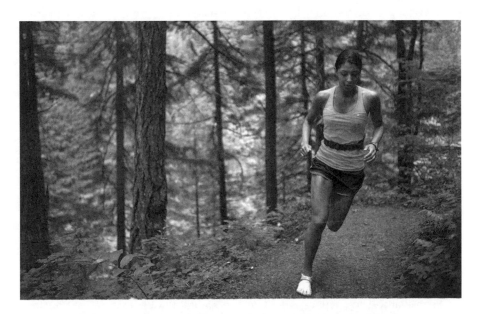

FiveFingers are used by many trail runners. Photo credit: Vibram

heels touch. The forefoot and mid-foot landings provide a natural springing action. You can also investigate Pose and Chi running, which advocate landing more on the forefoot. These two techniques teach movement techniques to enable athletes to position their body during exercises such as running, and teach better form and conditioning for reduced injuries (**www.posetech.com** and **www.chirunning.com**).

When venturing barefoot onto trails or even on pavement, you should take a few precautions. Start slowly with short barefoot excursions to give your feet time to adjust. Your feet are used to the support and cushioning of shoes, and going without will make a sudden change. Be attentive to the conditions of the path underfoot. Your feet can be cut or punctured by debris on the road or trail. If you want to run barefoot, start by walking.

Walking and running barefoot can be an excellent way to condition your feet in order to prevent blisters when you do wear boots or shoes. Your skin will be tougher and you may develop calluses. Yet, be forewarned: this is no guarantee that you will not get blisters. Remember that when it is raining, the moisture will soften the skin on your feet. That's a good time to switch to one of the minimalist shoes.

Aside from the possibility of cutting your feet on glass or metal, if you have any cuts or open skin on your feet, you run the risk of picking up an infection. Another concern is skin that calluses over. These calluses can split into fissures or cracks in the skin. This opens the inner layers of skin to a greater risk of infection. If you step on something sharp and get a puncture wound, seek medical care. Puncture wounds typically close up and this seals any debris, germs, or contaminants inside the wound. If you choose to go barefoot, it's smart to take care of your feet. There is no point in getting an infection through carelessness.

After reading about all the possible injuries from going barefoot, you may be worried. Going barefoot may be the goal of many athletes, but in reality, wearing minimalist shoes will provide protection and enhance the barefoot experience. Tellman Knudson likes FiveFingers, especially for people who:

- Don't want to deal with the pain of running barefoot,

- Want to minimize the risk of stepping on something that could hurt them,

- Run on hot surfaces where their feet would roast without protection, or

- Are in the process of transitioning from running in normal shoes to running barefoot.

Remember that switching to barefoot running or minimalist footwear does not mean that you can't ever run in shoes again. Many athletes employ a combination of going barefoot or wearing minimalist footwear or shoes. Running in minimalist footwear helps runners focus on good form, and for many, it will reduce injuries. If you want or need something more substantial than FiveFingers, consider using one of the minimalist shoes such as Inov-8, Nike Free, Newton, New Balance 800, or Terra Plana. These replicate the free and natural flexible motions of your feet better than the usual running shoe.

Avoiding Injuries

Running on any surface in bare feet exposes them to glass, rocks, nails, screws, twigs, wire, and roots—all typical debris in places we like to run. One misplaced step onto a rusty wire or a piece of glass can lead to an infected foot and, if not attended to properly, an even worse outcome. Learn to regularly check your feet for abrasions and cuts. Running on grass or trails offers a softer and more comfortable surface than asphalt or concrete. Wearing at least some degree of foot covering will protect the soles of your feet.

A strip of tape can be put on the ball of the forefoot for protection when running barefoot. Likewise, tape can even be added to the forefoot when wearing FiveFingers to reduce friction. Because the FiveFingers have individual toes, you could wear Injinji toe socks with them if you plan ahead and buy the footwear with room for the socks. That can provide an extra bit of cushioning, toe protection, and padding from any rough inside seams.

Scott Sanders uses FiveFingers and told me, "They are amazing shoes. My ITB [iliotibial band syndrome] and sore knee problems went away almost immediately. I wear them around town all the time, but I really can't run in them. Here are two problems I have had with FiveFingers:

■ They offer no protection from roots, rocks, stones, pavement, and concrete. An ultrarunner friend of mine broke her toe wearing them. I banged my foot on a root while training and have been forced to use them on the treadmill and elliptical pretty much exclusively. We have few soft trails to run on in Northern Georgia.

■ There is very little cushioning in the bottom of the sole. I tried inserting Dr. Scholl's Gel and regular shoe inserts to give me just a little more cushioning, but it didn't work."

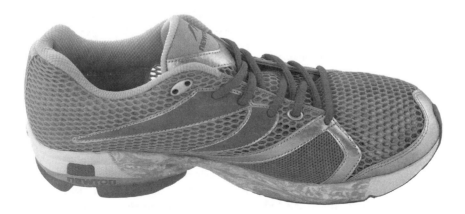

Newton shoes are made for a natural running form. Photo credit: Newton Running

Many athletes, like Scott, are buying FiveFingers and finding that the footwear is fine for walking, but athletes have a hard time running distances they used to run in normal shoes. Minimalist shoes are a good choice for these athletes. Inov-8 shoes are made for trails but not roads. Newton shoes offer a more normal-looking shoe designed for running on your mid-foot and forefoot, a natural running form.

Ice can help minimize swelling, especially as you are starting out. The "Cold & Heat Therapy" chapter has information on how to get the most benefits from icing.

When going out to run barefoot, add a few things to a fanny pack. Knudson, known for his efforts to run across America barefoot, suggests including tweezers, moleskin for padding, Gorilla Super Glue to seal wounds and help moleskin stick, duct tape, Band-Aids in case of cuts, and alcohol wipes to disinfect.

Barefoot Running Tips

- Go barefoot whenever possible—help your feet get used to it.

- Start slowly—give your feet time to strengthen themselves.

- When your skin gets sore, stop and wear something else.

- Strengthen your feet and ankles.

- Let pain be your guide—stop if your arches, top of your foot, or anything else hurts.

- Watch for abrasions and cuts on your feet and care for them.

- Be careful of hot and cold surfaces.

- Rest days are beneficial.

- Be attentive to roots and rocks, which can cause injury.

- Stand upright to stay on your toes and be light on your feet.

- Get over the social implications of going barefoot.

It is imperative that those wanting to try either barefoot running or minimalist footwear understand the importance of starting slowly and letting pain be your guide. Making the change to running barefoot and/or in minimalist footwear can easily lead to months of sore calf muscles, sore Achilles tendons, and various foot and ankle pains that could naturally limit your training. Even stress fractures can occur. Increasingly, many athletes ignore these warning signs and become injured. In mid-2010, articles started appearing about the epidemic of barefoot running injuries. Podiatrists and physical therapists reported a surge in injuries that seemed to be related to barefoot and minimalist footwear running. Heel and calf muscle injuries, Achilles tendinosis, and plantar fasciitis can happen when one does too much too soon. The transition from normal running shoes to running either barefoot or in minimalist footwear can take months. Most of us have been heel strikers

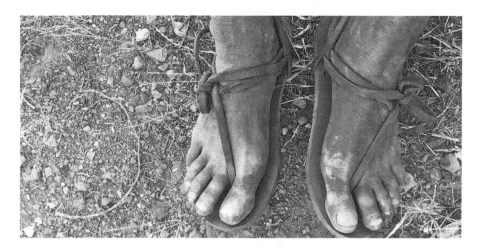

Barefoot Ted's Luna sandals. Photo credit: Barefoot Ted

for years. Changing to a mid-foot strike takes retraining our brain, which knows we are used to landing on our heels.

Be careful. Reduce your mileage. Start slowly. If you are older, be prepared for the transition to take even longer. Walk barefoot as much as possible. Let your bones, muscles, tendons, and ligaments get used to being free and unfettered from shoes.

Minimalist Footwear Choices

There are several choices in footwear when wanting a minimalist-type shoe. Vibram FiveFingers are the most commonly used. While athletes often try sandals, whether home-made huaraches or store-bought sandals, FiveFingers are seen on more feet than any other type of minimalist footwear. Inov-8 shoes are used by many runners because of their low profile and lightweight design—but are made only for trails. Newton shoes are becoming increasingly popular, especially for those running or walking on sidewalks and streets. The Nike Free and New Balance Minimus line are also good choices.

Remember that just because a shoe is marketed as minimalist doesn't mean that it is designed to accommodate a mid-foot or forefoot strike. Some are simply made with less support and structure, and a thinner outersole.

Consider your footwear needs based on the surfaces on which you run, how far you run, your running style, and your history of running injuries. Try the footwear on to make sure they feel right and run a bit in them—even if it's around the store. Ask the store for pointers and whether you can take them outside for a try.

Vibram FiveFingers

FiveFingers footwear was the brainchild of industrial designer Robert Fliri. He proposed the idea to Marco Bramani, grandson of Vibram founder Vitale Bramani, who invented the first rubber soles used on mountaineering boots in 1936.

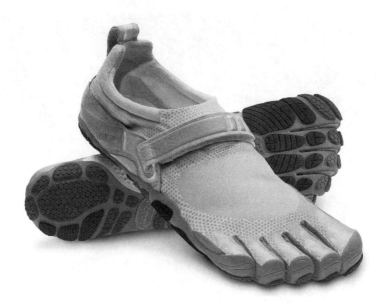

Vibram's FiveFingers Bikila. Photo credit: Vibram

Vibram FiveFingers are, simply put, little more than five-toed foot gloves for your feet. There is no arch support and no cushioning. The Vibram outsole is 3, 3.5, or 4 millimeters thick, depending on the style. Your feet and toes can spread out and bend and flex in a natural way, as they were intended to do naturally.

FiveFingers come in many styles. The best designs for running are those where the top of the shoes come up near the ankle. This keeps debris from getting inside and better secures the footwear to the foot. The KSO is one of the standard designs. A more rugged version, the KSO Trek, is designed for trails and trekking. Both have a Velcro strap that locks the shoe on your foot.

The Bikila is designed specifically for a more natural running experience with a more natural forefoot strike. Built on an entirely new platform, it features a 3-millimeter polyurethane insole (thickest under the ball) and a 4-millimeter anatomical pod outsole design that offers more plating protection and distributes forefoot impact without compromising important ground feedback essential to a proper forefoot strike running form.

For those wanting a more normal FiveFingers look, the Speed model, a FiveFingers' Bikila style with laces that resembles a shoe, may be worth looking at. For those wanting a lace style to avoid the tighter fit of the stretchy material over the instep, and/or those wanting a normal heel cup design, these may be the answer.

Getting Fit for FiveFingers

Gillian Robinson of www.zombierunner.com has fit many pairs of FiveFingers. She recommends them for people with toes that curl downward or upward, toes that overlap, hammertoes, and bunions. She suggests making sure that your toenails are trimmed and filed smooth to avoid poking through the mesh upper. Here are her tips on getting the best fit.

- Get fitted at a store that fits and sells FiveFingers.

- Wear them snugly against the foot, heel back in the shoe, but the toes should not be tight against the ends of the toe pockets.

- Size them to your longest toe (**www.birthdayshoes.com** has a section on modifying the second toe for Morton's foot).

- Get the right size: too big and they flop around and cause blisters; too small and your toes can't both flatten and flex.

The website **www.birthdayshoes.com** points out that FiveFingers do not come in American footwear sizing but in European sizing (that is, 34–48, depending on whether they're for men or women), and men and women can wear each other's FiveFingers, but women's are generally narrower.

Inov-8

Inov-8 footwear is worn by many trail runners because of its design, which allows the foot the freedom to move and function as nature intended, without interference from the structure of the shoe. The lightweight Inov-8 shoes protect the foot from the harsh external environment experienced by the off-road runner but maintain the feeling and function of barefoot running.

Newton

Newton running shoes are made to enhance the natural running gait of landing on your mid-foot or forefoot. Energy is absorbed and returned back to the runner through their patented Action/Reaction Technology. Runners I have talked to indicate the shoes help them land in a more natural position. For those wanting

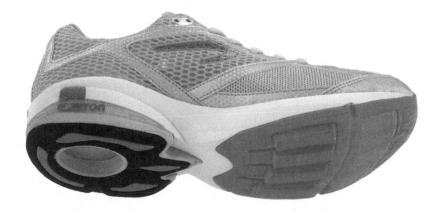

Newton shoes are made with actuator lugs in the forefoot for energy return. Photo credit: Newton Running

a minimalist shoe with protection and support that also provides a forefoot running technique, Newton shoes are a good choice. Newton footwear was the only minimalist footwear that I observed at the 2010 Badwater 135-mile ultramarathon through California's Death Valley.

Terra Plana's Evo

The Vivo Barefoot division of Terra Plana was developed specifically to produce shoes that replicate being barefoot. The Evo looks like a normal running shoe. Made with breathable mesh and lightweight micro fiber, they weigh in at 8 ounces. The outsole is 4 millimeters thick. Individuals who cannot wear FiveFingers because of fitting issues may do well in these shoes. The Evos allow for a greater variety of foot anatomy. As with FiveFingers, they allow a barefoot running experience with some degree of protection.

Other Minimalist Shoes

Because of the growing popularity of minimalist footwear, we can expect more companies to design footwear for this market. The websites and blogs listed at the end of this chapter are a good way to stay in touch with changes in the market. Following are several examples.

- **NIKE FREE SHOES** attempt to replicate the free and natural flexible motions of your feet. **www.nike.com**

- Based on the success of the MT100 and WT100 ultralightweight shoes made for a natural gait, New Balance is introducing **MINIMUS,** a new minimalist line of cross functional shoes for road and trail. **www.new balance.com.**

- The **KIGO SHEL** is a slip-on–style 5-ounce shoe made for trails, hiking, or walking. **www.kigofootwear.com**

- Saucony is introducing a lightweight **PROGRID KINVARA,** made to encourage a mid-foot strike. **www.saucony.com**

- Merrell is partnering with Vibram to introduce a new line of **MERRELL BAREFOOT** minimalist shoes. **www.merrell.com**

- Asics says its **SPEEDSTAR 5** "embodies the new minimalism." **www.asicsamerica.com**

We have to be careful and read reviews from magazine and websites dedicated to the barefoot and minimalist movement (**www.birthdayshoes.com** and **www.barefoot runningshoes.org** are two examples). Make sure the footwear is made for running, not just casual wear. Because of the growing interest in minimalist footwear, many companies are trying to enter the minimalist shoe marketplace, and those shopping for such shoes need to be informed.

As you might guess, wearing footwear without socks can lead to funky-smelling shoes. Wiping your feet with a premoistened antibacterial wipe is a good start. Kiwi Fresh Force, PediTech, and ZORBX Odor Remover are highly recommended on **www.birthdayshoes.com**, which has a great page of tips about keeping your FiveFingers (and any other shoes) stink free. Readers also give washing tips and offer suggestions ranging from powders, sprays, and soaks.

Barefoot Ted's tips on the next page can also be applied to those wearing minimalist footwear. It is about technique and form as well as whether we wear shoes or not.

Another popular barefoot runner, Barefoot Ken Bob Saxton, gave the following quote in an article on barefoot running in *Runner's World* (February 2010): "Barefoot running is actually something that's been tried and tested over millions of years of evolution. Feet have become the engineering marvel that they are because they work. We're just trying to help average runners become more mindful of how they're running and to enjoy it more."

Barefoot running and wearing minimalist footwear can help you get to that point. But remember, start slowly and let pain be your guide.

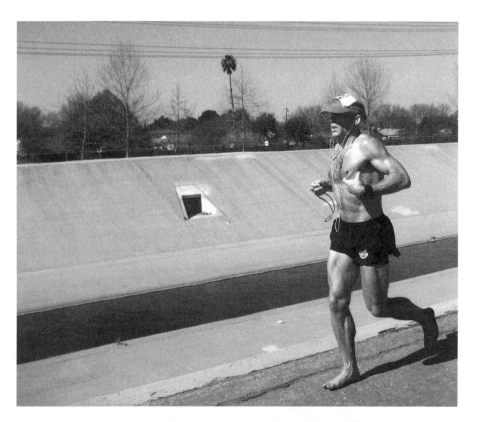

Barefoot Ted in typical running form. Photo credit: Barefoot Ted

Barefoot Ted's Tips to Getting Started

I asked Barefoot Ted to share from his experience. He has been running barefoot longer than most. Here is what he said.

So, you wanna start running barefoot? Firstly, before you begin, you want to evaluate what it is that is leading you to even accept the logic behind the concept of barefoot running. We all know that barefoot running has gotten a lot of attention lately. Much of it is valid and deserves your attention.

Yet, one must still ask: is this a viable option for me? Before you answer that question, let me explain why I think barefoot or minimal footwear running may not be good for you. It is not good if you are thinking it is some sort of cure-all that only requires taking off your shoes and starting to run injury free without radical changes in the way you may have been thinking of running up to now. If your running strategy has been about very specific time or distance goals, and you have been willing to push through pain to injury, then I would caution you: your bare feet will not allow you to continue this way.

Barefoot Ted's Barefoot Running Goals

So, what are the secrets I share with clients who take my Introduction to Barefoot Running Clinic? First, my aim is to get people to learn how to *feel* what good running feels like. One of the primary feelings becomes an awareness of the texture and hardness of terrain and of impact. This awareness is the beginning.

"o master this awareness, I have clients learn to move on hard surfaces *first*. Not focusing on distance or speed, I have my clients first walk and then trot on hard, fairly smooth surfaces. I work with them to focus on and begin to master three goals: quiet, quick, and in balance.

My Three Goals

1. QUIET Master gentle, quiet, forefoot-centric landings, silent and smooth. Learn to move with no hard edges and no pounding by learning how to have the impact of your landing flow through your forefoot and smoothly spread through the legs. Notice how silent your movement becomes. Imagine the movement of a big cat. Watch dogs trot. Let them be models for a flowing movement that wastes no energy.

2. QUICK Quicken your cadence. Running in bare feet encourages this naturally. Some shoe runners are plodders. You can hear them coming. Lots of wasted energy on poorly timed impact. Quicker cadence ends up making sense when you realize that your ability to absorb and recoil

Barefoot running is not about blocking or pushing through pain, or at least it shouldn't be. Rather it is about *tuning in* to your own body's highly sophisticated set of integrated awareness systems, systems that communicate through feelings and senses that are being collected in real-time as you move. From my perspective, learning how to run well means learning how to tap into the feeling of running well, which more often than not requires baring the foot to get the full feel of what happens when you move.

However, even if you decide that barefoot is the route for you, take one step backward and realize that you are most likely in the process of rehabilitating your feet and legs from years of being differently abled, shoed, and cast. Atrophy, loss of range of motion, weakness, neglect—the foot has not been treated well lately. All the padding and support and protection has not led to stronger feet, sadly.

So, the first key is to start slowly, incrementally, and avoid over-exuberance; avoid being driven by your ego. The hallmark of my barefoot running philosophy is regaining connectedness, mindfulness, and presence in your running and in your body.

energy through elasticity in your body dissipates quickly and is lost if not used. Learning how to get back in touch with the sweet spot of optimal recoil efficiency is easier to find when you can feel your feet, a feeling that encourages a landing phase with your foot more in line with your center of gravity. Overstriding is discouraged and nearly impossible when barefoot.

3. IN BALANCE The feeling of balance is a stable upright posture, balanced head, core engaged, belly button pulled into the spine, no waist bending, and head upright. I think that good running can be judged aesthetically. It should look good, not painful. When you see someone moving or running well, it looks smooth and fluid and graceful and efficient. The opposite looks painful, when someone is hunched and stiff, robotic and plodding. Indeed efficient running is tall and stable, the upper body acting as the fulcrum from which the legs and arms can move freely with a serious lack of bouncing or swaying of the head.

Ultimately my aim in coaching is to help people perfect what I call a persistent hunt trot . . . a gait not purely about speed, but about smooth, flowing, efficient, sustainable movement, movement that leaves you ready to play another day. Listen to your body. Learn what it is telling you. Then adjust and advance accordingly.

BAREFOOT & MINIMALIST FOOTWEAR WEBSITES

Note: Including the websites and books with this chapter rather than at the end is a bit of an anomaly, but we decided that it was important to keep these distinct resources with this chapter.

BAREFOOT RUNNING The daily barefoot digest by Tellman Knudson offers a place to have questions about barefoot running answered. Includes a forum, member's page, blog, chat, and more. **www.barefootrunning.com**

BAREFOOT RUNNING UNIVERSITY Barefoot ultramarathon runner Jason Robillard, author of *The Barefoot Running Book,* offers information about running barefoot, a blog, footwear reviews, links, and more at **www.barefootrunning university.com.**

BAREFOOT TED'S ADVENTURES The website of Barefoot Ted offers tips, a blog, a link to a Google group, his coaching page, and his custom-made huaraches or a do-it-yourself kit. **www.barefootted.com**

BIRTHDAY SHOES A website and blog dedicated to Vibram FiveFinger shoes, with tips and facts to help your minimalist experience. The Resource page offers an FAQ section, design reviews, running and walking tips, and barefoot research, and the site describes how to make modifications and repairs. **www. birthdayshoes.com**

DANIEL LIEBERMAN The Harvard researcher maintains a website about "Biomechanics of Foot Strikes & Applications to Running Barefoot or in Minimal Footwear." **www.barefootrunning.fas.harvard.edu**

HOW TO RUN BAREFOOT This website by Tellman Knudson offers e-mails with tips on running barefoot and a free *Fire and Ice Barefoot Runner's Survival Guide to Barefoot Running* e-book. **www.howtorunbarefoot.com**

BAREFOOT RUNNING BOOKS

McDougall, Christopher. *Born to Run: A Hidden Tribe, Superathletes, and the Greatest Race the World Has Never Seen.* New York: Alfred A. Knopf, 2009.

Robillard, Jason. *The Barefoot Running Book: A Practical Guide to the Art and Science of Barefoot and Minimalist Shoe Running.* Allendale, Michigan: Barefoot Running Press, 2010.

Sandler, Michael, and Jessica Lee. *Barefoot Running: How to Become Healthy, Fit, and Blissful by Getting in Touch with the Earth.* Boulder: RunBare Publishing, 2010.

BAREFOOT & MINIMALIST FOOTWEAR WEBSITES

HUARACHES Huaraches are the running sandals worn by the Taruhumara Indians, famed for their long-distance running. This website sells huaraches and gives instructions on making your own. **www.invisibleshoe.com**

INOV-8 FOOTWEAR The official site of Inov-8 Footwear has information on their products "designed around the natural functions of the foot." **www.inov-8.com**

NEWTON RUNNING is the website of the Newton line of running shoes. Good information on the science of natural running and articles on improving your running form. **www.newtonrunning.com**

RUNBARE The website of Michael Sandler and Jessica Lee, the authors of *Running Barefoot*. **www.runbare.com**

RUNNING BAREFOOT The website maintained by Barefoot Ken Bob is the original barefoot running site. Started in 1997, it offers tips and FAQs. **www.therunningbarefoot.com**

SOCIETY FOR BAREFOOT LIVING A website of resources, facts, and links about living barefoot. **www.barefooters.org**

TERRA PLANA Terra Plana's official site covering the EVO minimalist shoes. **www.terraplana.com**

VIBRAM FIVEFINGERS The Vibram website for their FiveFinger shoes. **www.vibramfivefingers.com**

ZERO DROP Approaching zero drop with your footwear will get you as close as possible to natural or barefoot running. The site offers shoe reviews and a shoe guide. **www.zerodrop.com**

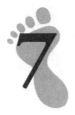

Socks

Socks perform four basic functions: cushioning, protection, warmth, and absorption of moisture off the skin. The sock fabric and weave will determine how well they do each. Socks made from synthetic fabrics wick moisture away from the skin and through the sock to its outer surface where it can evaporate.

Although I usually inform athletes of their foot care options and advise them to make the best choices for them, I have three absolutes. The first deals with socks. Serious athletes should avoid 100% cotton socks like the plague and always use moisture-wicking socks. The second absolute is covered in the chapter on gaiters (see page 150) and the third in the chapter on toe care (see page 299). And yet some athletes prefer common cotton crew socks, and others swear by synthetic socks or synthetic double-layer socks. If cotton crew socks work for you, continue using them. If, however, hot spots and/or blisters plague you, consider trying other types of socks. Some have discovered socks with individual toes and like these because they avoid dirt and grime collecting between the toes and causing friction.

For my first 24-hour track run, I wore thick cotton socks and used gobs of petroleum jelly on my feet. That was what everyone else seemed to be doing, so that was what I did. It didn't take long for blisters to develop on my heels and toes, which reduced me to a slow walk. Even so, I managed to get in a respectable 103 miles. Without the early foot problems, I am sure I could have done another 10 miles. I learned the hard way what did not work on my feet and set out to find what did work.

Not everyone needs a primer on how to put on your socks, but it is important to know a few tricks. Although it seems like a simple thing, it can make the difference between sore, blistered feet and happy feet.

Mindfulness: The Art of Putting on Your Socks

First, be sure your socks are clean and free of debris. Hold them by the cuff, pull them through the closed fist of the other hand, and then whip them in the air a couple times. Turn them inside out and then repeat. If the socks have a heavy seam at the toe, wear them inside out. Next, massage your feet and between the toes, making sure there is absolutely no grit or other debris. Then either roll or bunch the socks up, so the toes can be placed in the toe of the sock. Be sure the seam is across the top of the toes and, if possible, not lapping around the small toe. Now bring the sock up over the rest of the foot and up the leg; use a massaging motion to be sure there are no wrinkles and to detect any rough spots or debris.

Next, remove the insert from your shoe and inspect it. Remove any lint, toe jam, or other debris. Now bang the shoes together sole to sole a couple times and then tap the heel on the ground. Now shake out any debris and reach inside and feel all surfaces for debris or other problems. Replace the inserts and put on your shoes. It sounds complicated, but the whole process takes less than a minute and can prevent many foot problems.

—Rick Schick, ultrarunner and physician's assistant

Clean socks can feel heavenly. Wash your socks inside out to do a thorough job of cleaning the inside fibers and washing off any extra lint. When hiking, wash yesterday's socks and let them dry on the back of your pack. Try to change socks several times during a 100-mile run and once during a 50-mile run. During multi-day events, try to change socks several times a day. If clean socks are unavailable from your crew, try to wash the dirty socks so they are clean for later use.

You may be one of a growing number of athletes who wear socks inside out. Rob Langsdorf recommends turning your socks inside out to help prevent blisters: "Most socks have a rib near the toe where the sock is pulled together. The manufacturers put this on the inside of the sock, so it looks nice. Unfortunately it tends to rub the tops and sides of the toes and can cause blisters."

At summer's end, the usefulness of many of your shoes and socks may also be coming to an end. Go through your drawers and follow the quiz below. If you can answer "yes" to any of one or more of these eight questions, toss the socks. Socks are relatively inexpensive. Sure, some cost upward of $15–$20, but as with other gear, there comes a time when it is necessary to clean out your drawers. Just remember, when you go shopping for new ones, be sure to get moisture-wicking socks.

Tossing Socks

This is a quiz. Of all the socks in your sock drawer, how many should have been tossed out months ago? I'll bet you have at least two or three pairs of socks that should have been aimed at the wastebasket a long time ago. Maybe even more. So how do you know when to toss out a pair of socks? Actually, it's fairly easy. After washing socks, put your hand inside and feel around. Then turn them inside out and check them again. Here are eight tips.

- Can you see your fingers through the weave of the fabric?

- Can you see threadbare areas, typically on the heels?

- Are there holes in the toes, or anywhere else for that matter?

- Is the inside starting to unravel?

- Are any areas thinner in cushioning than the rest of the fabric around that area?

- Is the top cuff around your ankle starting to come apart?

- Is the toe seam bothersome?

- Is the top cuff no longer supportive, hanging down your ankle?

Here's an added tip. Don't check just your old socks. Check them all. I once ran in a fairly new pair of brand-name socks and developed a hot spot on one heel. Taking my shoe off, I discovered the sock was defective and the weave on the heel had separated. I had no more than 60 miles on the sock—but saved it for when I do foot care clinics as an example of a sock to toss.

When the weather gets colder and you switch to warmer socks, make sure they fit in your shoes. Warmer socks may be thicker socks, with a combination of fabrics and possibly a denser weave. The problem is that thicker socks squeezed into shoes not made for them can cause constriction of blood vessels and impede circulation to the feet. Be sure you can wiggle your toes in the toe box and your heels are not too cramped.

Sock Fibers & Construction

Socks come in a variety of fabrics: cotton, cotton blends, synthetics, silk, wool and wool blends, and fleece. An overview of these materials provides insights into their uses. Read the product information on the sock's packaging and try several types to find those that work best for you.

Natural, Synthetic, & Combination Materials

COTTON socks provide no wicking or insulating properties, and therefore moisture is retained against the skin. In damp or wet cotton, your feet are generally wet, cold, and more prone to blistering. Do yourself a favor and avoid 100% cotton socks.

COTTON BLENDS containing spandex, nylon, rayon, and acrylic offer a limited advantage over a pure cotton sock.

SYNTHETICS offer protection against blisters caused by moisture, poor fit, hot spots, slippage, and friction. These are made of hydrophobic materials, meaning they don't like moisture or water. Moisture-wicking fabrics such as Capilene, CoolMax, Olefin, and polypropylene wick moisture and perspiration away from the skin to the outer layer of the sock. Synthetic insulators such as Hollofil, Thermax, and ThermaStat help provide insulation. Some of these socks have a single layer, while others have double layers. Most synthetic socks use one of the above fabrics blended with cotton, nylon, spandex, or acrylic.

SILK socks are slick and are generally used as liners. Offering low wicking properties and low heat retention, they do not dry as fast as the newer synthetics.

WOOL wicks while retaining its cushioning but can be scratchy and rough.

WOOL BLENDS are comfortably warm in winter and cool in summer. Socks made from worsted wool are soft and durable. Merino wool, from sheep with a lighter and softer coat, is less resilient but very soft and comfortable. Wool may also be blended with other fabrics.

FLEECE socks are soft, provide exceptional warmth, and dry faster than wool, but can be looser in shape.

The weave of the sock will vary depending on the material. Socks will range from a loose weave to a dense weave. A loose weave feels coarse and provides less insulation. A dense weave feels softer and generally offers more cushioning. Put your hand inside a sock and stretch the foot portion with your fingers to see the weave. Denser-weave socks will show less space between the fibers.

Double-layer socks can help reduce or eliminate blisters. The two layers moving against each other instead of against the skin reduces skin friction. Most double-layer socks utilize wicking properties to move moisture away from the feet. Before wearing any double-layer sock, align the layers with your hand and then roll the socks onto the foot for the best fit.

Technology is moving faster than we can keep up—even in socks. The following are examples of socks utilizing technology to make them better fitting, better functioning, and longer wearing.

- More than a few sock companies are making anatomically correct socks for the right and left foot.

- Sock companies are making socks designed specifically for women. These socks have a more rounded toe and flex-stretch heels designed for a woman's feet.

- Many companies are making socks with either antibacterial or antimicrobial properties.

■ **DRYMAX** makes socks with a Moisture Removal System, which keeps feet dry with super-hydrophobic (water repelling) fibers. Moisture is lifted off the skin and moved to the outer sock layer. Tests show Drymax socks to be up to 25 times drier than other socks.

■ **INJINJI** makes toe socks with a four-point anatomical molding system. These Tetrasoks are constructed without seams. With individual toes to protect each toe, they help those prone to toe blisters. Made with CoolMax or wool, nylon, and spandex, they conform to the shape of your feet and toes.

■ **WIGWAM** has introduced a quick drying Pro sock with moisture-repelling fibers to transfer moisture from the bottom of the sock up and out of the shoe. Their Fusion line knits a liner sock and outer sock into one piece of fabric. The inner liner side of the sock wicks, while the outer layer is merino wool. The blend of the two makes for a sock that will keep your feet comfortable, dry, and more blister free.

■ Compression socks go over the calf and stimulate circulation in the muscles, providing support and enhancing stamina. By applying graduated pressure to the lower extremities, starting at the foot and up to the calf, blood is returned more rapidly to the heart and lungs. The patented technology shows a quicker return of oxygenated blood to the legs and reduces fatigue.

■ **BLISTER GUARD** technology utilizes Teflon as a low-friction fiber that prevent hot spots that cause blisters, abrasions, and calluses. The Teflon fibers are woven into the fabric of the sock at the toes, forefoot, and the heels. These socks have undergone strenuous tests, achieving an 80–100% reduction of blisters, and they are being marketed by various sock companies with combinations of traditional fibers such as acrylic, wool, nylon, and polyester, as well as performance fibers such as CoolMax and spandex. Look for the Blister Guard symbol.

Drymax sports socks are a great example of a leading edge sock company. Their socks' inner Drymax fibers are water hating while the outer polyester layer is water loving. This combination helps keep the skin dryer than other socks. In addition, they have incorporated friction-free Blister Guard technology, MicroZap antimicrobial technology, Moisture Removal System technology, color sizing marks, seamless design, five sizes for truer fit, and five density levels of protective padding. Their running-socks line offers socks for regular, trail, cold weather, hot weather, and maximum protection running. They are constantly tweaking their designs to increase effectiveness of ventilation, ankle protection, warmth for cold-weather socks, and more. And to top it off, their socks are made in the United States.

Buying Socks

Buy socks that fit your feet. The heels, toes, and length should fit snugly without sagging or being stretched too tight. Socks that are too big will bunch up and cause friction and skin irritation. Socks that are too small can cause the toes and joints to rub harder against the socks. Turn the socks inside out and look at the toe seams. Avoid those with bulky seams because they can rub, causing hot spots and blisters. Tube socks have no place in an athlete's sock drawer. After buying socks, be sure to try them on with your shoes or boots to be sure they fit together and are not too tight. Remember also to discard socks when they become threadbare and too thin to provide their advertised benefits. The heels of your socks are a good indication of the amount of padding and loft.

The correct sock is one that fits your foot and fills the inside of the shoe. Being too tight or too thick can constrict circulation and lead to problems, especially in cold weather. Rubbing can lead to hot spots, which lead to blisters. Changing to thinner socks can cause extra movement of the foot inside the shoe, leading to friction, hot spots, and, you guessed it, blisters.

Many stores offer a basket of socks to use when trying on shoes and boots. Avoid these if possible, and instead use your own socks when shopping. This way you will get to feel the fit with your personal socks and avoid picking up a foot fungus from another shopper.

Many people will pick a brand of socks and stick with them. That's fine, but remember, sock manufacturers have made tremendous advances in sock construction. There are many fantastic socks being made and you owe it yourself to check them out.

TIP: Go for the Garter

Sock garters can prevent socks from slipping and getting wrinkled inside of the shoe, which can lead to blisters and hot spots. This is especially true when feet are wet either from rain, stream crossings, or excessive perspiration. It also is more of a problem on trails with steep climbs and descents, although it can also happen when hiking on dry, level surfaces. Making a sock garter can help to prevent the problem.

Go to a craft store or sewing supply center and buy a couple feet of 1.25-inch-width elastic, the kind used in clothing. Be sure to get the ribbed or roll-proof variety. Measure around your leg at the narrowest point, just above the ankle, and then make a loop of the elastic about a half inch shorter. When placed over the sock at that point, the garter should feel snug but not tight.

Sock designs and the sock market change so fast that company websites are the best source of information for specific lines of socks. Each company introduces new versions of their socks each year. New fabrics and combinations of fabrics make the sock selection ever changing. Your local stores will have displays of many of these socks, or check out the websites listed below (and there are many more sock manufacturers out there). Investigate your sock options and talk to others about their preferences to determine which socks may be best for your sporting needs.

If you have a hard time finding the socks you want, check out **www.thesock company.com**.

Specialty Socks

The following sections identify specific socks for running and hiking, compression socks, sock liners, and high-technology oversocks. Many of these socks may be used for running, hiking, and adventure racing. Check them out at a store near you to feel them and read their packaging information. The products listing at the end of this chapter notes which companies make socks for each type of sport.

Running Socks

The list of companies making running socks seems endless. Even shoe companies are having socks made under their label. Most are moisture wicking and are offered in road and trail styles, a variety of heights, and a mix of fabric blends. Many runners swear by their favorite socks brand and style. Two innovative companies are Injinji with their toe socks, and Drymax with their unique interwoven fiber technologies that make up their moisture control system.

Hiking Socks

Hiking socks are different from running socks. Hikers most often wear crew or high-top socks. Some wear a wool outer sock with a liner that has wicking properties. Hikers could also try the thinner double-layer wicking socks in a crew style. These wear well, wick moisture away, and are made to reduce the possibility of blisters.

Pacific Crest Trail hiker Matthew Jankowicz used to get blisters, especially on long hikes over 20 miles a day. He tried tape, moleskin, and different kinds of boots. Finally, he switched to wearing three pairs of socks and it worked. He uses one pair of wicking socks over which he wears two pairs of boot socks. Matthew says, "I know some people think I'm crazy, but it works very well for me and I have hiked thousands of miles this way without getting any blisters on my feet."

Another hiker, going by the trail name of Morning Glory, found that wearing a thin liner sock, a Thorlos sock, and finally a wool-blend hiking sock worked well. She bought boots with enough room to accommodate the three pairs of socks. When wearing heavy socks for winter or otherwise, wear a boot a half size larger than normal. If you wear your normal size boot, it compresses the heavy sock and at best you gain little in the way of insulation. In the worst case, it is so tight that it inhibits blood flow to the toes and results in frostbite.

Sock Liners

Sock liners are thin and smooth, and they are usually worn under a heavier insulating or cushioning sock, typically wool. They are lightweight and quick drying. Most liners are made from hydrophobic fibers to wick moisture away from the foot and into the outer sock. A liner will perform in tandem with the outer sock the same way as double-layer socks; friction will occur between the two layers and not against the skin, reducing the chance of blisters. When shopping for liners, look for a style with wicking properties. While many runners are converting to the double-layer socks, some still prefer a two-sock system using liners.

Compression Socks

Compression socks have become popular in the past few years. These unique over-the-calf socks provide graduated compression that stimulates circulation in the foot and ankle with snug compression that tapers off higher up the sock. The improved circulation and reduced fatigue is reported to lead to better performance, reduced swelling, and higher VO2 (maximal oxygen consumption) levels.

Many users report a reduction in foot pain, swelling, and aches. Compression socks can also help in reducing post-exercise muscle soreness. Delayed onset muscle soreness (DOMS) is a common experience following unaccustomed "eccentric" exercise. In a study, subjects volunteered to perform a single bout of backward downhill walking exercise for 30 minutes. Following this exercise, subjects were required to wear graduated compression stockings for five hours per day for three consecutive days on one leg while the second leg had their normal sock. Muscle soreness and neuromuscular measures were taken pre- and post-walk, then 2, 24, 48, and 72 hours post-walking exercise for the two legs. There was a 28% reduction in DOMS on the leg wearing compression socks 72 hours after exercise. Additionally, the leg wearing the compression socks started to recover contractile properties within 24 hours, but not the other leg. It is theorized that in this study the compression socks might have had the effect of compressing the muscle tissue to such an extent that less structural damage occurred relative to a control condition. Compression socks accelerated the recovery of the muscle force capacity at 24 hours beyond that achieved by the control condition.[16]

There are many sock companies making compression socks for athletes. Oxysox was the early entry in this new field. Skins Sport Sox is a spandex compression sock with a stirrup under the foot rather than a whole-foot sock and is worn under other socks. CW-X's compression socks reportedly support the arch and calf and stabilize the ankle. SIGVARIS Athletic Recovery Socks offer graduated compression technology. 2XU's compression socks come in a Race Sock and a Recovery Sock.

Because of the height, compression socks can be warm when temperatures rise. Be observant for heat rash under the socks, especially at the top and bottom where there might be a constricting band. This is particularly important in extreme heat.

High-technology Oversocks

Oversocks are special high-technology socks that combine waterproof technology and the comfort of traditional socks into a somewhat baggy-looking sock. They were developed for anyone who participates in outdoor activities during which feet are exposed to water. They keep feet dry and comfortable even though the shoes or boots may be soaked and muddy. Even though the socks keep water out, your feet will sweat, creating their own moisture. Two tricks are to wear an inner, moisture-wicking sock and to use an antiperspirant on your feet to reduce the amount of sweat.

Be aware of moisture inside your shoes and socks in extreme cold conditions. Sweat and outside moisture can change to ice inside your socks, leading to frostbite.

National champion ultrarunner Roy Pirrung tested the high-technology oversock SealSkinz for a year in all kinds of weather. Roy recalls his win at the 100K Glacial Trail Run, a grueling race through the wet Kettle Moraine State Forest in Wisconsin: "It had rained the day before and conditions were sloppy. As other runners stopped every 10 miles to change their wet socks, I just raced ahead. I ended up finishing the race within 25 seconds of the course record and without any blisters." In wet and cold conditions, oversocks can work wonders. Roy found that SealSkinz have helped him to train outside in –25°F weather with a windchill factor of –80°F. His feet "stayed warm, dry, and comfortable."

SealSkinz socks are seamless waterproof socks that use moisture vapor transpiration (MVT) technology. The socks are made in a thin, lightweight, three-layer design. An inner CoolMax liner wicks moisture away from the skin while a middle layer of vapor-permeable membrane allows perspiration to escape and prevents water from entering. The outer layer uses nylon for abrasion resistance and durability. Their seamless design gives them a positive edge in preventing blisters. Their WaterBlocker socks are fully immersible and their revolutionary in-cuff seal ensures a tight, waterproof fit to keep out everything from water to grit. All-Season socks have a spandex cuff to ensure that the socks will stay up, but the cuff will allow water in. An over-the-calf sock is also available. Their ChillBlocker sock made to protect feet from extreme temperatures has a Polartec fleece liner.

Many adventure racers use SealSkinz socks to keep their feet free of blisters, abrasions caused by dirt and grime, and the effects of water immersion during their long, multiday competition. Adventure racer Rebecca Rusch was on Team Montrail at the Primal Quest Adventure race in Telluride, Colorado, where the team used SealSkinz to help them to a second-place finish. Rebecca says, "The only thing I've found for keeping out grit and sand (and leeches) are SealSkinz socks. I've used them in Borneo, Philippines, and Vietnam, and I will use them in Fiji. They're hot in these environments but keep your feet clean and healthy."

Rocky Gore-Tex oversocks from REI are waterproof, breathable, and designed to be worn over a pair of thin wicking socks. The socks have a Gore-Tex membrane laminated between inner and outer fabric layers. The inner seams are sealed with Gore-Seam tape. The sole and bottom panel are made of a nonstretch Gore-Tex fabric to increase durability and prevent slippage. The upper panels are stretchable Gore-Tex fabric for flexibility and conformity to the foot's shape. A spandex cuff helps the socks stay up. When wearing these socks, watch for skin irritations caused by the inner seams.

TIP: New Life for Old Bags

An alternative to oversocks is to put on a pair of thick socks and then a soft plastic bag over the feet, finally adding a thin outer sock. The inner socks, in the plastic bags, will get damp from body sweat and heat, but will stay reasonably comfortable compared to totally wet feet. The plastic bags that bread or newspapers come in work well, but check them first for leaks by blowing in them and squeezing them lightly while holding them closed.

Seirus Stormsocks rely on closed-cell insulation to provide warmth for winter activities. They are made from four-way stretch neoprene with breathable macroporous technology to prevent moisture buildup while sealing in body heat. These socks have a nylon fabric on either side of the neoprene that allows moisture to pass through. The regular Stormsock has an outer layer of Lycra and an inner membrane of high-technology Weather Shield that stops wind and water, and it is lined with Polartec fleece. The Hyperlite Stormsock reduces bulk by eliminating the fleece lining. Both socks have seams that should be checked for waterproofing.

S O C K   P R O D U C T S

In addition to the sock companies listed below, many shoe and boot companies, and even some insole companies, also offer their own brands of socks.

ACORN FLEECE SOCKS (hiking socks) **www.acornearth.com**

BALEGA INTERNATIONAL (running and trail running socks) **www.balegasports.com**

BAYSIX (running socks) **www.baysixusa.com**

BRIDGEDALE (running and hiking socks) **www.bridgedaleusa.com**

CW-X (compression socks) **www.cw-x.com**

DAHLGREN (hiking socks) **www.dahlgrenfootwear.com**

DARN TOUGH VERMONT (running and hiking socks) **www.darntough.com**

DEFEET (running socks) **www.defeet.com**

DRYMAX SPORTS (running and hiking socks) **www.drymaxsocks.com**

FEETURES (running and hiking socks) **www.feeturesbrand.com**

FOX RIVER (running, hiking, and liner socks) **www.foxsox.com**

INJINJI (running and hiking socks) **www.injinji.com**

LORPEN (running and hiking socks) **www.lorpen.com**

OXYSOCKS (compression socks) **www.oxysox.com**

2XU (compression socks) **www.2xu.com**

For more information about SealSkinz socks and Seirus Stormsocks, see the product listing on the previous page and below.

Try any type of oversocks before a competitive event. You may find that they do not work on your feet. Some athletes roll the tops down when not going through water to ventilate the feet. Oversocks work best when used with a CoolMax or other wicking material sock liner. This further enhances moisture dispersion as well as comfort. Care must be taken when pulling the socks on or off to avoid tearing the inner membrane. A torn membrane will allow water to penetrate at the tear site.

Unless you are wearing the SealSkinz WaterBlocker socks, your oversocks should not be submersed in water over the cuffs. If the cuff is loose fitting, water may get inside. Once water has gone down the leg into the sock, the wicking process slows or stops, depending on the amount of water in the sock. Over time, the body's heat combined with the wicking action of the CoolMax liner may dry the inside of the socks, but this depends on both the amount of water inside the sock and the degree of activity. Roy Pirrung recommends wearing tights over the cuffs to provide a covering seal.

SOCK PRODUCTS CONTINUED

PATAGONIA (hiking socks) **www.patagonia.com**

POINT6 (wool socks) **www.point6.com**

POWERSOX (running socks) **www.powersox.com**

REI SOCKS and **ROCKY GORE-TEX OVERSOCKS** (hiking socks and oversocks) **www.rei.com**

SEALSKINZ SOCKS (oversocks) **www.danalco.com**

SEIRUS STORMSOCKS (oversocks) **www.seirus.com**

SIGVARIS ATHLETIC RECOVERY SOCKS (compression socks) **www.athleticrecoverysocks.com**

SKINS (compression socks) **www.skinsusa.com**

SMARTKNITACTIVE SOCKS (running socks) **www.smartknitactive.com**

SMARTWOOL (running, hiking, and liner socks) **www.smartwool.com**

SOF SOLE (running socks) **www.sofsole.com**

TEKO SOCKS (running and hiking socks) **www.tekosocks.com**

THORLOS (running and hiking socks) **www.thorlo.com**

WIGWAM (running, hiking, and liner socks) **www.wigwam.com**

WRIGHTSOCK (running socks) **www.wrightsock.com**

X-SOCKS (running and hiking socks) **www.x-socks.com**

Going Sockless

In 1973 a running magazine advertised "new, lean, and luxurious—the first sockless athletic shoe." After three years of development, Bare Foot Gear offered the "original sockless shoe" with prime leather inside and out, no staples or nails, no seams or ridges, and no textiles to touch your foot, just unpainted and unsealed leather. Cupping the foot only at the heel and instep, it offered a large space up front for flexion and good air circulation. It claimed that with a drier foot, friction is minimized. Looking at the ad today, we might find humor in the ad's claim: "Most men prefer no socks because of the sheer maleness of the feel."

Some people prefer not to wear socks in their shoes. Matt Mahoney found that for him, the best way to prevent blisters was to train for them. Walking barefoot and sometimes running barefoot on grass, dirt, or sand toughened the skin on his feet. He does not wear socks with shoes but rotates between several brands of shoes to develop calluses at every spot that could rub. Matt found that socks caused his feet to slide around inside his shoes, and he couldn't grip the trail on steep hills. When he finds spots rubbing, he uses tape, petroleum jelly, or a blister pad.

Running in shoes without socks takes time and careful monitoring of your feet to avoid problems. Matt has conditioned his feet by walking a mile barefoot on roads every day. He estimates that he runs 15% of the time barefoot on grass and dirt and the other 85% in shoes without socks. He has strengthened the small muscles and tendons in his feet. The skin on the bottom of his feet has toughened to provide some degree of protection for running barefoot. If trying to go without socks, check your shoes for rough seams or ridges that can cut into your feet. Like Matt, use tape or a lubricant on areas that rub. Matt strongly believes that we need to "learn to run in simple shoes, sandals, or barefoot as people have done for thousands of years before Nike." Barefoot running and hiking is becoming more accepted. See the "Barefoot & Minimalist Footwear" chapter for more on this trend.

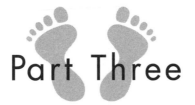

Part Three

Prevention

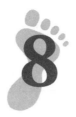

Making Prevention Work

The Sixth Law of Running Injuries:
Treat the cause, not the effect. Because each running injury
has a cause, it follows that the injury can never be cured
until the causative factors are eliminated.

—Tim Noakes, MD, Lore of Running[17]

Tim Noakes's sixth law of running injuries must be heeded—any running injury can be cured only after the cause is found and eliminated. All of us who run, hike, or adventure race at some point have problems with our feet or sustain foot injuries. The prevention chapters are numerous and lengthy because many factors contribute to foot problems and injuries, and for every factor, there is a preventive measure that can reduce or eliminate it. Prevention is the key to saving your feet. Dave Scott, a good friend and ultrarunner, put the foot problem in proper perspective: "When you don't take care of your feet during a long run or race, each step becomes a reminder of your ignorance."

"Be prepared." That's the motto of the Boy Scouts. "Be prepared for what?" someone once asked Robert Baden-Powell, the founder of the Boy Scout movement.

"Why, for any old thing," he answered.

It's very easy to relinquish our responsibility for preparedness and let someone else dictate what we should do. We tend to listen to those whom we look up to and to those who are more experienced. In many ways this is OK, and it is often the way it should be. However, only you can determine what works for your feet.

Knowing your prevention options is important. In the foreword to the first edition of this book, Billy Trolan, an emergency room physician and medical consultant to adventure racing teams, wrote the following:

> The one factor that continues to amaze me is that individuals and
> teams will spend vast amounts of money, time, and thought on training,

equipment, and travel, but little or no preparation on their feet. Too often the result has been that within a few hours to a few days, all that work has been ruined—ruined because the primary mode of transportation has broken down with blisters. This problem is universal with hikers, runners, [or anybody doing] any activity that requires feet. Most of these problems could easily be avoided with some preventive care. Other foot problems could have been taken care of with early treatment, stopping a small problem from becoming a costly one.

The most important factor is knowing what *your* feet need and how to do it before you have to do it. I have patched many feet at ultras and adventure races and have found that most racers have a fairly good knowledge base of what they should be doing. They know it's smart to wear the right kind of socks and to have footwear that fits well. Many have also made foot care kits for their crews. I would guess that about 30–40% are well versed in what their feet need and how to do it. The other 60–70% just wing it. They've read about foot care but somehow it falls lower on the priority list than does training, finding foods they can tolerate, locating the right flashlight for night running, and other choices. So they start their race and manage well for a while—until problems develop.

Ultrarunner Gillian Robinson shares a story from one of her long races that illustrates what all athletes need to learn:

> I sat for a shoe change and foot fix-up. I wasn't exactly sure what to do with my feet. I had taped the balls of my feet and my big toes. The big-toe taping wasn't working out so well. On the left, it had rubbed the next toe to cause a big ugly blister that had to be lanced. On the right, maybe the taping was too tight, because the big toenail was bruised at the base. I put 2nd Skin on the left toe and taped it up with Micropore tape. For the right toe, I just cut off the existing tape and hoped for the best. I sprayed my feet with Desenex to cool them down and dry them out, and then smeared them all over with Hydropel, which is a lubricant. I changed to new socks and different shoes. I felt a lot better. My toes didn't feel perfect, but better.

To have and keep healthy feet, you have to know what works for them in the sports in which you participate. You also have to know what to do when what worked no longer works—in other words, a fallback plan with the equipment to implement it and the knowledge to use it.

Hard-won Lessons

- Learn what lubricant works, but have a container of powder handy.

- Learn what socks work, but have one or two extra pairs of other types.

- Learn how to tape your toes, heels, and every other part of your feet just in case blisters form.

- Learn how to tape like a pro, and then practice taping, and then practice some more. Then start over until your taping is perfect.

- Learn how to lance blisters and patch over them.

- Learn what happens to your feet when you don't change wet socks. Your feet become macerated and feel as though one humongous blister is covering the bottom of each foot.

- Learn that something simple, such as properly trimming and filing your toenails, can prevent toe blisters and even black toenails.

The bottom line is that if you don't consciously learn what works for your feet, you will learn the hard way. Prevention is proactive. Time spent being proactive in preventing problems will pay off in the long run. Taking a proactive approach will mean that you spend less time being reactive to problems when you have neither the time to spare nor readily available materials.

The key to making prevention work is to find what works for you in the environment where you will use it. In other words, try the fix in the context in which it will be used. When you are trying to find what works for you on trails, running on roads will not typically provide the same results as actually running on trails. Walking around town wearing a backpack and your hiking boots is not the same as hiking on a rocky trail with uneven terrain. It may help to break in your boots but will not give the same feeling as a rough rocky trail. I made my own gaiters for trail running after determining that the dirt getting into my shoes was causing hot spots and blisters. Getting out on the trails will help you determine whether your footwear fits and if there are problems to correct. That's being proactive.

Mike Palmer has spent years finding what works for his feet: "This can be one hell of a frustrating process—you may have an overwhelming urge to throw in the towel and take up playing chess instead. One runner will swear on his mother's grave that such and such a thing solved his problem, but his solution won't work at all for you." It cannot be overstressed; you must find what works for your feet. Taking the time to learn what works for your feet is the key to being proactive.

Cathy Sassin knows what her feet need. One of the top adventure racers in the United States, she has trekked across the sands of Utah and South Africa, the volcanoes of Ecuador, and the glaciers of British Columbia and Patagonia. She has bushwhacked through Maine, went spelunking through Borneo, paddled and ridden through New Zealand and Australia, and raced across New England.

On the SealSkinz website, Cathy sums up the method behind her success. See her suggestions below.

Tried-and-true Foot Care

The four keys to winning any extreme sport are having a strong mental attitude, working as a team rather than as an individual, keeping hydrated, and having a great foot care regimen. After every race my team and I are generally the only ones without bloody, blistered feet. Everyone wants to know my secret, so here it is!

■ Spray feet with compound tincture of benzoin spray. This provides a tough protective layer where blisters usually form. Be careful not to apply too much or in the creases of the feet as it will crack and dry the skin.

■ Put a thin layer of Hydropel around the feet over the compound tincture of benzoin. Hydropel is a lubricant that offers both water repellency and lubrication without friction.

■ It is essential to keep feet comfortable and dry, so I put on a pair of liner socks (I recommend Wigwam) followed by a pair of SealSkinz waterproof socks. SealSkinz come in a variety of styles, but I recommend either the insulated socks (for colder conditions), over-the-calf socks, or their WaterBlocker sock with in-cuff seal to keep water out even when feet are submerged!

■ Wear a pair of boots or running shoes that are very lightweight but stable enough to handle rigorous terrain (every ounce counts in racing). When wearing running shoes, choose a lightweight model that allows water to squeeze out as you run.

■ Add a pair of gaiters to further prevent grit, dirt, and small rocks from getting in the boots, which will help prevent unnecessary friction and abrasions.

■ Use a pair of adjustable walking poles (I use Leki poles) to help distribute weight throughout the body every step of the way. Poles are great for balance on the downhills and help prevent feet from taking a pounding.

—Cathy Sassin, globe-trotting adventure racer

Components of Prevention

The one problem with our feet that we experience most often—which drives us crazy, costs us time, and, in some cases, leads to unfulfilled dreams—is blisters. Although the following chapters deal with all aspects of foot care, the prevalent theme is keeping our feet healthy by preventing dreaded blisters.

Blister prevention requires a combination of components: socks, powders, lubricants, skin toughening agent, taping, orthotics, nutrition for the feet, proper hydration, antiperspirants for the feet, gaiters, laces, and frequent sock and shoe changes, among others. You need to start with proper fitting shoes with a quality insole. No matter how well you tape, or how good your socks are, or how good any other component is, if the shoes fit incorrectly, you will have problems. The materials and compounds you apply to your skin (powder, lubricant, or tape) must work together with anything surrounding your feet (the insoles, orthotics, socks,

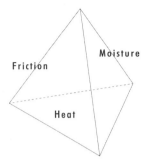

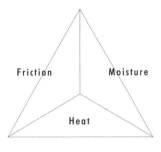

The three causes of blister formation

shoes, gaiters, and even your shoelaces) in order to prevent blisters. Cutting corners on any one of the factors can increase the chances of blisters.

Imagine a triangle with heat, friction, and moisture at its three sides. These three factors combine to make the skin more susceptible to blisters. David Hannaford, DPM, a podiatrist and runner, stresses, "If you eliminate any one of the three factors, you eliminate the blister."

Imagine that this triangle sits on a base that has two levels. Each level of the base is a circle made up of components that can prevent these three conditions from forming. Closest to the triangle is the upper circle of socks, powders, and lubricants—the first line of defense against blisters. Friction, which produces heat, can be reduced by wearing a sock with wicking properties or by using foot powders or lubricants. Moisture can also be reduced by wearing socks with wicking properties and by using powders.

Socks come in either single- or double-layer construction. Some single-layer socks, particularly those without wicking properties, allow friction to develop between the feet and the socks, which in turn can create blisters. Double-layer socks allow the sock layers to move against each other or the two materials to work together, which reduces friction between the feet and the socks.

Powders reduce friction by reducing moisture on the skin that in turn reduces friction between the feet and the socks.

Lubricants create a shield to protect skin that is in contact with skin and socks during motion. This lubricant shield reduces chafing, which in turn reduces friction.

Now, imagine another underlying circle made up of components that play a strong supporting role in prevention—the second level of defense against blisters. This lower circle is made up of skin toughening agents,

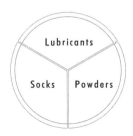

The first level of defense against blisters

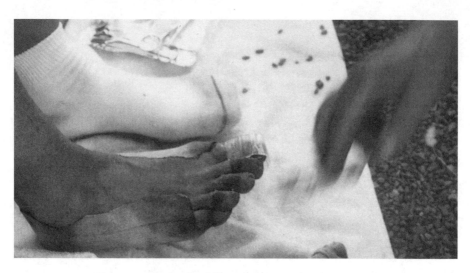

Taping can make the difference between finishing a race
and limping your way through (or dropping out).

taping, orthotics, nutrition for the feet and proper hydration, antiperspirants for the feet, gaiters, lacing, and frequent sock and shoe changes. Each can contribute to the prevention of blisters and other problems. You could argue that these outer components should be identified as major components, and to some extent you may be right. Some components may be more important for your feet than for mine. The trick is to determine what we each need to keep our feet healthy under the stresses of our particular sport.

Skin toughening agents form a coating to protect and toughen the skin. These products also help tape and blister patches adhere better to the skin.

Taping provides a barrier between the skin and socks so friction is reduced. Proper taping adds an extra layer of skin (the tape) to the foot to prevent hot spots and blisters. Taping can also be a treatment if hot spots and blisters develop. An alternative to taping, ENGO Patches go on the inside of your shoe or on your insole. These thin fabric-film composite patches can greatly reduce friction in targeted locations within your footwear by giving a slick, slippery surface to the area of your footwear or insole where friction is a problem. Jelly Toes are silicone gel devices that go over the toes and reduce friction.

Orthotics help maintain the foot in a functionally neutral position so arch and pressure problems are relieved. Small pads for the feet may also help correct foot imbalances and pressure points.

Skin care for the feet includes creams and lotions so dry and callused feet are softened. They result in softer and smoother skin. Proper hydration can help reduce swelling of the feet so the occurrence of hot spots and blisters is reduced.

Antiperspirants for the feet help those with excessively sweaty feet by reducing the moisture that makes the feet more prone to blisters.

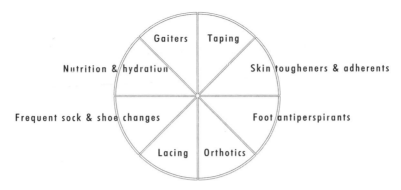

The second level of defense against blisters.

Gaiters provide protection against sand, dirt, rocks, and grit. These irritants cause friction and blisters as shoes and socks become dirty. Shoe and bootlaces often cause friction or pressure problems. Adjusting laces can relieve this friction and pressure and make footwear more comfortable.

Frequent sock changes help keep the feet in good condition. Wet or moist socks can cause problems. Changing the socks also gives opportunity to reapply either powder or lubricant and deal with any hot spots before they become blisters. Sometimes shoes are also changed as they become overly dirty or wet.

Finding the Right Combination

Each runner and hiker needs to find a prevention strategy that works for him or her. One may use a lubricant, another may use Zeasorb powder, and yet another may pretape his feet. They each may use one of many types and styles of socks. There are many combinations.

Ultrarunner Dave Scott claimed his feet are often "as soft as a baby's bottom" after the 100-mile Western States Endurance Run. Dave found that he rarely had foot problems. He trimmed his toenails, used a small amount of petroleum jelly, and regularly changed his shoes and socks. That is what worked for him. At the other extreme is the runner who has the skin falling off his feet from midsoles to heels. One hiker may end a six-day hike having had a few simple foot problems, while another may have suffered with major problems the whole trip—even if they wear the same shoes and socks. Determine what foot problems you normally experience, study this book, and then begin the task of finding what works best for your feet.

Ultrarunner Tim Twietmeyer has won the grueling 100-mile Western States Endurance Run five times while accumulating 23 silver belt buckles for finishes less than 24 hours. Over the past years, in addition to running ultras, he has enjoyed fast packing in the California High Sierra. He has found the differences interesting.

A week before running a 100-mile trail ultra, Tim trims his toenails as short as possible. The morning of the run he coats his feet with lanolin to reduce friction, provide warmth if running in snow or through water, and make his skin more resilient to getting wrinkled. Then he pulls on a pair of Thorlos Ultrathin socks. His strategy is "that the more sock you wear, the more moisture close to the foot. The more moisture, the more blisters and skin problems." He usually wears the same pair of shoes and socks the entire way. Tim acknowledges, "My feet don't usually have problems, and when they do, I'm close enough to the end to gut it out."

Tim has found that fast packing affects his feet differently. When he hiked the John Muir Trail in 1992 (doing 210 miles in five days and ten hours), his feet were trashed more than ever before. His group of five experienced ultrarunners averaged 14 hours per day on the rough trail. Tim remembers, "We covered the ground so fast that my feet swelled and I almost couldn't get my shoes on the last day." He used the same strategy of using lanolin and thin socks. Instead of running shoes, he chose lightweight hiking boots. Foot repair became the group's daily ritual as the 40-mile days took their toll. They realized that "an important strategy for keeping our feet from getting any worse was to get that first piece of duct tape on in just the right spot and make it stick. If we did that, our feet held up pretty well." By the end of the fifth day, the last piece of duct tape had been used on their feet. Tim's cardinal rule for fast packing is to "keep your feet dry." That can be hard to do when fighting afternoon thunderstorms, but when your feet are wet too long, it's only a matter of time before they blister. Whether running ultras or fast packing, Tim knows the importance of keeping his feet healthy, and he has experimented to find what works well for him.

We need to understand the importance of other elements that contribute to prevention. Proper strength training and conditioning will help make the foot and ankle stronger and more resistant to sprains and strains. Good care of the skin will help prevent calluses. Quality insoles and orthotics can help prevent or relieve the problems of plantar fasciitis, Achilles tendinitis, heel pain, metatarsalgia, Morton's neuroma, Morton's foot, sesamoiditis, corns, and bunions. Good-fitting footwear will help prevent problems with toenails, arches, and blisters. In short, everything you put on or around your foot becomes related to how well your foot functions.

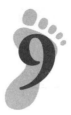

Compounds for the Feet

There are four compounds you can put on your feet. Some athletes will use only one, while others may use two, or at times, all four. The most commonly applied compound is lubricant, typically used to make the feet slippery to reduce friction. Powder is used more and more frequently as athletes learn how dry feet are subject to far less friction. Skin toughening agents and tape adherents are used by many involved in ultras and extreme sports. A small percentage of athletes use an antiperspirant to control excessive sweating of their feet.

One of the best ways of preventing hot spots and blisters is by using either powder or a lubricant on your feet. Both work well, but one may be better suited to your feet. If you have been using a lubricant on your feet and still get blisters, first try one of the newer, state-of-the-art lubricants. Lubricants will soften the skin and for some, this makes the feet more sensitive to the stresses of walking, running, hiking, and so on. In some cases, you might even feel the weave of the socks as an irritant. The softened skin can lead to painful feet and, in some cases, even blisters. If the blisters continue, try powder. Some skin will respond better to being dry, and powders that prevent moisture buildup on the skin are a good choice. For other athletes, lubricants are a better choice. If you have continued problems, try several of each.

As socks become more technical at transporting moisture away from the skin, athletes need to be aware of sock makers' advice. As an example, sock company Drymax recommends not using powders or lubricants with their socks because of the tendency to clog the Drymax fibers, inhibiting their ability to properly move moisture away from the skin, and not to put their socks in the dryer.

Powders

Athletes who find their feet become too soft and tender with lubricants can use powders as an alternative foot treatment. For these athletes, powder works better or as well as a lubricant.

P O W D E R   P R O D U C T S

ASICS CHAFE FREE POWDER is an antifriction powder made with Aceba, a dry lubricant. **www.asicsamerica.com**

BLISTERSHIELD POWDER made by TwoToms helps prevent hot spots, blisters, and calluses. Containing micronized wax and cornstarch, the very slick powder reduces friction and heat buildup. BlisterShield repels water by allowing vapor (perspiration) to pass through it, and it keeps moisture off your skin. To use the powder, just shake one teaspoon in each sock, distributing it evenly without bunching all of it at your toes. Add some extra in the heel after you put your sock on. **www.2toms.com**

BODYGLIDE LIQUIFIED POWDER is an advanced cream that transforms into a dry and protective skin lubricant. **www.bodyglide.com**

BROMI-TALC is made by Gordon Laboratories as a triple-action foot powder containing potassium alum, an astringent that retards perspiration, and bentonite, an absorption agent that absorbs 18 times its own weight in moisture. Bromi-Talc Plus powder contains additional properties to control excessive foot odor. Both powders are available by special order through your local drugstore, pharmacy, or podiatrist.

GOLD BOND is a medicated body powder that contains active ingredient zinc oxide as a skin protector and menthol to cool and relieve itching. Use the extra-strength powder for maximum benefits in absorbing excessive moisture. Gold Bond can be found in your local drugstore and pharmacy. **www. goldbond.com**

ODOR-EATERS FOOT POWDER is 25 times more absorbent than talc and also destroys foot odor. It can be found in most drugstores and pharmacies. **www. odor-eaters.com**

ZEASORB is a super-absorbent powder, which absorbs six times its weight in moisture—four times more than plain talcum powder. Zeasorb contains talc, a highly absorbent polymer-carbohydrate acrylic copolymer, and microporous cellulose. This powder is very efficient and works without caking. The talc provides softness and lubrication to reduce friction and heat buildup. Zeasorb-AF (which contains 2% miconazole nitrate) provides broad antifungal therapy and moisture control. Zeasorb-AF Lotion/Powder is a unique product for patients who need an antifungal lotion. Zeasorb is made by Stiefel Laboratories and can be found in your local drugstore or pharmacy. **www.stiefel.com**

There are powders and then there are powders. Cornstarch and talcum powder have been used for years as foot powders, but times and powders have changed. Having tried a super-absorbent powder, I would never again use a plain powder. Powders can be effective in reducing moisture on the feet, which, in turn, reduces friction and prevents blisters. Their effectiveness depends on their ability to absorb moisture while not caking into clumps, which can cause skin irritations and blisters. When using powders, remember to reapply the powder at regular intervals or after the feet have been exposed to water. If you have problems with athlete's foot or other skin problems, use an antifungal medicated powder.

After lightly powdering your feet, massage the powder between the toes. Then roll your socks on to the level of the heel and put some powder in the socks. Then squeeze off the top of the sock and shake your foot and repeatedly shake the sock until powder comes through the sock.

Several new powders are worth trying: BodyGlide's Liquified Powder is a technically advanced cream that transforms into a protective, powdery skin lubricant. Asics's Chafe Free powder is made with Aceba, a dry-skin lubricant.

Lubricants

As with powders, there are lubricants and then there are lubricants. Two of the old-time tried-and-true lubricants are lanolin and petroleum jelly. However, these are greasy, can cake up on socks, and tend to attract grit particles that can become an irritant and themselves cause blisters. Paul Romero, of adventure racing's Team SOLE, prefers good old-fashioned Vaseline. He likes it because it is easy to apply and good for other parts of the body. He says, "I've never been convinced the newer stuff works any better, and the other stuff is a hell of a lot more expensive and harder to find."

Technology has led to formulas such as BodyGlide, BlisterShield Roll-on, Asics's Chafe Free Endurance Gel, and Sportslick. Many of these are petroleum-free, waterproof, nonsticky, and hypoallergenic. Many athletes use Bag Balm or Udder Balm, while athletes whose feet are exposed to extended periods of moisture often prefer Hydropel or Friction Zone, advanced skin protectants that are water repelling and sweat resistant. Other athletes make their own special formulas.

Ultrarunner Robert Boeder used Andrew Lovy's formula (see next page) on his feet in 1994 when he completed the Grand Slam of trail ultrarunning, running four 100-mile runs in 14 weeks. Robert comments, "The idea is that these lotional charms will have the desired magical effect and blisters will not arise from my feet during the race."[18] This formula worked well for him. Since that time he switched to Bag Balm and then back to petroleum jelly, mainly because of its availability. Ultrarunner Jim Benike found success using Udder Balm on his feet and then wearing socks to bed. He used Udder Balm more as a skin softener and conditioner than as a lubricant. Udder creams may go by different names (for example, Bag Balm, Udder Balm, Dr. Naylor's Udder Balm, and Aunt Irma's Udder Balm).

Newer lubricants are being developed that utilize state-of-the-art ingredients to make them more effective. Hydropel contains 30% silicone and works effectively to repel moisture away from the skin. Michael Johnson, of **www.argear.com** who is also an adventure racer, reports on his website, "Hydropel seems to also protect your feet from water. I don't get soft, waterlogged skin on my feet when using it." Using Hydropel or Maximum Strength Desitin can help prevent macerated skin so common to feet wet for long periods of time. The newest lubricants that caught my attention are Blister Bomber and Trislide. Blister Bomber is applied via a dauber, leaving a coating that is silky smooth and virtually invisible. Trislide is applied in a continuous spray, leaving a silky emollient coating that is waterproof.

LUBRICANT PRODUCTS

ANDREW LOVY'S FORMULA was developed over several years and described in an article "New Blister Formula Revealed! Free!"[20] It helped him solve his blister and friction problems. Take vitamin A and D ointment, petroleum jelly, and Desitin ointment, and mix together equal amounts. To this add vitamin E cream and aloe vera cream (the thickness can be varied by the amount of these two ingredients). The result is a salve. For a thinner mixture, use vitamin E and aloe vera ointments instead of the creams. Andrew recommends applying a thin layer the evening before your run to clean skin where friction occurs. In the morning, before you run, apply a more generous amount to friction areas. Add more to problem areas as necessary during the run. Shop around to find the ingredients in sizes appropriate for the total amount you want to mix.

AQUAPHOR HEALING OINTMENT is a petroleum-based ointment that can be used as a lubricant on the feet and other body parts. As a healing ointment, Aquaphor can be used after events to return your feet to like-new condition. Available in a 1.75-ounce tube, it can be found in most drugstores. **www.aquaphor healing.com**

ASICS CHAFE FREE ENDURANCE GEL is an antifriction gel lubricant that is waterproof and nongreasy. It is made with Aceba, a dry lubricant, and it contains vitamin E and aloe. Once applied, it instantly dries to form a barrier against chafing. **www.asicsamerica.com**

AVON SILICONE GLOVE is a silicone cream for hands, but it works equally well on feet. Its nongreasy and nonsticky formula lubricates and softens while protecting against dryness and irritants. It is available in a handy 1.5-ounce tube. **www.avon.com**

BAG BALM comes in a green tin that has become familiar to many athletes. Bag Balm is made and advertised for use on cow udders, but it has found acceptance in sports circles. Consisting of a combination of lanolin, petrolatum,

Studies have shown that lubricants may initially reduce friction, but over long periods of time they may actually increase it. After one hour the friction levels returned to their baseline factor, and after three hours the friction levels were 35% above the baseline. As the lubricants are absorbed into the skin and into the socks, friction returns and increases.[19] Based on this study, we should learn to reapply lubricants at frequent intervals.

Use lubricants on your feet, hands, underarms, inner thighs, and nipples—anywhere you chafe. The important thing to remember about lubricants is to clean off the old coating before applying the new one. This is especially true during trail runs and hiking, when dust and dirt buildup can foul the lubricant with grit. Wipe off the old stuff with a cleansing towelette or an alcohol wipe.

Many athletes apply a lubricant the night before a long event. After applying the lube of your choice, put on socks. In the morning, your skin is soft and supple. With Hydropel or Desitin, this method will help the skin resist pruning

LUBRICANT PRODUCTS

8-hydroxy, and quinoline sulfate, it has proven to have healing properties. It can be used on cracked, callused, or sore skin, or simply as a lubricant for your feet or other body areas. Available in 1- or 10-ounce tins, it is usually found in drugstores, pet and feed stores, tack shops, and hardware stores. **www.bagbalm.com**

BLISTER BOMBER is a nonoily lubricant that is not affected by sweat or wetness. It leaves an almost invisible silky smooth coating on the skin. Available in a small 0.65-ounce dauber for easy application. **www.blisterbomber.com**

BODYGLIDE AND FOOTGLIDE FOOT FORMULA are petroleum-free lubricants that protect against friction and skin irritation. These products come in a glide-on applicator similar to a deodorant stick. These are hypoallergenic, waterproof, nonsticky, nongreasy (so they will not clog pores), and long lasting. **BODYGLIDE LIQUIFIED POWDER** is an advanced cream that transforms into a dry and protective skin lubricant. **www.bodyglide.com**

BRAVE SOLDIER'S FRICTION ZONE creates a water- and sweat-resistant shield that even under grueling conditions delivers long-lasting skin protection and superior anti-chafing properties. Its occlusive silicone/botanical barrier protects and conditions skin for hours while the antibacterial formula helps prevent minor skin irritations. **www.bravesoldier.com**

CHRIS KOCH'S SECRET FORMULA is made by an adventure racer. He suggests mixing a container of petroleum jelly, a tube of antibacterial ointment, and a tube of antifungal cream in a double boiler. Blend the ingredients and put the mixture in a small plastic jar, squeeze tube, or similar container. Chris has used this formula during multiday adventure races with good success. He usually uses it with a thin liner sock and a heavier outer sock.

---

when exposed to moisture. A clean way to coat your feet is to put a large amount of your lube into a large zip-top bag, then put one foot at a time into the bag, and massaging the lube onto the foot from outside the bag.

As always, try any new product before using it in a competitive event or taking it on a long hike. It is foolhardy to buy something and count on it in competition or on a six-day hike without trying it first. It may not work for you. Try any lubricant on a small patch of skin to be sure you are not allergic to the ingredients.

Skin Toughening Agents & Tape Adherents

Some athletes toughen the skin of their feet to prevent blisters. Often athletes think that toughened skin or calluses will always prevent blisters. For some it does. Others have found themselves with blisters under the calluses or toughened skin. These blisters are very difficult to treat. You still must use other blister prevention products such as moisture-wicking socks, lubricants, or powders.

LUBRICANT PRODUCTS CONTINUED

DESITIN MAXIMUM STRENGTH ORIGINAL PASTE has the highest level of zinc oxide available—40%—to help seal out wetness. It can be found in most drugstores or pharmacies.

HYDROPEL SPORTS OINTMENT is a maximum-strength skin protectant and lubricant. It is made with 30% silicone, petrolatum, dimethicone, and aluminum starch octonylsuccinate. Used by many adventure racers, it repels moisture away from the skin, helping to prevent blisters. It excels at protecting against friction and can be used anywhere on the body, and it is also rated effective as a protectant against poison ivy and poison oak. Hydropel is sold through many adventure-racing websites and is available in a 2-ounce tube. Available through **www.zombierunner.com.**

LANOLIN CREAM contains lanolin hydrous, a natural topical skin emollient that lubricates, protects, and sooths. It can be found in most drugstores or pharmacies.

SKIN LUBE is a lubricating ointment with a high melting point, which gives it longer-lasting protection against blisters and chafing than petroleum jelly. Its main ingredients are petrolatum, zinc stearate, and silicone. Colorless and nonstaining, it can be used on any friction-prone area of the body. It can be found in sporting-goods stores. **www.cramersportsmed.com**

SPORTSHIELD adds a smooth, thin, invisible coating to the skin that will not rub off. This coating eliminates or greatly minimizes the friction that causes blisters, chafing, and irritation. A silicone-based product, it is nonstaining, nontoxic, and nongreasy, and it can be used daily. Use it anywhere you chafe. Available in roll-on and towelettes. **www.2toms.com**

If you wish to try the skin-toughening approach, begin by spending time walking barefoot on various surfaces. Sandals, worn without socks, can build calluses, but be careful that the calluses do not become too thick or rough. As the skin is irritated through exposure to rough surfaces, it thickens and calluses develop. Remember to keep calluses and roughened skin surfaces smooth by using creams, a pumice stone, or a foot file (see "Skin Care" on page 162 and "Skin Disorders" on page 326).

When I was in Chile in 2004, I met a runner who used a unique and clever way to toughen his feet for the dry desert. For months before going to Chile, he filled a large tub with rice and walked in place. The coarseness of the rice against his moving feet helped to prepare his skin for the seven days and 150 miles of the Racing the Planet's Atacama Crossing. Give it a try—you have nothing to lose except a few bags of rice.

Tom Gets Tough—Why Shouldn't You?

Tom Crawford's Tea & Betadine Skin Toughener was developed by an ultrarunner who has completed numerous ultras, including the challenging Death Valley to Mount Whitney, both one-way and as an out-and-back

SPORTSLICK, created by a sports physician, is a multipurpose lubricant made for athletes. The gel is easily applied to the toes, feet, inner thighs, underarms, nipples, and lips. SportSlick prevents blisters and chafing with antifriction polymers, silicone, and petrolatum that create a silky feel. It also enriches the skin with vitamin E and C, soybean oil, the antibacterial agent Triclosan, and the antifungal agent Tolnaftate (1%). SportSlick is available in two sizes. **www.sportslick.com**

SPORTWAX provides relief from friction and skin irritation. It is made with a natural beeswax-based formula, and it is hypoallergenic and waterproof. Available in a twist-up stick in two sizes. **www.sportwax.com**

TRISLIDE was developed for triathletes. It is a antifriction/anti-chafing continuous spray skin lubricant. It sprays on evenly and leaves a silky feeling that allows skin to breathe. Waterproof and sweatproof, it works on all areas of the body, including feet. Trislide is available in a 4-ounce canister. **www.trislide.com**

UDDER BALM has a lemon fragrance, is nongreasy, and is quickly absorbed by the skin. Similar to Bag Balm, Udder Balm was first made for cow udders. With ingredients including lanolin, aloe vera gel, and vitamins A, D, and E, this cream is ideal for relief from rough and cracked skin, and also for corns, cracked cuticles, and sunburn. Udder Balm is available in 4-ounce tubes and a 1-pound jar. **www.udderbalm.com**

VASELINE is available in two formulas. The old-time standard is 100% pure petroleum jelly; the other is Creamy Vaseline with Vitamin E. Vaseline is available in most drugstores. **www.vaseline.com**

run. Tom's method begins with mixing ten tea bags and 1 cup of Betadine into a half gallon of water. For one week, dip your feet 20 times over the course of a day, letting them air-dry between dips. The second week, add 1 cup of salt to the water, tea, and Betadine mixture. Then for one week, soak your feet for 20 minutes at a time, several times daily. Betadine can be found in drugstores and medical supply stores.

Richard Benyo recalled how he used Tom's method to prepare his feet for the Death Valley 300. "Each night I'd pour the solution into a plastic foot bath and keep my soles and toes in the solution for 15 minutes; then I'd alternately raise one foot out of the brew for three minutes, allowing it to dry, then lower it and bring the other foot out. I'd do that for a half hour. Then I'd let them dry and I'd go to bed with orange soles. When I showered the next morning, it would wash off. But little by little, it made my feet more resistant to blisters."[21] Even with this preparation, Richard sometimes found his feet susceptible to blisters.

You can use several products to toughen your skin or choose the tea and Betadine soak (mentioned on the previoous page). After applying the last coat of the toughening agent, apply a light coating of either one of the lubricants or powders to cut the stickiness. Skipping this step may cause your socks to stick to your feet.

You can use several of the products as tape adherents to help your choice of tape or moleskin better stick to your feet. Without the adherent, most tapes and blister products will begin to peel off after an hour or two. After applying a blister patch or taping your feet, apply a light coating of powder over any dry sprayed area to counteract the adhesive.

Allow the compound tincture of benzoin or any sticky tape adherent to dry before applying any tape. Generally one to two minutes' drying time is sufficient. Wet benzoin is very sticky and slippery. Tape and blister-care products can move around on the foot and fold over on themselves, creating problems. Socks can become stuck to your feet and toes can stick together if you do not allow the benzoin time to dry.

Antiperspirants for the Feet

According to the American Podiatric Medical Association, our feet have approximately 250,000 sweat glands and produce as much as a pint of moisture each day. An

SKIN TOUGHENING AGENTS & ADHERENTS

COMPOUND TINCTURE OF BENZOIN is available in liquid, swabs, or squeeze vials. Commonly used as a tape or bandage adherent, it is sometimes used as a skin toughener. After applying the tincture, let it dry for about two minutes before applying tape. Compound tincture of benzoin leaves an orange-brownish color on the skin. Avoid getting the tincture into any cuts, abrasions, or open blisters—it can burn! Usually available in liquid form at drugstores, pharmacies, or medical supply stores. Order swabs or ampules from **www.zombie runner.com** or **www.medco-athletics.com.**

CRAMER TUF-SKIN has been used for years by athletic trainers as a taping base. It is ideal for pretaping and skin toughening. Its main ingredients are isopropyl alcohol, isobutane, resin, and benzoin. **www.cramersportsmed.com**

MASTISOL is a clear, nonirritating liquid adhesive that is not water soluble and is routinely used in hospitals for dressing wounds. It is advertised as stickier than compound tincture of benzoin. Order from **www.zombierunner.com** or **www.medco-athletics.com.**

MUELLER TUFFNER CLEAR SPRAY is used as a base for athletic taping, but it is also identified as a skin toughener. Its main ingredients are acetone, 1,1,1-trichloroethanem isopropanol, resin, and compound tincture of benzoin. Look for this product at sporting good stores. **www.muellersportsmed.com**

increase in body temperature will increase the perspiration level. Some people experience excessive perspiration of their feet. Hyperhidrosis is a medical term meaning excessive moisture. This moisture often increases the chance of blisters. Individuals with this condition may find that applying an antiperspirant to the feet reduces the amount of perspiration, which in turn prevents the formation of blisters. David Zuniga is one runner who has found that the use of an antiperspirant has helped his feet. He started using an antiperspirant on the recommendation of his podiatrist and finds his feet stay "dry as a bone."

Aside from antiperspirants, problems associated with excessive moisture can often be reduced by wearing moisture-wicking socks, changing socks frequently, and changing shoes if the moisture is particularly excessive.

Certain Dri and Gillette Clinical Strength antiperspirants offer perspiration control that will also work on feet that sweat excessively. If something stronger is needed, ask your physician for a more powerful solution, such as Drysol Solution, available by prescription.

To save your shoes from faster than normal deterioration from the excess moisture, here a few tips. Stuff newspaper into your wet shoes to dry them out overnight. Sprinkle a bit of baking soda powder into each shoe after using them. Remove the insoles and shake the shoes to get the powder evenly distributed. The baking soda will also help control the harsh smells that are common with

SKIN TOUGHENING AGENTS & ADHERENTS

NEW-SKIN LIQUID BANDAGE comes in either an antiseptic spray or liquid that is useful as a skin protectant or toughener to prevent hot spots and blisters. It dries rapidly to form a tough protective cover that is antiseptic, flexible, and waterproof, while letting the skin breathe. Clean the skin, spray or coat, and let dry. A second coating is recommended for additional protection. Keep toes bent when applying and drying. There is no residue or stickiness. Do not apply to infected or draining sites. It is strong-smelling stuff, so use with good ventilation and avoid breathing too deeply. Its main ingredients are pyroxylin solution, acetone ACS, oil of cloves, and 8-hydroxyquinoline. Look for New-Skin at drugstores or online. **www.medtechinc.com**

RUBBING ALCOHOL was the preference of renowned walker Colin Fletcher as a skin toughener.[22] Use it on your toes, soles, and heels several times daily. He recommended almost hourly applications of rubbing alcohol followed by foot powder while walking and hiking with sore feet. Rubbing alcohol is available in drugstores.

TUF-FOOT is made from nature's healing balsams and other ingredients. Dr. Andrew Bonn created this unique and original compound in 1935. Made exclusively for feet, either human or animal, Tuf-Foot is guaranteed to toughen soft, tender, or sore feet by working on the tissues. This protects against bruises, blisters, and foot soreness. Recommended use is daily until feet are in good condition and then twice weekly. **www.tuffoot.com**

FOOT ANTIPERSPIRANT PRODUCTS

ANTIPERSPIRANTS that can work on your feet are available in drugstores. Check the shelves at your local store and try one or two. Certain Dri Feet, Gillette Clinical Strength Antiperspirant, and Ban Roll-On are all worth trying. Drysol Solution is a prescription-strength antiperspirant that is applied daily and, after a couple days, virtually eliminates all perspiration.

ASICS CHAFE FREE POWDER is an antifriction powder made with Aceba, a dry lubricant. **www.asicsamerica.com**

BROMI-LOTION is a unique antiperspirant formulated as a soothing lotion, rather than as a spray or roll-on. Made by Gordon Laboratories, it is available only by special order through your local drugstore, pharmacy, or podiatrist.

BROMI-TALC PLUS is an antiperspirant powder from Gordon Laboratories containing a deodorizing powder, sodium potassium, alumino silicate, bentonite, and talc to eliminate odor instantly and help reduce sweating of the feet. *See "Powder Products," page 118.*

CERTAIN DRI FEET is available in either Moisture Control Pads or Microsponge Powder with 12% aluminum chloride, the active ingredient used in prescription antiperspirants. Because Certain Dri is water-based (instead of alcohol-based, like its prescription competitors), it is available without a doctor's prescription at drugstores nationwide. **www.certaindri.com**

DRYSOL SOLUTION is made with 20% aluminum chloride hexahydrate, a strong antiperspirant for excessive perspiration. Available through a prescription from your doctor.

heavy sweating inside shoes. Rotate between two pairs of shoes to give them a chance to dry out. Use one of the odor control products: Penguin's Fresh Twist Shoe Deodorizers and Sneaker & Shoe Deodorizer, and Sof Sole's Odor Control Peppermint Mist.

Blisters & Antiperspirants

Ultrarunner Mike Palmer has worked at resolving blister problems related to sweaty feet. He wears sandals as much as he can to keep his feet dry during the day. A couple of weeks before an ultra of 50 miles or more, he uses alcohol at night to dry his feet. He has also found coating his feet with compound tincture of benzoin dries the skin and provides a protective coating. In the month before a 100-mile run, if the weather allows, he tries to frequently walk about a mile barefoot in an attempt to further toughen the skin. Then before the run he uses an absorbent foot powder and puts dispensers of this powder in his drop bags for every point where he will make a sock change. Mike also recommends frequent sock changes during long races. Even though this is time-consuming, it's better than trying to run on hot spots and blistered feet. For Mike, the moisture promotes blistering. Since using benzoin, the

FOOT ANTIPERSPIRANT PRODUCTS

DRYZ INSOLES help the feet stay dryer and cooler while eliminating odor. *See "Insole Products," pages 72–73.*

FOOT SOLUTION by Onox is a spray solution made to control excessive moisture and foot odor. A combination of mineral salts decreases excessive sweat and foot odor symptoms. The spray also helps reduce blistering and itching while repelling athlete's foot fungus. Ingredients include zinc chloride, deionized water, sodium chloride, sodium nitrate, boric acid, and sodium silco-fluoride. Be aware that the salt solution will sting if you have cuts or breaks in your skin. Foot Solution can be ordered through FootSmart. **www.footsmart.com**

GOLD BOND is a medicated body powder. Use the extra-strength powder for maximum benefits in absorbing excessive moisture. *See "Powder Products," page 118.*

HAND SENSE is a protective cream that bonds with the skin to create a soft shield that prevents irritations and rashes and reduces perspiration. **www.hand sense.com**

ODOR-EATERS FOOT POWDER is 25 times more absorbent than talc and also destroys foot odor. It can be found in most drugstores and pharmacies. **www. odor-eaters.com**

ZEASORB is a super absorbent powder, absorbing six times its weight in moisture and four time more than plain talcum powder. *See "Powder Products," page 118.*

maceration (the whitish, flaky condition of moist skin) has been eliminated and blistering is not so frequent or extensive.

In an interesting study, cadets attending the U.S. Military Academy were separated into two groups that used either an antiperspirant or placebo preparation. Each group was asked to apply their preparation for five consecutive nights before completing a 21K hike. After the hike, only 21% of the cadets who reported using the antiperspirant preparation for at least three nights before the hike were diagnosed with foot blisters. The placebo group reported a 48% incidence of foot blisters. Joseph Knapik, ScD, the lead author of the study that appeared in the August 1998 issue of the *Journal of the American Academy of Dermatology* reported, "Blisters are usually minor problems, but they can cause great discomfort for the patient. Typically they only require simple first aid and a short period of limited activity. It is possible, however, for them to lead to more serious problems such as local or systemic infections."

Researchers theorized that reduced sweating might reduce friction and consequently lower the occurrence of blisters. The cadets applied the preparation to completely dry feet, up the ankle to the top of the boot line. Before the hike, each cadet was examined for existing foot conditions. Immediately after the hike, the feet of each cadet were inspected for blisters using the same criteria as the prehike examination. Researchers found that sweat reduction was a key mechanism for the reduction of blisters.

While the antiperspirant was found to be very effective in reducing blisters, some side effects did occur. "Itching and rashes occurred in 57% of the antiperspirant group, but only 6% of the placebo group," Dr. Knapik noted. "This suggests that a large portion of the population may have problems with the antiperspirant used in the study. However, reducing the amount of the active compound or applying the antiperspirant every other night, rather than every night as the cadets did, may reduce the irritation."

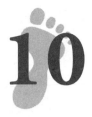

Taping for Blisters

If your feet are prone to blistering, taping may be a lifesaver. After 12 hours of a 72-hour run, my Vaseline-coated feet were almost too sore to run on, and I had a blister between two toes. Nancy Crawford, an experienced running friend, taught me how to prepare my feet for taping and use duct tape to both fix the blister and tape the tender balls of my feet, which would likely blister in the hours ahead. I completed the next 60 hours without a foot problem!

While you may consider taping an extreme, consider the benefits of taping if you are highly susceptible to blisters. You can tape before your event as a proactive preventive measure or in a reactive mode after hot spots or blisters develop. Tape can be applied to more than feet. Rich Lewis finds that applying duct tape to his socks over where he typically develops hot spots or blisters, particularly in new shoes, is a good prevention measure. Others use duct tape inside their shoes or boots to cover irritating seams in their footwear.

Ultrarunner Gillian Robinson usually tapes her big toes because the skin underneath the toe almost always rubs. For a long ultra (100 miles) she tapes more extensively—all of her toes, the balls of her feet, and the arches. She typically does not have heel trouble. Don Lundell usually follows a specific regiment for short ultras: taping the places where he gets blisters (left foot: heel and inside of the foot behind the big toe). When he pretapes, he prefers using Elastikon and Micropore tapes.

Keep in mind that the overall goal of taping is prevention. While taping is a great skill to learn, you need to be sure the shoes you wear are the best fit possible for your feet. With shoes that fit well, your taping needs will hopefully be minimal.

I recommend that runners first train in the conditions for the race intended. Once a runner has trained in this environment, it becomes evident what areas of the feet are prone to problems and they can then be pretaped. Just as training for the distance is vitally important, so is trying the technique of taping in training prior to the race.

Taping is useful for pre-run preparation as well as for fixing newly developed problem spots. If you typically blister on the balls of your feet, consider taping

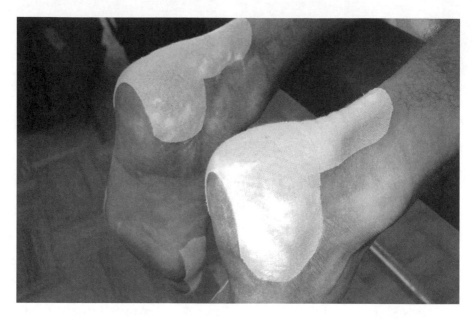

Preventive taping over the Achilles tendon, heel, and side of the foot

before the run when you have the time to do it right rather than at an aid station when you need every minute of time. Practice taping to learn how best to apply the tape to meet your particular needs. Determine how much time is needed to do a complete application. If you are going to have crew support for an event, teach them how to do the taping. It is usually easier to tape the night before an event than wait until the morning when time is rushed and you may do a hurried job.

If you are bothered by blisters and have found that powders and/or lubricants do not work, try the different tapes to find a tape and taping method that works for you. In the chapter on foot care kits (page 340), you will find a list of taping materials to carry during your runs and hikes.

Beginning on page 135 are three methods of taping the feet. The first, developed by Badwater Blister Queen Denise Jones, uses a combination of Kinesio Tex and Hypafix tapes. It is the method I use. The second method, devised by Suzi Cope, uses Johnson & Johnson Elastikon tape. The third uses duct tape. Following a description of each of these methods are descriptions of how to tape different parts of the feet. Remember, any tape that moves or shifts is worse than no tape at all.

Tapes

There are many types of tape available to try. Duct tape was the standard for years, but Kinesio Tex, Leukotape, and Micropore have become popular with ultrarunners and adventure racers. Elastikon, Hypafix, EnduraSports, and EnduraFix tapes can be used as well. Athletic white tape is not well suited for taping feet because of its lack of quality adhesive. While you might find other tapes, the ones below are the most commonly used and have withstood the test of time. They can be found at or ordered through most medical supply stores or ordered online.

Types of Tape

The following tapes are available through drugstores unless otherwise noted.

DUCT TAPE is a 2-inch-wide, very sticky silver tape with a fabric core that has excellent adhesive qualities. It does not breathe but is very strong and tough. Buy high-quality duct tape, which is available at any hardware store.

ELASTIKON from Johnson & Johnson Medical Inc. is a medium-thickness, stretchy, breathable tape that comes in 1-, 2-, 3-, and 4-inch widths. It is thicker than most tapes and requires an edging tape such as Micropore. It has excellent adhesive qualities but leaves serious tape residue when removed. Because of its rough surface, it is not recommended for toes, and on tender feet, the weave can be felt. It does not hold up well in extreme heat. Available at **www.zombierunner.com.**

ENDURAFIX is a 2-inch, thin, soft, and breathable tape, with a removable backing, that provides extra comfort and protection especially to sensitive skin. It works well on toes, over hot spots, on heels, and for anchoring tape between the toes. It is similar to Hypafix. **www.optp.com**

ENDURASPORTS tape is breathable and has a specially formulated zinc oxide heat-sensitive adhesive that is triggered to ensure secure adhesion—even with perspiration, water, or cold weather. This 1.5-inch tape is strong and similar to Leukotape, working well on the balls of the feet and heels. **www.optp.com**

HYPAFIX is a 2-inch, thin, woven, soft, and breathable tape with a removable backing. Works well on toes and between toes and around the heels. It is good for quick patching jobs and for anchoring tape between toes. Available at **www.zombierunner.com.**

KINESIO TEX tape is a ribbed tape that stretches longitudinally and has a paper backing that is removed when applying. Designed for muscle taping, it comes in 2-, 3-, and 4-inch widths and in a variety of colors. This tape is very smooth, soft, breathable, and water resistant. It can stay on for three to four days and leaves no tape residue when removed. **www.kinesiotex-tape.com**

LEUKOTAPE P is a breathable tape in one width, 1.5 inch. It is strong and very sticky—a good choice as an alternative to duct tape. It has a very strong adhesive. It works well on the bottom of the feet and heels. Available online.

MICROPORE is a soft paper tape made by 3M that comes in 0.5-inch and 1-inch widths. It's often used for toes. Available at **www.zombierunner.com.**

OTHER TAPES include two tapes similar to Kinesio Tex, including **KTTAPE** from **www.kttape.com** and **ROCKTAPE** from **www.rocktape.com**; **RELIAMED ELASTIC TAPE,** similar to Elastikon, from **www.zombierunner.com**; and **MEDIPORE** and **MICROFOAM** tapes available online. While there are many types of tapes, the ones mentioned individually above have stood the test of time.

The best tape depends on what your objective is. If you want to save money, duct tape is cheap. But duct tape does not mold well around the curves of heels, sides of the feet, and toes. Elastikon has been around for years and is used by many athletes because of its stickiness. But it is on the thick side and has a definite weave that can bother tender feet. On the roll it sticks to itself and has no backing. In extreme heat, this makes its adhesive qualities less effective. Leukotape and EnduraSports tape are also sticky but come in only one width, don't shape well to the curves of the feet, and simply have not caught on as well as other tapes. Hypafix and EnduraFix are thin and are good on and between toes. Micropore's use is limited to toes. That leaves Kinesio Tex.

Kinesio Tex tape is my tape of choice for 90% of my taping jobs. The other 10% is done with Hypafix between toes. I have become a proponent of the "less is better" theory. Kinesio Tex is thin, easily applied, and sticks exceptionally well. The thicker the tape, the more it is felt. If it doesn't lay smooth, it can be uncomfortable. If you add 2nd Skin or any other patch under a thick tape, you stand the chance of it being uncomfortable. This can change the runner's gait, potentially leading to other problems.

Kinesio Tex is made with an elastic polymer and cotton fabric, is very thin and very porous, and has a heat-activated medical-grade acrylic adhesive, which bonds with the skin. The tape comes in 1-, 2-, and 3-inch widths and in a variety of colors. It is commonly used in physical therapy. Because it has a paper backing, pieces can be measured and precut. It is best applied to clean, oil-free, dry skin, preferably an hour before being exposed to moisture. The more body heat in the taped area, the faster the bonding.

Denise Jones says of Kinesio Tex, "This tape has superior sticking powder, breathability, and stretch." Here are her reasons, including a couple of tips:

- Kinesio Tex has a paper backing, which is peeled off before applying and prevents it from sticking to itself in extreme heat.

- It's much easier to work with.

- The tape is latex free.

- It has a much smoother texture and is far easier to apply.

- It's very sticky, has a nice 30–40% longitudinal stretch, and is resilient.

- It can be used on the toes, unlike Elastikon, which is too abrasive for toes and may blister the toe next to it.

■ On the larger areas of the foot, seal it around the edges with a tape adherent so it won't roll.

■ After applying, briskly rubbing the tape from the center toward the ends for 30–40 seconds generates heat, which bonds it to the skin.

Some tapes are smoother than others. Duct tape is smooth but does not breathe or conform to the curves of the foot. Elastikon is coarse as well as thick. Leukotape and Endura-Tape are somewhat smooth. Kinesio Tex is the smoothest. Try to picture the following: your skin's outer layer typically moves against the inner layers—then you apply a tape that is not smooth to the skin, pull on a sock, and finally put your foot inside a shoe. The tape sticks to the skin. As you run, the foot naturally moves a bit inside your shoes. However, the sock cannot move freely against the coarseness of the tape. This forces the tape to move with the sock, which stresses the outer later of skin against the inner layers. The result is very sore feet. Others may not agree, but I have seen too many runners with sore feet, many at the point of not being able to run any more, and the common denominator has been tape that is not smooth. A story will illustrate this.

One year at Badwater I removed tape from the bottoms of a runner's feet and repatched them. He had run 90 miles and had another 40 to go. Over and over he told me, "My feet hurt. I can't run. I can't walk." The balls of each foot were hurting him so badly that he wanted to quit. As I carefully removed the Elastikon tape I discovered he had a small hard-cored callus on the ball of each foot. I put a small Spenco gel patch over the hard core of each callus and used two 2-inch strips of Kinesio Tex tape across the ball of the foot, from the toe crease to mid-foot. He went on to earn a 48-hour finisher's buckle. The smooth Kinesio Tex tape worked where the Elastikon did not. That said, I still think Elastikon is a good tape for some runners' feet. I just happen to like Kinesio Tex more.

Working the Tape

There are three important steps to know about working with tape. The first, skin preparation, is important to provide a base for the tape to adhere to. The second, tape application, is important to reduce problems later. And third, knowing how to remove the tape will save your skin.

Skin Preparation

Athletes who decide to try taping should purchase a tape adherent that provides a taping base to hold the tape to the skin (see "Skin Toughening Agents & Tape Adherents," page 121). The best adherents are compound tincture of benzoin in a liquid or swabs (a blush makeup brush is a good size if applying the liquid benzoin), Cramer's Tuf-Skin spray, or Mueller's Tuffner Clear Spray.

Preparation involves several steps. Before taping, clean the feet of their natural oils, dust, and dirt. This is vital to getting a good stick with the tape. If you have used any lubricant on your feet, wipe it off with a towel first. Rubbing alcohol works well to clean the feet and it dries quickly. For fanny-pack use, buy alcohol wipes in small disposable packets. Next, apply the tape adherent to the areas needing tape and let it dry so it becomes tacky. Then apply the tape based on your specific needs or problems.

You can use a thin dab of a lubricant under the tape at problem areas such as the ball of the foot or the heel. This will help when you later remove the tape. When tape has been on awhile, removing it sometimes takes the skin off underneath it as well because that skin has softened. Duct tape and Elastikon are harder to remove and are more likely to take off the skin, especially if they have been on a long while.

Tape Application

When applying the tape, keep it as smooth as possible. Ridges in the tape can cut into the skin and lead to irritation that can cause blisters. If the tape must be overlapped, be sure the overlapping edge of the tape is in the same direction as the force of motion. For example, if taping the ball of the foot, the force is toward the rear of the foot, so the most forward piece of tape should overlap over the piece toward the back. If taping the heel, the force is toward the rear and up the back of the heel, so the tape on the bottom of the heel should overlap the piece higher up on the back of the heel. This will keep the tape from catching on the sock and peeling up. The less overlap the better. Applying the tape too tightly may cause circulation problems. If, after application, the skin becomes discolored, cool, or numb, loosen the tape. If there is any indication of skin irritation (itching, redness, or rash), discontinue use of the tape immediately.

Place a single layer of toilet paper or tissue over any existing blisters where the outer skin has pulled loose from the inner skin. This keeps the adhesive from attacking the sensitive area and protects the blistered skin when the tape is removed. You can also substitute a piece of duct tape against the tissue, sticky side to sticky side, allowing the slick side of the duct tape to face the hot spot or blister. Do not use gauze because it is too abrasive.

After the foot is taped, several finishing touches should be made. Run a thin layer of lubricant over the tape and around the edges. This reinforces the tape's status as part of your foot by providing a barrier that neutralizes any adhesive leaks and allows the taped surface to slip easily across friction points without snagging. Another option is to apply a sprinkling of powder to the sprayed areas that are not taped to counteract any adhesive left uncovered. Jane Moorhead saw a podiatrist using a votive candle and, after taping, rubbing it over the edges of the tape. The small amount of wax reduces friction and helps prevent curling. This is less messy than using a lubricant.

You may be able to tape all areas of your feet yourself. If you have problems reaching the outer edges of your feet, your heels, or any other awkward area, find someone to help with the taping.

As important as taping the feet is, all those benefits can be lost if the athlete is not careful in putting on or taking off his or her socks. The socks should be rolled on and off. All the time and value of a good tape job can be ruined when changing socks too fast. The use of a shoehorn is recommended to keep additional fiction off the heel as it is lowered into the shoe.

Removing the Tape

When removing the tape, work slowly and carefully. You do not want to pull off a layer of skin or a toenail with the tape. Work from the sides to the center, using the fingers of one hand to hold the skin tight or taunt while pulling the tape with the other hand. Ultrarunner Suzi Cope suggests using baby oil and gentle massage to roll off the tape and excessive adhesive. You can use fingernail polish remover to get rid of any leftover adhesive on your skin or toenails. After a race, Will Brown gets in the shower with the tape still on. After it's wet, he lifts one side of the tape up so more water can get in. After a few minutes, it's easy to remove. Nik Weber has found that ethyl rubbing alcohol removes tape the best, but warns it will sting until it evaporates when applied to open wounds. But it still hurts less than lifting the blister skin up with the tape. He says, "I use a long cotton swab with a wooden stick and soak through the tape if it is porous like Elastikon, then use the soaked cotton swab to peel the edges of the tape loose. You sort of push at the tape-skin interface with the cotton swab until the tape releases."

Three Taping Techniques

Denise Jones's Taping Techniques

Denise Jones has taped feet in one of the most grueling environments—the extreme heat of California's Death Valley for the Badwater Ultramarathon. Her method uses Kinesio Tex with compound tincture of benzoin or Mastisol as an adherent and HypaFix to anchor tape between toes. She also uses a thin layer of lubricant (Hydropel) and sometimes foot powder. Denise and I are constantly discussing tapes and taping techniques and have fine-tuned these techniques. When I tape feet, I use these same techniques.

To prepare feet for taping, Denise insists that you have to file down any calluses with a pedicure file so that if a blister develops, it can be treated. If thick calluses are allowed to remain, they can prove next to impossible to get underneath to drain blisters, and those blisters become larger and more painful. Before taping, also make sure toenails are trimmed square and filed so no rough edges remain.

Kinesio Tex tape can be easily applied. It is very sticky, smooth, and stretchy; and it breathes. Applied well, it forms a bond with the skin. Denise has found that in extreme heat conditions, Elastikon and duct tape will not work. Any tapes used need to be porous, which Kinesio Tex is. Denise uses the following taping method:

> Most important, when I use Kinesio Tex tape on the larger areas of the foot, it's imperative that compound tincture of benzoin is first swabbed onto the area where the tape will be applied. This sticks the tape to the foot. Allow the tincture to become tacky, and then tape as flatly and neatly as possible. After taping, I reapply tincture around the edges of the tape to help seal the tape.

If the ends of the toes blister, then I tape over the top of the toe first, then around the toe to encase it like a glove. I make sure that all areas of the toe are secure with no gaps and no ridges. If a corner is bulky, I cut it off and secure it with more tincture. If one toe is taped and the toe next to it is not, I make sure the tape is absolutely smooth so that the rubbing that occurs in running will not blister the untaped toe. After taping, I use foot powder to keep feet dry within the socks.

If taping over a blister, Denise first uses Zeasorb foot powder to dry the feet before taping, and then she cleans the feet with an alcohol wipe. She cuts a hole in each blister for draining, and then applies either zinc oxide or a piece of toilet tissue. This allows the runner to continue with little pain. It's the fluid in the blister that causes the pain.

Finally, Denise recommends pretaping the night before a race and wearing socks to bed to help the tape conform to the foot. If anything comes unstuck during the night, it can then be restuck the next morning.

Suzi Cope's Taping Techniques

Suzi Cope, an ultrarunner, developed this taping technique while completing the Grand Slam of trail ultrarunning, five 100-mile runs in one summer, with only a couple of small tape blisters. Suzi's technique involves taping the bottom of each foot up to the heel and around the sides of the foot and each toe. She recommends taping the night before an event, after taking a shower. She has often had the tape on up to 36 hours without a problem. River and stream crossings are not a problem because the tape dries as fast as socks and shoes. Suzi stresses this technique will not work for everybody. Individual footprint and running style can affect the taping.

Suzi uses Elastikon tape in 2-inch and 4-inch widths. Do not stretch the tape; simply form it to the foot and press firmly. All points where the tape folds or is pinched together should be folded like gift wrap and cut flush with the skin. This is truly preventive maintenance, creating a sock-type effect. Determine your specific hot spot or blister problems and try taping as needed. When cutting the tape flush with the skin, be careful not to cut the skin. Suzi's technique uses three steps to tape the whole foot. First she tapes the bottom of the foot, and then the sides, followed by the toes. If you only have problems on the ball of the foot, the heels, or the toes, use the appropriate taping strategy.

Duct Tape Techniques

Athletes who have found other tapes won't hold, especially in wet conditions, often use duct tape. I have seen duct tape stay on for days. Its adhesive is one of the best around! For some athletes, the silver duct tape is a staple of their foot care kit.

Many runners have successfully used Gary Cantrell's article "From the South: The Amazing Miracle of Duct Tape"[23] to learn how to prevent and also to treat blisters. Gary's basic principle is to cover the spot that's injured with a patch, and in some cases then anchor the edges and corners of that patch. The powerful adhesive of duct tape holds it close and true to the outline of your skin and the tough plastic outer tape reinforced with fabric can withstand almost unlimited friction. The friction points on your skin will then have what amounts to an additional layer of skin—the duct tape.

Remember a few general duct tape rules. Choose a good quality duct tape with a visible fabric core, not a cheap plastic imitation. Many hardware stores carry several different types of duct tape. The standard grade is typically 9 millimeters thick, while the contractor and professional grades are generally 10 millimeters. Duct tape is available only in a 2-inch width. Although the tape is sometimes available in a variety of colors, the common silver tape works the best.

Apply the tape over the danger spots where blisters frequently occur. Don't apply tape where it is not needed. Use only a single thickness because additional layers become too hard and unyielding. When the tape is applied, that part of the foot should be flexed to its maximum extension. Cut the ends of the tape so they are rounded. If your feet are hairy, shave the parts where the tape will be applied.

Generally speaking with duct tape, do not tape all the way around toes or the foot because of possible circulation problems. If, after applying tape, the skin or portion of the foot farthest from the body becomes discolored, cool, or numb, loosen the tape.

Taping the Feet

A good tape job is an art. It takes practice. It also cannot be rushed. Doing it the night before an event when you have time can result in a better tape job than doing it at an aid station, when you are anxious to get back in the race. Denise Jones warns:

> If taping isn't done properly, it's almost worse than no taping. Any rough edge can become a subsequent blister. Some of the athletes I've worked on have used Elastikon, but they either didn't seal the edges with Micropore or didn't use a tape adherent. Then the tape rolled. I've tried so hard to get the message out there, but often when I see the job of taping that is done, it's less than adequate and is sometimes even a setup for blistering; for example, when the tape is too close to the toe junction on the balls of the feet, blisters can develop between the toes once the feet swell.

So practice early, and practice often. Develop taping skills with each part of your foot. And then practice on your friends and with your teammates. Taking 10–20 minutes to patch a blister and tape feet during a race may seem hard to do. However, it can get you back on your feet and able to run more efficiently.

Remember when applying tape to the bottoms of your feet or heels to grasp the toes of the foot and pull back to stretch the skin to its fullest. Otherwise as you run or walk, the shear forces will loosen the tape and may cause additional blisters.

All the images showing the techniques on the following pages are done with Kinesio Tex tape. It is my tape of choice, along with an occasional strip of HypaFix, for all my taping jobs.

The taping methods described on the following pages can be done directly over blisters if you apply a dab of zinc oxide or a Spenco 2nd Skin patch over the top of the drained blister. If the blister's roof is torn off, a dab of zinc oxide will help dry the skin and protect the new skin from the tape.

Ball of the Foot

Taping the ball of the foot can be tricky. You may find it easier to make a card template in the shape of your foot, from the ball of the foot to the base of the toes. Then cut the tape according to the template. This makes trimming easier, if needed at all, especially if you are taping your own feet.

Kinesio Tex and Elastikon tapes are stretchy and will shape to follow the crease where the toes meet the ball of the foot. Other tapes have to be cut to fit this curved area.

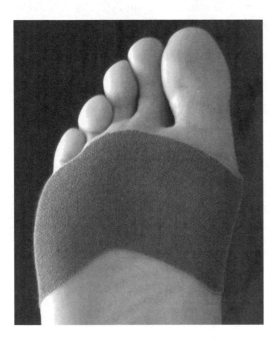

Shape a piece of tape at the toe crease and up the side of the foot. To tape the ball of the foot, cut a long strip of full-width tape and lay it on the ball of the foot, with the forward edge following the shape of the forefoot as it transitions into the toes. Pull the ends of the tape up, cutting them an inch up on either side of the foot. Cut or shape the tape at the forward edge of the ball of the foot so it does not contact or cut into the crease at the base of the toes or the toes themselves. Be sure to apply the extra figure-eight tape between the toes to anchor the forward edge of the tape. See the section "Between the Toe & Foot" later in this chapter.

Bottom of the Foot

Taping the bottom of the foot from the ball of the foot to the heel can be done with one piece of 3-inch tape. Apply the tape from just behind the bend of the toe base, centering the tape on the bottom of the foot from front to back. Have equal edges on the inside and outside of the foot. Trim the front edge to follow the contour of the toe base, avoiding the crease. Form the tape to the foot's arch. Bring the back edge up the heel and fold over on each side, like a gift wrap, making a dart. Cut the fold flush with the foot, leaving two edges just meeting in a V pattern. Then tape the sides of the foot as described below. Be sure to add two figure-eight pieces of tape according to instructions in the section "Between the

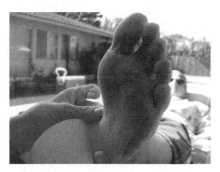

Run a three-inch strip of tape from the
toe crease to the back of the heel.

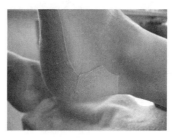

Shape the tape up the heel
and trim the folds flat.

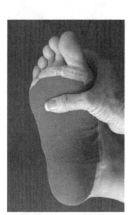

An alternative method
to tape the bottom
of the foot is using
strips side to side
from the toes to heel.

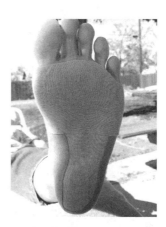

In the third step, run a strip
side to side around the heel.

Toe & Foot" on page 141. A second method of taping is to run strips of tape side to side from the base of the toes back to the heel. This usually requires three to four overlapping strips.

Sides of the Foot

Once the tape is affixed to the bottom of the foot, apply tape to the sides of the foot. Apply a 1- or 2-inch piece around the foot from one side, around the back of the heel to the other side. Slightly overlap the edge of the bottom of the foot tape. Trim the edges to avoid rubbing at the toe crease and anklebone. This also provides protection to the sides and back of your heel. This strip can be done independently from the strip on the bottom of the foot.

If you find the bottom edge of the tape catching on your socks, put this layer on before taping the bottom of the foot. Then tape the bottom of the foot so that tape overlaps the side of the foot tape. This method keeps the overlapping tape in the direction of the force of motion. You can also add an optional strip across the ball of the foot for added protection.

Sides & Bottom of the Heel

Many times, feet blister at the area where the insole meets the inside of the shoe. The side of the heel can be taped by either running a piece of tape around the back of the heel or under the heel from side to side. Start with a strip of 2-inch tape, applied side to side around the back of the heel. Try and keep the top edge under the anklebone and end just forward of the anklebone. To tape the bottom of the heel, place a strip of tape under the heel, anchoring it to the tape running around the sides. If you are taping only the back part and/or the bottom back of the heel, pinch the folds and trim them with scissors. If you need two pieces on the bottom, apply the forward piece first and the back piece last. When applying the tape, Kinesio Tex and Elastikon can be slightly stretched. If you have a roll of 3-inch tape, an alternative method is to use one strip going side to side, under the heel.

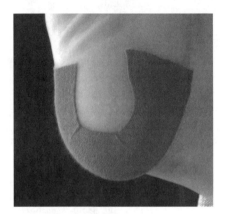

Run a strip of tape side to side
around the back of the heel.

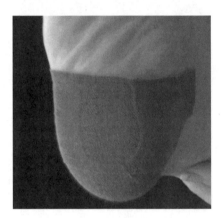

Then run a strip under
the heel side to side.

The Toes

Toe taping can be done with Kinesio Tex or Micropore tapes. Even though Micropore is paper tape, it sticks well and is strong, even when the foot gets wet. The best method of taping toes is a two-piece tape job. First, apply a strip of 1-inch tape over the top of the toe, going over the toenail and around the tip to the bottom of the toe, even with the end on top. Pinch the folds and trim with scissors. Wrap another strip around the toe, from one side to the other, over the tip of the toe. Then pinch any folds and trim with scissors. This puts a smooth section of tape against the neighboring toe—not the edges, had you reversed the order of the pieces applied. Never extend the edge far enough down that it will dig into the tender skin between the toes. If taping for toenail pain, you can apply a piece of Spenco 2nd Skin over the nail and tape directly over that. This provides a bit of cushion to the nail.

A proper taping on toes or larger areas should appear like an extra layer of skin on the foot—no lumps or bumps. If any folds bunch anywhere, pinch them together and cut the excess flush with small scissors. Sometimes tincture needs to be applied again to keep corners and edges down.

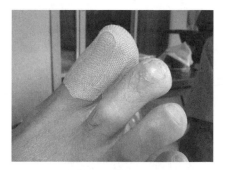

This shows the two strips of tape: top to bottom and side to side.

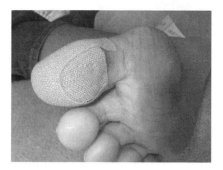

The side-to-side tape won't curl when rubbing on neighboring toes.

Between the Toe & Foot

This important method comes in handy for those hard-to-tape areas at the base of your toes or between the toes. Cut a figure eight from a piece of tape and, spreading the toes, anchor the bottom of the figure eight on the ball of the foot, pull the top of the figure eight between the toes and anchor it on the top of the foot. A soft tape such as Hypafix, EnduraFix, or Kinesio Tex works best. This figure-eight taping is also important to use when taping the ball of the foot. Use two figure eights, one between the big and second toes, and another between the third and fourth toes. The figure eight anchors the forward edge of tape on the bottom of the foot and keeps it from curling as the foot moves through its stride.

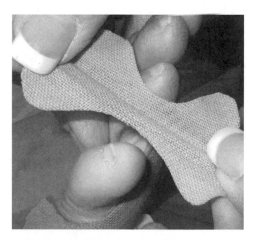

A simple piece of tape cut in a figure 8 runs between the toes.

Other Areas of the Foot

Any part of the foot can be taped. For instance, a blister in the crease of the big toe can be covered by running a strip of tape from the top base of the toe, in between the big and second toe, and under and around to the outside of the toe. The strip will be thinner at the top and wider as it runs under the toe. The arch can easily be taped side to side, under the foot with one or two 2-inch strips or one 3-inch strip.

TAPING ALTERNATIVE PRODUCTS

BUNGA TOE PADS AND TOE CAPS are made from a medical-grade polymer material. **www.bungapads.com**

BUNHEAD GEL products are made of a nonsilicone polymer, formulated with medical grade mineral oils to cushion and protect those areas of the foot prone to friction trauma. They are washable, supple, comforting, hypoallergenic, and nontoxic. Styles include Jelly Tips, Jelly Toes, the Big Tip, and Clearstretch Tips. Locate a retailer through their website, **www.bunheads.com.**

ENGO PATCHES are low-friction patches uniquely applied to blister-prone areas of footwear, insoles, socks, and athletic equipment—not skin—for easier, longer-lasting, blister-free protection. Ultra-thin patches leave footwear volume virtually unaltered. Strong, latex-free adhesive prevents migration and movement, even through moisture and sweat. Scientific and field tests show ENGO's slippery blue surface significantly reduces rubbing, providing immediate relief. Several sizes are available: small ovals for toes; large ovals for the ball of foot, arch, and heel areas; rectangles for custom trimming; and a back-of-the-heel patch. **www.goengo.com**

HAPAD offers Pedifix Visco-Gel Toe Caps that can be used over toes to prevent blisters. **www.hapad.com**

PRO-TEC'S TOE CAPS, made from custom-grade silicone, are soft and stretchable and designed to fit all toes. You can locate a reseller through their website. **www.injurybegone.com**

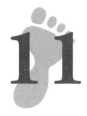

Orthotics

Orthotics are custom-made or over-the-counter insoles that replace the generic, removable insoles in store-bought shoes and boots. Their purpose is to cure athletes' lower extremity ailments. Many runners wear an orthotic device in one or both shoes to help maintain the foot in a functionally correct position. Orthotics may be prescribed for the treatment of plantar fasciitis, tendinitis, knee pain, shin splints, lower-back pain, Morton's neuromas, and other conditions. Orthotics can correct gait irregularities and provide support for flat feet and pronation problems. They can also relieve pressure by providing support behind a problem area such as a callous, neuroma, or metatarsal injury. Malalignment problems such as leg-length inequality can also be corrected. Typically prescribed by a podiatrist or orthopedist, orthotics are medical devices made from cast impressions of your feet. A properly fit orthotic will control arch and pressure-point problems. A custom-made orthotic will position the foot in the ideal position in every stage of motion—whether walking, running, or pivoting.

Signs that you may need an orthotic can include repeated overuse strains or injuries, excessive fatigue in your legs and feet, or genetic structural problems (over- or underpronation, bunions, differences in leg length, arch problems, and so on). Other signs are your shoes showing different wear patterns or wearing out more quickly than usual. The need for orthotics may begin with pain in your feet, repeated blistering in the same place on your feet from pressure, or even problems in your knees or hips as your gait is changed due to biomechanical stresses. Doug Mitchell says, "I had substantial pain in the ball/metatarsal area many years ago. I was doing about 60 miles a week and heavy lifting too, including very heavy calf raises. It turned out that I had a minor structural problem in the foot that created a lot of stress on the ball of my feet. After a while, I went to see a podiatrist, which resulted in my first orthotics. They solved the problem." Doug uses his orthotics almost exclusively in his running and athletic footwear. Check with your health care plan to determine if it covers orthotics.

An added benefit of orthotics is the way they support the body's natural movements. This reduces the demands placed on the muscles when the body is out of alignment. The result is less work by the muscles, which translates to less fatigue, fewer injuries, and higher performance.

When you work with your pedorthist, podiatrist, or orthopedist to determine the right orthotic for your feet, remember several key points:

- Talk to your podiatrist about soft, semirigid, and rigid designs.

- Fiber-reinforced orthotics are typically stronger than other types.

- Make sure that your shoes will accommodate the orthotics. This may depend on the depth of the uppers and the design of the shoe's inside.

- Determine whether your orthotics are to be used alone or with your shoe's stock insole.

- If possible, have a padded layer of material added to the top of the orthotic or use a flat Spenco insole on top of the orthotics for cushioning.

- If you change the model of shoes you wear, have the orthotics adjusted to fit the new shoes.

- Ascertain whether the orthotics are for short- or long-term use. This will depend on your reason for needing them.

Typical Orthotic Modifications & Alterations

- Extra-deep heel seat for more rear-foot control

- Extra heel cushioning

- Soft forefoot extensions at the end of toes

- Metatarsal pads, either soft or pressed into the shell, which can take pressure off neuromas and metatarsal pain

- Morton's extension for a short first metatarsal/long second

- Extra varus (roll out)/valgus (roll in) forefoot or rear foot posting, which inverts or everts the foot more

- Cutouts in the extension for relieving pressure

Bob Williams shares an important point about having orthotics made:

The foot can change over time, just like other parts of the body. Particularly prone to change are our arches because they will drop as one ages. When the arch drops, the foot elongates and you may be forced to get larger or longer shoes. Orthotics can make the difference in simply allowing one to be able to run again. However, when I first started noticing some sagging arches and had orthotics made, it wasn't until I was on my third different pair that I found comfort. If you do choose to get orthotics, make sure that you have a satisfaction guaranteed arrangement with the podiatrist.

It is worth trying a pair of inexpensive inserts before spending the extra money on much more expensive custom-made inserts or even orthotics. Researchers at Hadassah University Hospital in Israel found that made-to-order inserts were no better than generics at helping solve Israeli soldiers' foot and gait problems. Author Charles Milgrom, MD, said semirigid insoles were the most comfortable.

Another study, by the American Orthopaedic Foot and Ankle Society, found that inexpensive off-the-shelf insoles are more likely to be effective than pricey, custom-made products. According to the society, many foot problems can benefit from the cushioning of a cheap insert more than the repositioning provided by a custom-made insert. Many of these insets are made from foam, silicone, plastic, wool, or combinations of different materials.

Custom-made Orthotics

Custom-made orthotics may be soft, semirigid, or rigid, and are made specifically for your feet. Materials may include felt pads, cork, foam, viscoelastic, silicone, closed-cell rubber or closed-cell polyethylene, fiberglass, carbon fiber, or leather. Orthotics can be made in various lengths and include metatarsal pads or heel wedges. They are made to work in partnership with your boots and shoes. Poor-quality boots and shoes may alter the corrective action of an orthotic.

In the article "The Ideal Running Orthosis: A Philosophy of Design,"[24] the authors build a case for the ideal orthotic. They recommend a custom fit in either semirigid or semiflexible design, lightweight, yet inexpensive, with a covering to decrease shear while giving control to both the forefoot and hindfoot, all while retaining memory in its shape and being adjustable at a later time. It also needs to be transferable to most of the client's shoes. They place orthotics in two categories of design: corrective and accommodative. A *corrective* orthotic should attempt, with a rigid design, to correct the foot's position so that its abnormal anatomy will mold to the corrected position. An *accommodative* orthotic should attempt to relieve areas of high stress or reposition the foot to better deal with its stress, usually with a soft or semiflexible design. The most common type of orthotic is semiflexible.

Getting Orthotics

Orthotics can be ordered and cast by many professionals: physical therapists, trainers, physician's assistants, pedorthists, orthopedic techs, chiropractors, and podiatrists, to name a few. Given a choice, I would recommend a pedorthist or sports podiatrist to do the ordering and casting. In reality, pedorthists are the only professionals trained in the actual fabrication of custom foot orthotics. Other health care professionals have to order from a supplier. Finding the professional who has the patience to listen to your history is important. There are some other professionals who do a fine job diagnosing and casting for orthotics, but feet are not their primary interest.

All Orthotics Are Not Alike

Custom-molded orthotics are devices made from an actual mold or cast of the foot. There are two media to cast in, foam and plaster splints. Foam is neater but is inaccurate. Impressions are usually taken with the patient seated. Once the material is compressed, it cannot be changed. Too much pressure in one area and the casting is flawed. Plaster splints allow for the foot to be manipulated into the correct position while the material is still soft. The cast then hardens over the next two to four minutes. Impressions are either taken with the patient sitting with the legs straight out to the caster or lying prone (stomach down) with feet dangling off the end of a table. This author prefers the latter.

The majority of orthotics that are used for sports are made from white polypropylene or any one of the many varieties of carbon fiber. Carbon-fiber orthotics may be flexible or ultrarigid. If adjustments such as raising or lowering the arch or removing a high spot are needed, the carbon-fiber varieties are easily adjusted by heating with a heat gun and then manipulating. They hold their adjustment much better than the polypropylenes that have a lot more memory. These devices tend to go back to their original shape after attempted heat adjustments. Permanent adjustments have to be made by the maker of the orthotic.

The stiffness of the orthotic is an important feature. The more flexible devices provide less control but can be more comfortable. These are ideal when an accommodative forefoot or metatarsal pad is used. Though if control is what is needed to prevent excess movement such as overpronation or over-supination, then a rigid device will normally be well tolerated. I can't even begin to count the number of times I have replaced another doctor's flexible orthotics with a pair of semirigid or rigid ones with great success.

—podiatrist Tim Jantz

Whoever makes your orthotics needs to ask the right questions and order the right tests to make the correct diagnosis about which type of corrective orthotic is necessary. The typical process includes a detailed injury history, complete lower-extremity biomechanical examination including a gait analysis, and a check of your shoes or boots. The aim is to identify the cause of your injury and try to prevent its continuation or recurrence. *Patient compliance in wearing the orthotic is the dominant issue in resolving foot problems.* Modifications to the orthotics may be necessary to ensure a proper fit—if the orthotic is uncomfortable, chances are that you won't wear it. Once you are using orthotics without any pain, continue to use the orthotics as long as they work for your feet. Some injuries that require orthotics will be relieved after a short period of time; other gait, support, and foot-function problems will require long-term use.

Mail-order orthotics need to be checked out thoroughly and purchased only through reputable companies. Adjustments to mail-order orthotics can be difficult. Arch supports sold in sporting goods and drugstores should not be mistaken for orthotics. The Hapad, Lynco, and Spenco orthotics identified below are just three of many low-cost orthotics that can be helpful as an alternative to custom orthotics and quick-fix drugstore remedies.

Over-the-counter Orthotics

Not everyone needs a custom orthotic, and it may be worth your while to try one or two over-the-counter insoles. They may work. Some of these insoles are designed for specific foot problems. Ultrarunner and podiatrist Tim Jantz explains:

> Store-bought orthotics are just that—they are purchased at a store such as Walmart, Kmart, Osco, Walgreens, or running specialty stores. These devices I refer to as arch supports. They support the arch, which can provide relief of mild arch strain and heel pain to name a few. But they don't address the biomechanical problems that often are the cause of many maladies. They are simple, soft, and flexible. After all, they are made to fit every foot type that is a size 8 or 10 or 12. Some examples are Sof Sole and Dr. Scholl's DynaStep. These types of devices consist of soft to firm foam, and some even have a thin layer of carbon fiber for more support. They range in price from $5 to $35.

Nick Williams tells how he "had tried hard orthotics, soft orthotics, Spenco orthotics, and just about anything else to keep my feet from hurting." Then an orthopedic surgeon told him about Hapads and gave him a pair. They have kept him pain free for the last five years and are flexible on trails. Nick now swears by Hapads and via e-mail told ultrarunner Ed Furtaw about them. Ed wore custom-made orthotics for ten years but now uses the Hapad's Comf-Orthotic three-quarter–length insoles without heel pain. He says, "They are definitely more comfortable than wearing orthotics." Ed added Hapad Scaphoid Pads for extra arch support. Now Ed's wife has switched from custom orthotics to the Comf-Orthotic. After an area on one arch got a little sore, they peeled away some of the wool material to make it fit better. Ed believes, "With something such as Hapads, a person can take more responsibility for their own orthotic adjustments, which would be very difficult or impossible with custom-molded rigid orthotics." An orthopedist told me that if he had only one product to offer his patients, he would choose Hapads!

Using Your Orthotics

Ask your pedorthist, podiatrist, or orthopedist what you need to do to help the orthotics work. You should receive complete instructions on the use and care of your orthotics. He or she might give you a detailed treatment schedule of stretching and strengthening exercises and advice on shoe or boot selection. You may also

O R T H O T I C   P R O D U C T S

Many custom-made orthotics are available, and your pedorthist, podiatrist, or orthopedist will help select the correct one for your feet. The product lines of custom-made orthotics and insoles are constantly changing.

ARCHCRAFTERS CUSTOMCOMFORT INSOLES are computer machined to the exact shape of your foot. Placing your feet into a specially designed "footprinter" captures the imprint of your feet. A scanned image of your feet is then made from the imprint and is used to make your custom insoles. **www.archcrafters.com**

The insoles listed below are proven alternatives to the more costly custom orthotics. Your podiatrist or pedorthist can show you other types.

AETREX FULL-LENGTH ANTI-SHOX SPORTS ORTHOTICS are molded with patented heel cushion, medial posting, longitudinal arch support, and metatarsal relief. Gel protects calcaneus and metatarsal heads. An antishear top cover holds the foot in place. **www.aetrex.com**

THE EZ RUNNER ORTHOTIC is a lightweight, thin-profile, fluid orthotic. Silicone fluid is sealed into a polyurethane pouch with a viscosity matching that of the foot's fat pad. Gel flows precisely with each stride from heel strike to push off. It provides cushioning and correction at the forefoot and metatarsal heads. **www.footpainfree.com**

HAPAD ORTHOTICS are either full-length or three-quarter–length insoles. Both are made from Hapad featherweight wool. The coiled, springlike wool fibers provide firm and resilient support while offering arch, metatarsal, and heel cushioning. The full-length contoured Comf-Orthotic Sports Replacement Insole is made in three layers: a moisture-wicking suede top, a ventilated Poron middle layer for shock absorption, and a bottom of Microcel Puff, a self-molding

be advised to wear the orthotics for several hours a day and gradually work your way up to longer periods.

If your foot seems to slip on your orthotic, ask about changing the surface material. A thin layer of Spenco insole material or your favorite insole material can usually be glued to the orthotic using rubber cement. The use of Spenco's Slip-In Insoles can add needed cushioning to your orthotics. Check with the maker of your orthotic before adding anything to the surface because doing so can change your gait and affect the purpose of the orthotic.

If you have orthotics that are three-quarter length, basically stopping at the ball of the foot, you need to use a thin insole, similar to the green Spenco flat insoles, under the orthotic. Usually running or hiking on the exposed bottom of the shoe is uncomfortable. Ask the maker of your orthotic how to add cushion under the forefoot and toes.

O R T H O T I C   P R O D U C T S

footbed. The insole includes a metatarsal bar to relieve pressure at the ball of the foot, a medial arch support to limit pronation, and a heel cup for stability and control of the foot and ankle. **www.hapad.com**

LYNCO BIOMECHANICAL SPORTS ORTHOTICS, made by Aetrex, offer a ready-made triple-density orthotic system that comes in enough variations to accommodate 90% of foot disorders. After identifying your foot type as normal, high arched, or flat/overpronated, they create a model. Each model comes with either a neutral-cupped heel or a medial posted heel, and with or without a metatarsal pad. Additional Reflex self-adhesive pads can be added to the orthotics to relieve pain from Morton's toe, sesamoiditis, and leg-length discrepancy. **www.aetrex.com**

POWERSTEPS INSOLES, by Dr. Les Appel, offer a unique four-phase design to relieve heel and arch pain. With a heel cradle and platform, a strong prescription-like arch support, an antibacterial top fabric, and a double layer cushion casing, they provide optimal arch and heel support and stability. **www.powersteps.com**

SOLE CUSTOM FOOTBEDS, which use heat-to-fit technology, offer an excellent, inexpensive alternative to custom orthotics. They come in regular and ultra-cushioning versions. The footbeds have Poron cushioning, a deep heel cup for stability, and an aggressive arch for support. When you heat the insoles in your oven, put them into your shoes, and stand on them, they mold to your feet. **www.yoursole.com**

SPENCO ARCH SUPPORTS are offered in several designs ready made for your foot size. **www.spenco.com**

Once you have your orthotics, you need to put them into your shoes. Full- and partial-length orthotics are meant to replace your current insoles. Partial length insoles, ending just behind the ball of the foot, may be more comfortable with a thin flat insole over the top or underneath to avoid less of a drop off at the end of the orthotic.

It is not unusual for orthotics to require a tune-up every few years. If you start having foot pain or other problems, contact whoever made them and ask about having them checked. Sometimes all that needs fixing is a resurfacing of the top fabric.

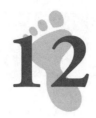

Gaiters

I usually tell athletes of their foot care options and advise them to make the best choice—however, I have three absolutes. The first: You should always use moisture-wicking socks. The second: You need properly trimmed toenails. The third: If you are going out on trails, you need to wear gaiters.

A few years ago when I was working an aid station at a 50K trail run, I was amazed at how few runners wore gaiters. One thing was certain—all had muddy shoes and many had muddy socks. And I don't mean a few drops of mud. I mean the gooey, down your shoes and between your toes type of mud. The mud hardens and causes friction and hot spots, and blisters form. The pace slows, good running form dissolves, your biomechanics alter your stride, and the downhill spiral begins.

Gaiters have been proven to be functional trail gear that all dedicated trail runners and adventure racers should use on trails. Hikers wearing low-top boots could also benefit from using gaiters. Forming a barrier around the leg and the top of the shoe, gaiters keep rocks, dust, and waterborne grit from getting into socks or between the socks and shoe. Gaiters can mean the difference between finishing a trail run or long hike with feet in good shape or feet plagued with hot spots and blisters. Some gaiters slip over the foot, while others close on the side or in the front with Velcro.

My infatuation with gaiters began in 1989. Before my third Western States 100-Mile Endurance Run, I knew I had to do something extra to help my feet. Because I was prone to blisters and the trail was known for its dust and rocks, I decided to make a pair of gaiters out of socks. While I realize the gaiters alone did not make the whole difference, I did lower my personal best time by 1.5 hours. The bottom line was that my feet were protected from the dust, grit, and rocks of the trail, and I had minimal problems.

John Wood has tried a number of gaiters and has learned a few tricks. He comments:

> The ones that strap under the shoe are a nuisance if you need to change shoes or socks in a 100-mile race. First of all, you are likely to be a bit stiff at the later stages of the race, so unless you have a pit crew, trying to

loosen the strap and get it re-fastened is liable to put you into a cramp, let alone cost you a bunch of time. Also, the strap under the shoe can get chewed through and break if you are running on trails with sharp rocks. The gaiters that have a Velcro fastener in the back are very easy to loosen and pull back so you can change socks or shoes. The disadvantage is that you have to affix the Velcro to the back of all shoes that you plan on wearing. The self-stick Velcro is pretty worthless. Instead, get the nonadhesive Velcro at a fabric store and some Liquid Nails glue to stick the back of the Velcro to your shoe. To help hold the Velcro while the glue is drying, just tape it down. Some people use Super Glue, but I have even had that come off. [Another strong glue is Gorilla Glue.]

Whether you are an adventure racer, a simple short-distance trail runner, a hiker, or an ultrarunner, you owe it to yourself to cover your socks and shoes with gaiters.

In an innovating design, Inov-8 makes a sock with a gaiter. Their Debris Gaiter is a gaiter while the Debrisock is an anatomically designed single-piece gaiter sock. Many runners like this gaiter/sock design because it is simple to use.

Making Your Own Gaiters

You can find any number of gaiters at your local stores. But sometimes, homemade ones work just as well or even better. Homemade gaiters can be easily made by anyone willing to try.

Ultrarunner Raymond Zirblis wore women's knee-highs over his shoes during the Marathon des Sables. The nylons stretched well, covered the whole shoe and up the leg, and kept sand and pebbles out, but the mesh was too open to keep dust out.

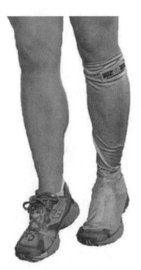

They tore and wore away, but they stayed on all day. Ray used a fresh pair each day, reporting that while not perfect, they worked better than most of the gaiters he saw there during the six days of the desert run. Cathy Tibbetts-Witkes has also run the Marathon des Sables, and after much experimenting, she, too, designed her own gaiters.

Custom-made Gaiters

Cathy Tibbetts-Witkes and Lisa de Speville are two athletes who make their own gaiters. Both have made two sizes: ankle-length for the ordinary ultra and knee-length for sand dunes. They fit snugly over the shoe and attach to the outside with Velcro glued near the bottom on the sole of the shoe. Their gaiters are held up with elastic sewn into the top that is sized

Lisa's homemade gaiters provide sand protection.

for the circumference of the leg either above the ankle or calf. "It took a few tries to work the bugs out," Cathy says, "but now I have totally sandproof gaiters. Just keeping the fine dust out has cut down tremendously on blisters." Lisa calls her gaiters the most crucial piece of equipment she takes to a sand race. A critical component of gaiters worn in sand events is to have them attach to the sole of the shoes. The 4 Deserts Gaiters from Racing the Planet are made to attach to the shoe's sole to provide sand protection. With a little time and minimal expense, you can also make a set of gaiters. Lisa offers instructions on her website **www.adventure lisa.blogspot.com/2009/11/make-your-own-mini-gaiters.html.**

Kent Holder tells of using the arms off an old nylon jacket with elastic sleeves. He cuts the sleeves off about 6 inches up the sleeve from the cuff. He simply pulls the arms, elastic end first, onto his legs over his socks. The loose nylon covers the top of the shoes, and Kent reports that it keeps all of the usual trail debris from entering the shoe. With this type of gaiter, there are no straps, so changing your shoes and socks is a breeze. Rodney Hammons has found another way to get a gaiter effect. He wears a pair of knee-high–type nylons under his Ultimax socks and then pulls the nylons down over the socks and tops of his shoes. Improvising can work wonders.

Repairing Gaiter Straps

The nylon straps or cords that come with most gaiters go under the shoes and boots and will wear out over time as the trails and rocks take their toll. Wrapping the straps with duct tape can help extend their life span. Then simply replace the tape when it wears through.

TIP: A Simple Slit Saves the Strap

Some athletes use a serrated-edge file or a knife to make a slit in the sole into which the strap or cord fits. This can protect them from fraying or being worn through as quickly. If you choose to make this modification to your shoes, be careful not to cut too deeply and compromise the integrity of the sole.

There are several methods to replace the worn-out straps. The first method simply uses 0.25-inch nylon cord. Cut the old strap 0.75 inch from its attachments to the gaiter. Use a lighted match to slightly melt the ends of the straps to prevent fraying. Be careful to not touch the melted nylon until it cools. Punch a small hole in the middle of the 0.75-inch section, and use another lighted match to slightly melt the edges of the hole. Thread the nylon cord through the holes and knot securely so the length is the same as the old strap. Slightly melt the ends of the cord to avoid fraying.

Another method recommended by Mike Erickson uses swagged (pressed around the edges of the cable) 0.0625-inch stainless steel cable instead of the nylon cord—he reports that these have held up for more than five years. Put a piece of duct tape over the swagged ends. Mike also reports using thin nylon cord doused with super glue and then wrapped with a couple layers of duct tape. Others use Kevlar shoelaces or picture-frame wire. Improvise to find other creative methods. A tough polyurethane strap that attaches to gaiters with adjustable fasteners can be found online at **www.dgioutdoors.com.**

Do-it-yourself Strap Replacement

To replace the nylon strap itself, use the method recommended by ultrarunner Kirk Boisseree, using the following materials, which are usually found in fabric stores: 1-inch-wide nylon webbing, size 24 (0.625-inch) metal large snaps (four sets of male and female pieces), and a snap installation tool. The snap tool can usually be found in craft or sewing stores. Make the new straps as follows:

1. Using the old strap as a guide, cut two pieces of webbing the same length. Use a lighted match to slightly melt the ends of the straps to prevent fraying. Be careful to not touch the melted nylon until it cools.

2. At each end of the replacement straps, install a female snap. Use a center punch or a nail to make a hole in the center of the strap 0.75 inch from each end.

3. Push the snap through the hole and set the snap using the tool, following the instructions on the package.

4. Repeat for all four female snaps, making sure the snaps face the same way on each strap end.

5. Install the male snaps on the old straps about 0.5–0.75 inch from the gaiter. Using the center punch and installation tool, center the male snap in the hole, facing the outside of the shoe and set the snap.

6. Remove the middle portion of the worn strap, cutting it down to about a 0.5 inch from the new snaps.

7. Snap on the new straps and check for a proper fit.

G A I T E R   P R O D U C T S

DIRTY GIRL GAITERS are made by ultrarunner Chrissy Weiss and are popular for their groovy color and patterns. Her design is a soft, comfortable, four-way stretch spandex unisex gaiter that attaches to the front shoelace with a hook and secures to the back of the shoe with a self-adhesive Velcro strip—thus avoiding the strap under the shoe. **www.dirtygirlgaiters.com**

EASTERN MOUNTAIN SPORTS offers three types of gaiters. The Scrambler is a low style while the Spindrift and Summit styles are made higher for boots. All use a strap under the shoe's arch. **www.ems.com**

EQUINOX makes a line of gaiters, which can be used by hikers and adventure racers. Styles include mini- to mid- and high-gaiters featuring a strap under the shoe's arch. **www.equinoxltd.com**

4 DESERT GAITERS from Racing the Planet are made from nylon and spandex and are ankle high. Their uniqueness is the design, which attaches to the shoe's sole to provide sand protection. They suggest having a cobbler sew the Velcro onto the sole for strength. Make sure the stitching can't be felt inside the shoe. Also available is a Velcro strip and glue. **www.racingtheplanet.com**

The **INOV-8 DEBRI GAITER** and **DEBRISOCK** are two different gaiters. The Debris Gaiter is a typical gaiter while the Debrisock is a combination gaiter and sock made as a single unit. Both are anatomically designed for total debris control and fasten securely against the shoe. The Debrisocks are offered in Merino wool or CoolMax. Both styles have a ring that fits under the shoe's sole. **www.inov-8.com**

JOETRAILMAN GAITERS are made without the usual strap under the shoe. They attach to the shoelaces closest to the front of the shoe via a hook and to the rear with a Velcro tab. The tension of the four-way stretch material holds the gaiter in place. Joe Dana's gaiters are offered in small and regular to fit all types of shoes. This style slips on your foot before putting on your shoes, which also makes it easy to change shoes or socks. **www.joetrailman.com**

GAITER PRODUCTS

MONTBELL STRETCH GAITERS are made for rugged wear. They have a hook that attaches to your shoelace up front, and a stretch cord runs underneath your shoe to keep everything nice and tight. The stretch cord is adjustable for length and is user replaceable. They are made out of durable Schoeller Dynamic stretch fabric that offers permanent stretch, durability, water and dirt repellent, and great breathability. **www.montbell.com**

MOUNTAIN HARDWEAR GAITERS are offered in a variety of styles, high and low, strap and strapless. They are made with stretch nylon and fit easily over boots and trail shoes. **www.mountainhardwear.com**

OUTDOOR RESEARCH makes several gaiter styles appropriate for running and hiking. The one-size-fits-all Flex-Tex Low Gaiters are made from stretchy Spandura fabric, suited for hiking boots or running shoes. One-size-fits-all Rocky Mountain Low Gaiters are made from vapor-permeable uncoated pack cloth, and the full-length Rocky Mountain High Gaiters are available in either Gore-Tex fabric or pack cloth. All gaiters open in the front with Velcro, have an eyelet on either side for a lace that goes under the shoe's arch, and a metal hook that fastens to a shoelace. **www.orgear.com**

RACEREADY TRAIL GAITERS are made for running shoes and low-top hiking boots. Made in a combination of colors from quick-drying and breathable Supplex nylon, these gaiters have a "space-age tough" cord that goes under the shoe's arch. They fasten with the usual Velcro closure on the outside of the shoe. They could be used on other hiking boots by lengthening the strap. **www.raceready.com**

REI makes several designs of gaiters. Their Desert Gaiters are made from Solarweave fabric for coolness. The Trail Gaiters are made with Cordura nylon. Each style has a side Velcro closure and an instep cord. Find them at local REI stores or at **www.rei.com.**

13

Lacing Options

There are many options for lacing shoes or boots. The way you lace can accommodate many common foot problems or foot types: narrow or wide feet, high arches, localized foot pain, heel control, toenail and corn problems, and more. According to Australian mathematician Burkard Polster, there are 43,200 possible ways to tie a shoe with two rows of six eyelets. For those intrigued by shoelaces, Mr. Polster is the author of *The Shoelace Book: A Mathematical Guide to the Best (and Worst) Ways to Lace Your Shoes.*

Tying laces too tightly can create pressure on the bony, thin-shinned tops of your feet. This can be worse if you have high arches or your shoes have thin tongues. Some athletes have problems with laces causing friction and pressure. After a long run or hike, some runners and hikers experience bruising over the instep where the laces tie. This sore, red spot is often called shoe-related neuritis because the laces irritate the nerves on the top of the foot. Occasionally, this can cause numbness of the toes. Laces can be adjusted to fine-tune the fit of the shoe or boot and to relieve pressure over the instep.

The lacing variations described below can make a shoe fit better and allow for needed spacing in the tongue area or provide for better heel control. The conventional method of lacing—crisscross to the top of the shoe—works best for the majority of people. But in some cases, other lacing patterns may alleviate trouble arising from the shape of a foot or the construction of the shoe. In the illustrations on the following pages, dotted lines show where laces are hidden from view.

Other than changing your lacing patterns, you might consider several lacing products that work well for running shoes, some boots, and many types of shoes. Easy Laces have been around for more than 25 years and are a favorite with many athletes. These products replace the normal shoelaces and end the problem of laces coming untied or breaking. Experiment with stretch laces to find the most comfortable degree of lace tightness that does not cause undue pressure on the instep and yet controls the heel. A tongue cushion can help with instep irritations.

Lacing Tips

To prevent laces from untying, don't double-knot at the top. Instead, gather the loops and lace ends and tuck them through one or two of the cross strands toward the toe of the shoe. This prevents laces from coming untied as effectively as double-knotting and is easier to untie. Also, when you're running through brush, it keeps the laces from getting snagged or picking up debris.

Physician's assistant and ultrarunner Rich Schick suggests another method for keeping laces tied. First, make your laces as short as possible so the loops are not too long. Then add a simple knot at the ends of each lace. When tying your shoes, instead of leaving extra lace, pull on each of the loops until each end knot is snug to the bow. Finally, tuck the loops under one or two of the lace crossings.

Ian's Shoelace Site (**www.shoelaceknot.com**) describes and shows a variety of knots for tying shoes. Ian's Secure Shoelace Knot is the best for active athletes. His website is a wealth of information about shoelaces and he even offers an iPhone app showing lacing configurations.

If you will be in wet or cold weather, steer clear of loosely woven or cotton laces. Check your local outdoor store for laces made of polyester, nylon, or a blend of materials. Many athletes find their round laces come untied faster than any other design. Kevlar laces are very strong but may have to be double-knotted to stay tied.

Try flat instead of round laces, use one of the elastic laces below, or lace your shoes according to the foot-appropriate pain illustration (see below).

Many shoes and boots are made with speed lacing hooks instead of eyelets. To keep laces secured with these hooks, wrap the lace over the hook, around it again, and then to the center for the knot.

Lacing Methods

Flat feet, high arches or not enough support in the arches, narrow or wide feet, and heel-control problems can be helped, to varying degrees, by lacing techniques. Several of the lacing techniques described on the following pages work best with shoes having alternating eyelets spaced in a zigzag pattern, rather than in a straight line.

For Narrow Feet

For narrow feet, use the eyelets farthest from the tongue of the shoe. This will bring up the sides of the shoe for a tighter fit across the top of the foot. This method works on shoes with variable-width eyelets.

Lacing pattern
for narrow feet

For Wide Feet

For wide feet, use the eyelets closest to the tongue of the shoe. This gives the foot more space by leaving more width across the lace area. This method works best on shoes with variable-width eyelets. An alternative

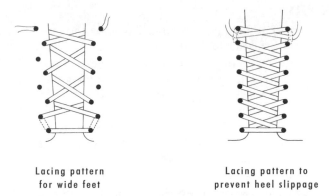

Lacing pattern
for wide feet

Lacing pattern to
prevent heel slippage

method is to pass back under the lace as it emerges from the second eyelet. This prevents the lace across the first eyelets from getting tighter as you run.

To Prevent Heel Slippage

For heel slippage or heel problems, use every eyelet, making sure that the area closest to the heel is tied tightly and that the area nearer the toes has less tension. When you have reached the next to the last eyelet on each side, thread the lace through the top eyelet of the same side, leaving a small arch of lace between the eyelets. Then thread the opposite lace through each opposite arch before tying the laces together at the top. Wendy Holdaway found a solution by having a shoe repair shop put in a second set of eyelets from the top-most eyelet, around the heel at the top of shoe. She says, "It looks odd but gives me room in the toe box while holding the shoes to my very narrow heels."

For High Arches

For high arches, lace the shoes so the laces go straight across. After lacing the bottom two eyelets on the outer side to the inner two eyelets, lace up two eyelets on the same inner side and cross over to the outer side. Lace through these two eyelets and move up two eyelets on the same outer side. Continue this alternating

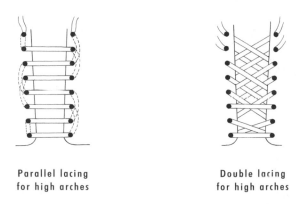

Parallel lacing
for high arches

Double lacing
for high arches

method until one set of eyelets is left. Continue lacing up to the top eyelets on each side.

A high-arch lacing alternative is to string one lace through the first two bottom eyelets and then every other eyelet to the top. A second lace is threaded through the remaining eyelets. This allows tighter lacing at the ball of the foot and the ankle while the mid-foot is laced more loosely. With this method, quick adjustments are easily made for uphills and downhills.

For Narrow Heel & Wide Forefoot

For a narrow heel and wide forefoot, use two laces per shoe. Lace one through the bottom half of the eyelets tied loosely. Lace the other through the top half of the eyelets tied more tightly than the bottom lace. Another option is to lace the first few loops loosely, tie a knot, and then lace the rest of the way up the shoe. Doug Freese suggests skipping the first one or two bottom most eyelets rather than deal with two sets of laces.

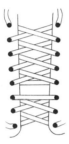

Lacing pattern for narrow
heel and wide forefoot

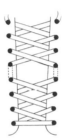

Avoid lacing over
the painful area.

For Foot Pain

To alleviate foot pain, lace as normal for your foot type but skip the eyelets over the area of pain.

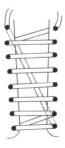

Alleviate pain caused by
toenail trouble or corns

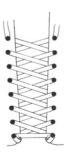

Locking the lace maintains
constant pressure at the toes.

LACE PRODUCTS

EASY LACES are lockable shoelaces featuring a stretchy elastic cord with a lock where the usual bow is tied. You can slip your foot into the shoe or boot without releasing the lock, or you can release the lock to open the shoe farther. The laces are available in a myriad of colors. **www.easy-lace.com**

HAPAD TONGUE CUSHIONS prevent rubbing and alleviate other irritations at the instep. If you have narrow heels, they also hold the foot back into the heel of the shoe for a better fit. The coiled, springlike wool fibers provide firm and resilient support. The pad attaches to the underside of the tongue of the shoe. **www.hapad.com**

LACE LOCKS, sometimes called cord locks, are simple plastic cylinders with a button that locks or releases a lace run through a center hole. Two laces easily fit through the hole, which secures the laces at the desired tension. These are usually found in sporting goods stores.

THE LACE-STICK is for athletes whose laces come untied. Offered in a small tube, Lace-Stick is a sticky, waxlike, invisible, and safe substance. Use it to coat laces to prevent them from untying. **www.lacestick.com**

LOCK-LACES feature specially designed elastic laces combined with a spring-activated locking device. The high-tension springs are made from a metal alloy that won't rust or corrode. The locking device holds the laces (when knotted) in place so they stay secure and maintain the same constant tension on the foot. Available in a variety of colors and lengths. **www.locklaces.com**

SPEED LACES consist of six plastic eyelet fittings, laces, a cord lock, and a lace pull. The risers fasten into the lace holes and allow the laces to tighten evenly above the surface of the shoes. The cord locks and lace pulls allow self-adjusting equal tension of the laces. **www.speedlaces.com**

ULTIMATE SHOELACES are unique elastic laces with small, soft, collapsible knots about every half inch. This unique lace allows different tensions between eyelets of the same shoe. When you stretch the lace, the knots disappear. Simply stretch the laces to feed them through the eyelets of your shoes. After lacing, adjust the tension between eyelets. There are five knot sizes to fit all types of shoes and boots. Laces come in a variety of colors and lengths. **www.xtenex.com**

THE YANKZ SURE LACE SYSTEM includes expandable cord laces and locking devices with two points of adjustability, providing a custom fit. A toe-clip hook holds the extra loop of lace. Shoes can be changed without unlocking the laces. **www.yankz.com**

For Toenail Problems or Corns

For toenail problems or corns, lace down from the top eyelet opposite the problem toe to the bottom eyelet on the side of the problem toe, leaving enough end to tie the laces together. Then lace from the bottom up, side to side, until the top eyelet is reached. This method creates an upward tension on the bottom eyelet over the problem toe, relieving pressure. See page 159 for an illustration.

For Constant Toe Pressure

To maintain constant pressure at the toes, lace the bottom eyelets as usual. Then lock the lace in place by looping the lace around and back through the same eyelet. Continue lacing as normal. Locking the lace at the second or third eyelet can modify this technique. This allows you to tie the laces as tight as you want above the lock while keeping the laces as loose as desired below the lock. See page 159 for an illustration.

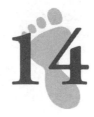

Self Care for Your Feet

Skin Care

In order to keep our feet healthy, it is necessary to take care of them, and that includes giving them the attention they need. But then how many of us know what our feet really need? Jillian Standish, a certified massage therapist, feels that many runners simply don't think about using lotions or creams on their feet.

It's relatively easy to tell how healthy someone's feet are—for me anyway. I just run my hands up and down their feet, and over and between their toes. That's about as up close and personal as you can get. The skin on healthy feet will feel soft and supple. The skin feels somewhat smooth and moist as opposed to feeling dry and flaky. I'll allow only one or two patches of small calluses per foot—if any at all. Many people treasure their calluses and do everything to keep them while others work hard to rid themselves of the rough skin. No corns, plantar warts, or athlete's foot will be seen or felt—just soft and supple skin. Notice how I come back to that again?

I'll also look closely at their toenails. These are a great indicator of the health of the feet. Are they properly trimmed and filed? Have the nails been picked at, which leads to ingrown toenails? Are the nails soft, flaky, thickened, and discolored? Is there nail fungus? Nice healthy nails are firm and strong and are trimmed well.

Because our feet have more than 250,000 sweat glands, the mixture of sweat and bacteria in our shoes and socks are what make our feet smelly. Clean, dry feet and clean shoes and socks can lower the risk of foot odor and fungal infections.

Take the time when showering to use soap and a washcloth on your feet. The rubbing exfoliates dry skin and helps do a thorough cleaning. Then dry your feet, taking extra care on the toes and between the toes. If you tend to forget washing your feet, get Soapy Soles. It's a foot-shaped cushion that adheres to your shower floor and has 1,500 soft scrubbing bristles to clean your feet (**www.soapysoles.com**).

In the summer when we are most active, our feet are often abused. They become hard, callused, or blistered by our multiday hikes, long training runs on back-to-back days, or cross-sport training, as well as by going barefoot or wearing sandals without socks. We repeatedly stress our feet without giving them time to recover and heal. In dry, cold weather our skin becomes dry, resulting in cracks in the skin. Deep cracks are called fissures and are often accompanied by calluses.

The Heel Smoother Pro is the perfect tool for reducing calluses. This two-speed battery-operated pedicure appliance smooths calluses and removes dry skin on heels and toes—anywhere on your feet. It stops when too much pressure is placed on the skin, preventing overexfoliating, which can damage the skin. The DuraCrystal Power Tips is made with the same crystals used in professional microdermabrasion treatments. This leaves the skin very smooth. It is the only pedicure appliance to receive the American Podiatric Medical Association Seal of Acceptance.

Use creams or lotions that help improve the skin's texture and tone by exfoliating dry and dead skin and allowing newly rejuvenated skin to emerge. Some creams contain alpha hydroxy acids, which are all-natural substances found in fruits and sugar cane that generally speed up the exfoliation process.

The use of a deep-penetrating hydrating cream twice a day will help your feet stay soft and supple by restoring your feet's natural oils. Ultrarunner Roy Pirrung uses flaxseed oil products to keep his skin well conditioned. Pay close attention to your heels and the balls of your feet, two of the places where fissures and calluses typically form. To help the cream work its magic, at bedtime rub in the cream and place plastic wrap over your heels. The wrap seals in the cream to enhance the moisturizing effect. In the morning after showering, use the Heel Smoother Pro, a pumice stone, or callus file to buff the skin and reduce calluses. After this buffing, rub in a small amount of cream to keep them soft during the day.

A good testimonial for soft feet comes from racewalker Dave Littlehales:

> I used to think that tough, callused feet were the way to go. But after the '97 Vermont 100, where I developed huge full-bottom-of-the-feet blisters bilaterally, my podiatrist convinced me to go 100% in the other direction—soft and supple. Now I get a pedicure at least once a month, which smooths out all calluses and rough spots. I also put creams on my feet on a daily basis. When I hit the trails or roads, I use foot powder. Things have improved greatly.

Keeping Feet Fresh

It's very easy to keep your feet and shoes fresh by using a small amount of baking soda. Use it as a powder on your feet or sprinkle a bit into your shoes to control odor. A short spray of Lysol into each shoe is another option to help control odor.

Long-distance hiker Brick Robbins finds that after several months on the trail, he has a hard time with "stuff" growing on his feet. He has solved this common problem by soaking his feet for 20 minutes in a solution of about a gallon of water and 2–4 ounces of povidone-iodine every week or so. He says that it has kept his "feet from smelling too bad and seemed to kill the stuff that had started to grow under one of my big toes." Betadine can be used as an alternative to povidone-iodine.

If your shoes get stinky or have a mildew smell after getting soaked in rain, wash them with soap and water and let them dry naturally. After they have dried, give each shoe a couple shots of Lysol. Do not put your shoes in the dryer.

By the end of summer many athletes are suffering from dry and cracked feet—usually from going barefoot or wearing sandals. If you have not had success with your current choice of foot lotion or cream, try Vicks VapoRub. Larry E. Millikan, MD, a professor of dermatology at the Tulane University School of Medicine, says the petroleum in VapoRub holds in moisture, may have antifungal properties, and can reduce itching.

SKIN PRODUCTS

A wide assortment of skin products that are useful for athletes is readily available at your local health-food store or drugstore.

ALL TERRAIN'S THERAPEUTIC FOOT RUB, RECOVERY RUB, and FOOT BAR sooths, relaxes, and refreshes tired and aching feet.

AQUAPHOR HEALING OINTMENT can be used for dry, cracked, and blistered skin.

BURT'S BEES COCONUT FOOT CREAM

Dr. Scholl's makes an **ULTRA OVERNIGHT FOOT CREAM and ROUGH SKIN REMOVING FOOT CREAM.**

FLAXSEED OIL products contain sources of essential fatty acids for proper skin conditioning.

FOOTHERAPY NATURAL MINERAL FOOT BATH for soaking and softening corns and calluses.

FOOTSMART carries a complete line of skin-care products made for the feet. Total Foot Recovery Cream comes in three formulas: Original, Tea Tree Oil, and Shea Butter. Callus Treatment Cream with Urethin breaks down painful, hardened skin. Callex Callus Ointment and the Credo Callus Rasp reduce thick calluses.

HAND SENSE is a protective cream that enhances the natural lipid system by penetrating the outer layer of skin and bonding with the skin to create a soft shield that prevents irritation of the sensitive living tissue underneath. It works to reduce the incident of rashes on the feet plus it reduces perspiration. **www.handsense.com**

THE HEEL SMOOTHER PRO by Artemis Woman is the best tool made for callus control. With two speeds, it stops when too much pressure is put on the skin. The DuraCrystal Power Tips do quick work on heel, toe, and other calluses. It comes with two tips for curved areas of the foot. Choose between a battery-operated and rechargeable model.

Occasionally check your feet and ankles for small areas of pigmented skin, moles that have changed in size or appearance, and any unexplained discoloration under a toenail. These could be early signs of melanoma and need to be checked by your doctor. Melanomas on the feet or ankles have a higher mortality than other melanomas because they are usually discovered at a later stage.

Pedicures

I asked Denise Jones, the Badwater Blister Queen, to write about pedicures. She shares her insights:

Why would an athlete or runner consider getting pedicures? Surely such a lavish bubbling foot treatment in a spa or salon might sound way too frilly

SKIN PRODUCTS

JOHNSON & JOHNSON'S NO MORE RASH, a unique three-in-one formula that promotes effective healing, soothes red, irritated skin and forms a protective barrier. It contains zinc oxide and skin conditioners such as lanolin, petrolatum, and vitamins E and B5.

KATHY'S FAMILY FOOT BALM, FOOT SCRUB, and FOOT BATH is made with 100% natural and organic ingredients.

KERASAL ULTRA20 EXTRA STRENGTH FOOT CREAM for dry heels softens even the driest feet.

KINESYS SPORT'S SOOTHING FOOT SPRAY has peppermint and menthol.

NEUTROGENA FOOT CREAM, a Norwegian formula, both moisturizes and softens dry skin.

ON YOUR TOES works as odor control and an antibacterial foot powder.

PRETTY FEET & HANDS ULTRA MOISTURIZING CREAM and PRETTY FEET & HANDS ROUGH SKIN REMOVER

SKINMD NATURAL, a shielding lotion that adds moisture while stopping the loss of your natural moisture to heal dry and damaged skin.

TINEACIDE ANTIFUNGAL SHOE SPRAY for eliminating fungi and bacteria in footwear.

TRIPOD LABS' HYDROSTAT foot cream works on dry, rough skin on heels and feet.

VOGEL'S HOMEOPATHIC 7 HERB CREAM, a combination of herbs and oils in a natural base, is formulated to soften and smooth rough, dry, or cracked skin.

ZIM'S CRACK CREAM helps to moisturize, soothe, and soften dry, cracked, and painful skin. You can choose between two formulas: a nighttime liquid or daytime cream. The creams are formulated with their unique herbal base of arnica and myrcia oil.

and out of the ordinary for such a sport. Think about it this way: your feet get you there in ultras. If your feet are in bad shape, they can greatly hinder your long-distance adventures.

Consider getting a pedicure for the health of your feet, not just for the aesthetics. You may think that the callus you've developed is your insurance and a means by which your foot protects those friction areas better. Quite the contrary, calluses are never normal. Rather, they are a sign of poor biomechanics or ill-fitting footgear.

Unless a callus is troublesome, most runners tend to ignore it. Once you have experienced a deep blister underneath a callus, you are more likely to rid your feet of it or at least minimize it. So consider getting pedicures. Also, warn your manicurist/pedicurist that you are a runner and you do not want your callus shaved off, but rather you'd prefer having them gently removed a little at a time with a pumice stone, or even better a buffing pad. Getting feet in better shape is a process, not instantaneous.

Additionally, problems can arise from poorly filed and trimmed toenails. Many runners have paid a high price for untrimmed nails, where an edge can catch on the sock and thus cause the entire toenail to lift after enough miles. Not only is this painful, but most of the time, it's also preventable. So get those toenails in good shape too with a pedicure. Then there is the foot massage. Ahhhh, it is therapeutic and just plain feels good! Until I get a good foot massage, I don't even realize how sore my feet are.

When you get a pedicure, your toenails are often cut and shaped before being soaked; however, some salons do this after soaking. Make sure, as a runner, that you get those toenails short enough and filed down smoothly. Then your feet will be soaked in a large basin of warm water. One foot at a time is removed from the water, a cuticle lotion is applied to the edge of the toenails, and your cuticles are trimmed and returned to soak. Then one at a time, each foot is removed from the water, and a rough piece of rock called a pumice stone is used to remove calluses and dead skin from the base of the foot. Both feet are patted dry with a clean towel. Finally, toenails may be buffed or polish applied and lotion is massaged into each foot and leg.

If you are not sold on pedicures, listen to a few athletes.

Karen shared her perspective: "I love my pedicures. I'm with the others in that regular upkeep of my nails makes them less prone to have issues. The biggest issue for me is nails that get too long banging against the end of my shoes. [The pedicurists] seem to be able to cut them short but not too short. Although I never let them touch the calluses on my toes, they do a great job of bringing down the ones on the backs of my heels, which get quite painful when I run. I also like that they make me stick to a moisturizing regimen on my feet, which generally keeps the calluses down to a dull roar."

Terri Schneider wrote: "I try and get regular pedicures for several reasons: 1) I have very tough feet, which isn't necessarily a benefit for ultras as I get thick calluses, then blisters under them (very deep and painful) in 100-milers. The pedicure cuts away all thick areas and dead skin, nail pieces, and things that might dig in and cause blisters or problems. It keeps your skin a healthy and even thickness. 2) My feet look and feel much healthier when I get pedicures regularly. Dead skin is scraped away, allowing for a continual natural sloughing of skin. It also keeps the shoe smell down dramatically!"

Before getting a pedicure, ask how the spas are disinfected. Typically, the disinfectant takes ten minutes to work. For several days after the pedicure, check your feet for infection. Don't get a pedicure if you have cuts or abrasions, even open blisters, on your feet. Women should not shave their legs, wax, or use hair removal creams within a day before getting a pedicure.

Pedicures for Men

A local newspaper, the *Modesto Bee* in central California, carried a story about Nails by Lee, a salon in Modesto. It seems the owner, David Lee, has discovered a great way to get men into his salon.

Once a month, Lee has been holding pedicure/manicure nights for men. Although women are welcome, most of the clients on these nights are men. For $15, you'll get a full pedicure. Lee provides food and drinks. On a recent night, tables held bean burritos and Mexican rice. Drinks included Jose Cuervo Gold tequila and margaritas.

This is a great opportunity to get toenails properly trimmed, skin exfoliated, and calluses managed. While most men choose to get only a pedicure, many businessmen also get manicures because their hands have to be nice and manicured. Others use waxing services to reduce excess hair, or get a facial.

Many of Lee's clients splurge and have their nails done in burgundy, in fire-engine red, or even in a French style topped with gold and/or silver sparkles.

Foot Massage

Massage is great for the feet. It helps increase circulation to injured areas, and the increased blood supply helps speed recovery while reducing swelling. Sports massage focuses on releasing tight, contracted, or overworked muscles used in your sport or activity to restore them to their optimum condition.

Inflexibility associated with tightness can hinder efficient training and performance. When muscles are relaxed and receiving better circulation, they are stronger and tolerate higher levels of training with less pain and breakdown. Tight muscles can lead to strains and soft-tissue injury. Chronic tightness can cause muscle and connective tissue injury and inflammation, resulting in biomechanical imbalances, back pain, Achilles tendinitis, and plantar fasciitis. This is where massage and stretching can help.

Jillian Standish is a certified massage therapist whose typical clients are average athletes who need the benefits of massage to enhance their running. She devotes time during her massages to the feet since the lower leg muscles attach into the feet. As a prerace conditioner, the massage helps loosen the muscles, often lengthening the runner's stride. As a post-race conditioner, she massages knots out of tired and stressed muscles.

Healing from many injuries can be speeded with massage. Mild strains can be eliminated with a few sessions of deep-tissue muscle massage. When a serious strain involves torn muscle fibers, scar tissue develops, which can cause pain when the muscle contracts. Stretching and joint movement combined with deep longitudinal massage strokes can help break down this scar tissue. Chronic tendinitis associated with scar tissue and adhesions in tendons may be resolved with sessions of deep cross-fiber friction massage. Some practitioners use active release techniques (ART) for soft-tissue treatments. This treatment softens and stretches fibrous scar tissue, resulting in improved circulation, increased range of motion, and increased strength.

Robert F. Rusnak, DC, a certified chiropractic sports physician and ART practitioner, explains ART: "The ART technique consists of specific movements of the body to make layers of soft tissue slide over one another, while at the same time, specific pressure is applied to split and strip away the scar tissue that is sticking structures together like glue. The 'release' is accomplished by lengthening muscles, ligaments, and tendons or freeing a nerve along its path."

Look for a licensed massage therapist in the phone book, ask other athletes for referrals, or check your local sports stores for practitioners in your area. Likewise, physical therapists, sports-medicine chiropractors, and specialists in sports and orthopedic rehabilitation often incorporate massage into their practices.

Self-massage

To do a self-massage of your feet, start by warming your feet in a bath or with warm, moist towels. Cross one leg over the other with the sole facing you. Use both thumbs to massage your feet in a deep, circular motion, working small areas at a time. Work from your toes toward your heel, and then to your ankle. Use various movements and pressure to find what feels best. All movement, and pressure, should be toward the heart—moving the old, stagnated blood back to your heart. The use of massage oil or creams can help with the kneading of the skin and can soften dry heels and calluses. Self-foot massage is easier if you're limber, but even if you're not, you can manage it. If possible, have a partner massage your feet.

Foot Massage Techniques

- **BOTTOMS OF THE FEET** Place your thumbs on the heel of one foot. Apply pressure to the underside of the foot, starting at the bottom and slowly moving toward the toes.

- **BALLS OF THE FEET** Make small circles using your thumbs. With fingers on top of the foot and thumb on the ball of the foot, push from toes toward the heels to roll the metatarsal heads.

■ **ARCHES OF THE FEET** Massage the center of the arch with mild to moderate thumb pressure. The correct point is halfway between the heel and the ball of the foot and halfway between the inner and outer edges of the sides of the foot.

■ **HEELS** Massage the bottom and sides of the heel using thumbs or knuckles.

■ **TOES** Stroke between the toes upward toward the heart.

■ **TOP OF THE FEET** Using your fingers, massage the top of the foot, focusing on soft points between the bones of the forefoot upward toward the ankle.

■ **STROKING THE FEET** Using both hands, place your fingers on the top of the foot and the thumbs underneath. One hand at a time, stroke upward (slide your hands toward the ankle).

■ **WALKING BAREFOOT** Especially if done outdoors on a variety of surfaces, walking barefoot stimulates the muscles, nerves, and joints of the feet.

MASSAGE PRODUCTS

THE STICK is a massage tool that can be used on any major muscle groups through clothing or directly on the skin. It provides instant myofascial release, which promotes healthy and relaxed muscle fibers and good circulation. It comes in four sizes and can be used before and after exercise to aid strength, flexibility, and endurance. **www.thestick.com**

Tourles, Stephanie. *NATURAL FOOT CARE: HERBAL TREATMENTS, MASSAGE, AND EXERCISES FOR HEALTHY FEET.* Pownal, Vermont: Storey Books, 1998. This book presents a holistic approach to caring for feet, introducing alternative and natural treatments for good foot health.

Hydration, Dehydration, & Sodium

A subject often overlooked by athletes is the effect on the skin of dehydration and the loss of important electrolytes. Long periods of physical exercise cause stress to the extremities as fluid accumulates in the hands and feet. Fingers and toes often swell as they retain fluid because of low blood sodium (hyponatremia). This causes foot problems as the soft, waterlogged tissues become vulnerable to the rubbing and pounding as we continue to run and hike.

Make sure that you replace electrolytes, especially on long events. Drinking water or even sports drinks may not provide the proper replacement of sodium and other important electrolytes. The popular energy bars and gels may also be low in the electrolytes needed by the body.

Karl King, developer of the SUCCEED! Buffer/Electrolyte Caps, points out that the maintenance of proper electrolyte levels will reduce swelling of hands and feet even after many hours of exercise, and reduce hot spots and blisters on the feet. "When there is heat and humidity, the sweat rate is high and sodium is usually lost in significant amounts," he says. "The sodium comes from the blood stream, and when the plasma gets too low, the body reacts to maintain the minimal tolerable level by pushing water from the blood into extracellular spaces. Thus, hands and feet swell. When the tissue on the feet swells, the feet become soft and more susceptible to blisters and damaged toenails. The feet swell inside the running shoes, putting extra pressure on the tissues, and those tissues can be rubbed to the point of physical damage. We see blisters form as layers of skin separate, and we see toenails move more, damaging the weakened tissues that normally anchor them." Many times the water that creates blisters is underneath the skin, not on the surface.

HYDRATION & ELECTROLYTES

E-CAPS ENDUROLYTES are formulated to counteract the effects of electrolyte depletion and imbalances of hot weather. The caps can be taken as a supplement or mixed in any fluid replacement drink. The Endurolyte caps contain calcium, magnesium, potassium, sodium chloride, L-tyrosine, vitamin B-6, and manganese. **www.hammernutrition.com**

SUCCEED! BUFFER/ELECTROLYTE CAPS replenish in the proper proportions electrolytes commonly found in blood plasma, supporting hours of exercise. They are designed for individuals engaging in physical activities where people sweat heavily. The caps contain a chemical buffering system of sodium chloride, sodium bicarbonate, sodium citrate, sodium phosphate, and potassium chloride, which neutralizes the acids formed during heavy exercise. This both reduces nausea associated with exercise, particularly in the heat, and reduces the swelling of hands and feet common after many hours of exercise. Using the caps often leads to a reduction in hot spots and blisters. They should not be used when water is in short supply. **www.succeedscaps.com**

THERMOTABS are buffered salt tablets that can be taken to prevent muscle cramps or heat prostration due to excessive perspiration. The active ingredients are sodium chloride and potassium chloride. Look for Thermotabs at your local drugstore or pharmacy.

As ultrarunner Jay Hodde notes, "The terms *proper hydration* and *well hydrated* should not be used interchangeably. Being well hydrated with fluids says nothing about the sodium content of the fluid; both are important." When you are well hydrated yet have low sodium, extra fluid accumulates in the tissues of the feet and the likelihood of blister formation increases. When you become fluid-deficient, the skin loses its normal levels of water and in turn loses its turgor. Then it easily rubs or folds over on itself, which leads to blisters.

Rod Dalitz comments, "I am now convinced that electrolyte balance may be a big factor in blisters. With too much or too little salt, the layer just under the skin swells, and your skin is easier to disconnect from underlying tissue—which makes a blister." Many athletes have found out the hard way that simply drinking a fluid replacement drink often will not provide the necessary electrolytes in the proper concentrations that the body needs. The use of a sodium replacement product in prolonged physical activity can help in the prevention of blisters.

Electrolytes and Black Toenails

Karl King emphasizes, "Black toenails are often a result of insufficient electrolyte management. Too little sodium makes hands *and* feet swell. You can see your hands, but you can't see it happening with your feet because they are in your shoes. When the tissues swell because they have excess water, the mechanical strength of the nail footing goes down. Then any movement will do tissue damage. Most of the damage is done in the second half of an ultra when electrolyte status is often thrown off if you don't take care of it. Not many people get black toenails from a 15-mile run. Before I figured out electrolytes, I had black toenails like all of my ultra friends. After improving the way I handled electrolytes, my toenails gradually healed and black toenails were a thing of the past."

Changing Your Shoes & Socks

Whether you are close to achieving an age-group win, reaching a personal best, simply finishing within the time limit, or reaching a specific trail destination, the three to ten minutes necessary for foot care may seem like a lifetime. Only you can make the decision on taking the time to care for your feet. I have seen many runners take off their shoes and socks to reveal skin that falls off the bottoms—not small pieces but enough to cover half their foot! It cannot be emphasized enough—take the time necessary to manage your feet or they will manage you.

When possible, change shoes and socks before problems develop. You

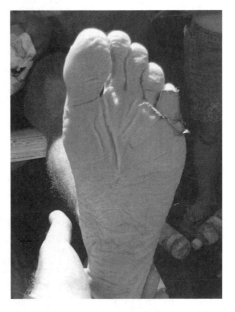

The skin creases on this severely macerated foot resulted from not changing shoes and socks.

may opt to carry an extra pair of socks and a small foot care kit in a fanny pack, allowing for road or trailside foot care as necessary. Dry skin is more resistant to blister formation than skin that has been softened by moisture. Depending on the event, you may choose to change at predetermined points or predetermined times. At these times, you should inspect your feet for problems and treat them appropriately. Powder and/or lubricants should be reapplied when changing socks.

For long runs, determine in advance how often you will change your shoes and socks. Aid stations that are accessible to crew support or aid stations that have your drop bags are the best places to change shoes. On a 24-hour run having additional half- or full-size larger shoes available may save your feet.

Changing shoes can help tired feet become refreshed. Because cushioning and support is different in each style of shoe, your feet may feel better in changed shoes. Each shoe's fit and dynamics has the potential to alter your gait and bring relief to your feet, ankles, knees, hips, and back—but a change can cause problems too. If you are changing shoes to get rid of a hot spot, be aware that sometimes relief new shoes bring to one area can result in other problems elsewhere. Simply pay close attention to your feet as you start out in your changed shoes. Sometimes it is necessary to go back to the old shoes.

TIP: Horning In

Whenever you change shoes and/or socks, be sure to smooth your socks to avoid problem-producing wrinkles. Run your hand inside the shoe to smooth the shoe's seams and check for any irritating debris. When changing socks or shoes, too many athletes simply shove their feet into their shoes. This puts pressure on the heels and tender skin. Use a shoehorn when changing shoes to ease sore feet back into the shoe. The shoehorn will also help keep intact any taping you may have done to your feet. If you have an untaped blister on your heel, the pressure can tear the skin off the blister. Plan ahead and add an inexpensive shoehorn into each drop bag or aid station foot care kits.

Trail running and hiking often make for wet shoes and boots that become dirt-caked. Change shoes and socks as soon as possible after getting wet. Even though shoes and socks do dry out after a stream crossing or in rain, continuing to run or hike may cause the skin on your feet to become overly soft and tender and more prone to blisters. Softening of the skin, called maceration, can cause skin over and around blisters to separate. Where the blister is already ruptured, the skin then opens up. When the skin has been wet for long periods of time, it is not uncommon, when removing socks, to find the skin as shriveled as a prune and the skin separating. The use of high-technology oversocks (see page 101 in the "Socks" chapter) to keep the feet dry can help reduce maceration and blisters.

Hikers need to carry a basic foot care kit as part of a first-aid kit. They should wash their dirty socks daily and dry them on the back of their packs. Some hikers will wisely choose to change socks several times a day. If possible, take a few minutes for a short 5–10 minute soak in a cold stream or lake to refresh your tired feet. Before putting socks that were washed in a stream back on your feet, turn them inside out and fluff up the fabric to restore some of their loft.

In extremely cold weather, it is important to keep feet dry and warm. Socks and footwear that are too tight can cause constriction and impede circulation. Changing from wet into dry socks helps keep the feet warm. The use of moisture-wicking socks also is helpful.

Keeping Your Shoes Fresh

We have all been around them at one time or another. Or maybe you are one too! You know, those who can't shake smelly feet. You can take steps to control your smelly shoes.

There are many products on the market to control odor, from baking-soda balls to absorbent volcanic stone. Results are often so-so. For the absolute best treatment, try what many bowling alleys use on their often-worn-shoes: Lysol disinfectant spray. Try the Crisp Linen Scent for a less Lysol-y smell. To use, pull out your shoe insoles and spray the entire surface, giving a spritz inside the shoes too. Let all parts air out for a few hours before wearing.

The unique and innovative Fresh Force upside-down aerosol dispenser blasts odor in both the forward and rear part of the shoe, heel to toe. Simply insert Fresh Force into the shoe and press down, and the dual-action spray effectively controls odor on contact all day. I like the easy application (**www.kiwicare.com**).

A more natural approach is taken by **www.aromaweb.com.** They give instructions to make a shoe deodorizer from natural ingredients. They suggest 4 tablespoons cornstarch, 4 tablespoons baking soda, 20 drops tea tree oil, 10 drops lemon oil, and 10 drops lavender oil. Sprinkle the deodorizer lightly into shoes in the evenings or at times when the shoes will not be worn for a few hours. You will not see a cure for smelly shoes the first time you use the deodorizer. The magic occurs after regular uses.

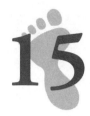

Extreme Conditions & Multiday Events

Cold and wet, frostbite, heat, jungle rot, sand, snow and ice, trench foot, and multiday events are conditions that adventure racers, ultrarunners, and travelers need to understand. The interesting thing is that many of these conditions can be experienced in the same event. The interesting thing is that many of these conditions can be experienced in the same event.

During the ELF Adventure Race, Steve Gurney's team had to deal with many foot care issues: hot spots, blisters, grit, water, swelling, water, jungle rot, water—all common elements in a multiday adventure race. Some sports test and challenge us in different environments. These events will also challenge your foot care skills. Because of the uniqueness of each event, there are tips that will work in one environment and not in another.

"Cleanliness was important, and as I started to get jungle rot, I used copious quantities of that magic Betadine. We cleared grit out frequently but quickly. Several times our feet started to swell to the point that we could feel damage occurring, so we stopped to allow the swelling to go down. When we did move, we moved quickly and efficiently so as to reduce time on feet.

"I used insoles that molded to my feet and shoes, which also helped to reduce blisters, and they proved easy to modify with a knife to relieve hot spots. Several teammates used SealSkinz socks to keep the grit and infection out. We used a silicone lubricant to attempt to seal out moisture and to lubricate. I guess the ultimate key is to thoughtfully think about the conditions and plan smart."

—Steve Gurney, on winning the ELF Adventure Race

Jane Moorhead worked on participants' feet at the 2003 Primal Quest Adventure Race. Her experiences second Steve Gurney's points about planning for foot care under various conditions.

"I *personal experience*

n the day I worked we saw almost 20 racers. Close to 75% of them had at least some degree of immersion foot, and they all had blisters in various stages. One racer told me that he had taken three pairs of socks and changed them religiously when his feet got wet. Another team cut the toes out of their $90 shoes in order to promote draining. Most of them had applied tape, moleskin, or some other type of dressing.

"So why were their feet in such bad condition? My husband worked the race as the support team leader for an Australian team. Out of the four people on his team, two had badly macerated tissue from broken blisters on the balls of their feet and two did not. Why? I wish I had an absolute answer, but I think there are many factors.

"Keeping feet dry is a must. One racer had such bad immersion foot that when he removed the tape from the bottom of his foot, he took a couple of layers of skin with it. We began turning people away from the tent until they had washed and dried their feet and let them bake in the sun awhile to dry the tissues out. The best taping in the world wasn't going to work on wet feet.

"*Know your feet!* Those who had used taping or moleskin going into the event fared better than those who didn't. If a racer knows that he or she tends to get pinch blisters on their little toes, they need to tape at the start of the race, not during.

"Racers should stop at the first sign of foot trouble to tape their feet. This was a demanding race, so even the most experienced racers may have underestimated the toll it would take on their feet. However, my impression was that many teams just wanted to keep moving and didn't take the necessary ten minutes to tape.

"And finally, sometimes you are just blessed with tough feet. Sorry, but it's true."

—Jane Moorhead, after working on feet
at the 2003 Primal Quest Adventure Race

Never assume that you are blessed with such tough feet. Use the following tips based on the event's location, weather, terrain, and length, as well as how your feet have held up in past events. Read the whole section on multiday events because extreme and multiday events are often related.

Cold & Wet

At one time or another, every one of us has trained or competed in an event in which our feet were cold and wet for long periods of time. In a short event, these conditions could persist for a couple of hours. In a one-day event, they could last four to eight hours, and in a long event they may last four to eight hours a day for continuous days. However long the period, this wet condition can have a negative effect on our feet. Blisters may go from being minor inconveniences to major problems. Maceration can happen. In severe cases, trench foot can become a real medical issue. When these conditions set in, you will be at the mercy of your hurting feet.

Wet, cold feet can lead to long-term or even permanent disability. Even at temperatures above freezing, the combination of cold and moisture can lead to serious injury. Trench foot can occur even when temperatures are in the mid-60s in such activities as backpacking. The care of your feet in cold weather is crucial in many sports.

Rich Schick, an ultrarunner and physician's assistant, gives important advice about being cold:

The first thing to remember is that at any level of activity, you only have a limited total amount of heat produced by the body. The body is going to give priority to the vital organs and only send what is left over out to the hands and feet. This is why the first step to keeping the feet warm is to make sure that the torso and especially the head and neck are kept warm. Likewise, if the legs are bare or inadequately protected, a lot of heat will be lost before it ever reaches the feet. Next, you must understand the principal of how insulation works. Clothing traps air and allows the body to heat it. If insulation is compressed, it is no longer insulation. In the feet this translates to you can't have tight footgear and expect your feet to stay warm.

[A key problem is that] feet either get wet from environmental conditions of rain or snow or as a result of wet snow or especially slush on the ground. Terrain factors of stream crossing and standing water also are sources of wet feet. Surprisingly, the most common cause of wet feet is the enemy within, perspiration. This combination of factors usually makes the reality of the situation a matter of how to deal with wet feet rather than how to keep your feet dry.

The choice of socks is crucial. The basic principle is that the thicker the sock, the more moisture it can hold and the longer it will take to dry. Furthermore, heavy socks are most often overkill and will lead to continuously wet feet from excess perspiration. For any activity of greater intensity than a leisurely walk, bulky socks are not necessary. For stop-and-go activities carrying a pair for use when at rest is a good idea. I recommend a very light sock liner of a hydrophobic material such as Thermax or Capilene. Over this a lightweight sock of similar material, wool, or even nylon can be worn for additional warmth if needed. This combination won't pick up much weight and will dry quickly.

So what happens when your feet are wet and cold and how can that affect your racing? As your skin becomes wet, it softens and becomes more susceptible to blisters. If a blister forms, it is more likely to rupture. The skin then separates further. Maceration happens when skin becomes soft and wet for long periods of time. When you take off your socks and find that your feet look like prunes, this is what has happened. The skin is tender and can fold over on itself, separating and creating problems. As layers of skin separate, blisters spread, the skin becomes whitish in color, and it can split open and bleed. It is very hard to patch feet when this has happened. Feet become so tender that every step is painful.

Again, Rich offers good advice: "You must protect the feet from maceration or skin breakdown. A light coat of Vaseline or other petroleum jelly is inexpensive and quite effective. I find that a beeswax and lanolin preparation such as Kiwi's Camp Dry is even more effective. It is designed to waterproof footgear but has more durability than the Vaseline-type products. For those with especially sweaty feet, a quick spray with an antiperspirant prior to the application of the barrier ointment can be very helpful." Another

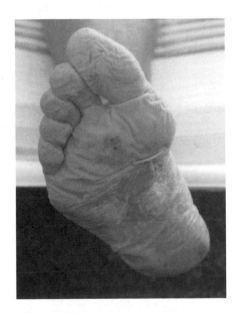

A macerated foot resulting from exposure to moisture

good choice is Hydropel Sports Ointment, which is used by many adventure racers because of its moisture-repelling capabilities. Podiatrist Rob Conenello likes either Gordon Labs' Forma-Ray or Pedinol's Formalyde-10 Spray to dry the skin. Commonly used diaper-rash treatments such as Desitin Maximum Strength Original Paste or Boudreaux's Butt Paste are inexpensive options to control moisture and can be found at drugstores and pharmacies.

Many athletes with macerated feet feel as if the whole bottom of their foot is blistered. In fact, there are often no blisters. The skin is so soft and tender that every step is painful. Many times the skin has folded over on itself or has lifted to form deep creases. These feet need to be dried as much as possible by removing them from the moisture source, applying drying powders, and exposing them to air. On occasion I have used a large 3-inch 2nd Skin circle over the ball of the foot in an attempt to relieve the pain. But there is no quick fix for macerated feet.

Drying your footwear can help your feet. Drying products are made to cut the drying time of wet footwear, quickly absorbing moisture from your footwear, which improves your comfort, prolongs their life, and reduces the likelihood of mildew forming. Stuffitts Shoe Savers are filled with cedar chips and absorb 60% of the moisture from shoes in one hour and 80% in six hours. Stuffitts go inside your shoes and can be used anywhere to absorb moisture and eliminate odors. For home use, check out the Peet Dryer or the Go! Peet Dryer with adapters for home and car use (**www.peetshoedryer.com**).

Also remember what you may have learned as a child. When your head is cold, the rest of you will be cold. So warm your head with a hat or cap, knit cap, or some form of headgear. Keeping your head warm will help warm your feet.

Tips to Avoid Pruned Feet (Maceration)

Maceration of the skin can cause a great deal of pain and interfere with walking and running. These steps should be taken prior to exposure for the best effect. Also pay attention to the Tips for Managing Cold & Moisture on the opposite page.

- Apply a beeswax and lanolin preparation such as Pro-Tech-Skin from Atsko, Kiwi's Camp Dry, or Hydropel Sports Ointment, which is used by many adventure racers because of its moisture-repelling capabilities.

- Coat your feet with Desitin Maximum Strength Original Paste.

- Reapply the skin protectant at frequent intervals or when changing socks, making sure to clean the feet first.

- Make sure your footwear drains moisture out of the inside of the shoe.

- Warm your feet when stopping, resting, or sleeping.

- When resting or sleeping, remove footwear, dry your feet, and allow them to air.

Tips for Managing Cold & Moisture

Consider the following pointers when planning any training or competitive event in which cold and moisture will be an issue.

■ For high-intensity, fast-paced sports, lightweight and fast-drying shoes are the best bet.

■ If you wear shoes with a Gore-Tex fabric, remember that your feet will sweat and create moisture inside the shoe—therefore moisture-wicking socks should always be worn. *Note:* Once a Gore-Tex fabric shoe has water inside from a stream crossing or other water source, it will stay wet inside for a long time.

■ Treat your shoes with a waterproof spray to protect the shoes from the elements and, in turn, keep your feet warmer.

■ If your shoes have a breathable upper, a layer of duct tape over the upper can keep the wind and moisture out.

■ Wearing shoes that do not have adequate draining capabilities will subject your feet to extended periods of moisture. Use a heated nail or a drill to make a few small holes where your upper attaches to the lower part of your shoe or boot. Make one on each side of the heel and one on each side of the forefoot. Some athletes prefer holes in the sole of the shoe for faster draining.

■ Wear socks that have moisture-wicking capabilities. Choose synthetic fabrics such as Drymax, CoolMax, Olefin, or a blend of materials. SmartWool socks, made from wool, are good in wet conditions. Whatever socks you wear, change them frequently and dry the old socks.

■ Consider wearing waterproof socks. You have two choices. SealSkinz socks are designed to keep water out. Seirus Stormsocks are made from neoprene and are designed to hold warmth in, but some water can get inside. Even with these socks, if your feet get wet from sweat, they will still suffer, albeit to a lesser degree.

■ Some recommend using a plastic bag over your socks or between two pairs of socks. While this can keep your feet from getting soaked, your feet will get wet from sweat.

■ In humid conditions, make a cuff out of a highly absorbent, microfiber towel (such as those sold in backpacking stores). A 3-inch-wide cuff around the top of your socks will catch much of the moisture running down your legs. Made with elastic or a Velcro fastener, it can easily be removed, rung out, and reapplied.

■ Foot powders that absorb moisture can help keep your feet dry. Put small containers of powder into your drop bags and in your pack. Reapply powder when changing socks. Zeasorb or Odor-Eaters both make a good moisture-absorbing powder that does not cake up into clumps. Wipe off the old powder and grit before applying new powder.

■ When resting or sleeping, always take off your wet shoes and socks to allow your feet to breathe.

Trench Foot

The name *trench foot* originated during World War I when the troops stood in cold, wet trenches for days without relief. It is sometimes known as immersion foot.

Trench foot, officially called pernio chilblains, is a serious nonfreezing cold injury that develops when the skin of the feet is exposed to a combination of moisture and cold for extended periods. Tissue death can occur in feet exposed

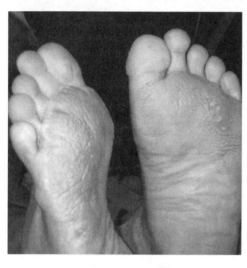

A bad case of trench foot

to moisture and cold in boots or shoes that constrict the feet for periods of 12 hours or longer. It can occur in temperatures as high as 60°F if the feet are constantly wet—in other words, it does not have to be in winter conditions.

Trench foot is caused by factors common to athletes participating in extreme sports: dehydration, wet shoes and socks, poor nutrition, inadequate and too tight footwear, and cold. Many of the multiday ultramarathons and adventure races can create conditions right for trench foot. Under the right conditions, even a one-day event could jeopardize your feet. Similarly, hik-ers can find themselves in the same conditions. Footwear that does not breathe or drain can lead to moisture inside your shoes and socks, which can result in trench foot. Wearing any kind of vapor-barrier sock or shoe can lead to trouble.

Due to the cold, wet, and constricting environment inside the shoe, vaso-constriction (blood vessels constricting) reduces circulation to preserve heat loss. With the resulting lack of oxygen and nutrients in the blood, toxins build up and skin tissue begins to die. The skin reddens and becomes numb. Swelling fol-lows with associated itching and tingling pain. When the skin rewarms, blisters form, and when they fall off, ulcers develop, and then open and weep or bleed. If trench foot is left untreated, ulcerations and gangrene may occur and amputa-tion may be required. It's a consequence of how damp and cool your feet are, no matter what you wear on your feet.

It can take 24–48 hours before the severity of the damage is fully apparent. If your feet are painful, swollen, and blistered, you need medical attention.

Tips for Avoiding Trench Foot

Trench foot is caused by factors common to athletes participating in extreme sports: dehydration, wet shoes and socks, poor nutrition, inadequate and too tight footwear, and cold. There are specific ways to reduce your chance of getting trench foot.

■ Wash and dry your feet, massaging them after drying.

■ Do not sleep in wet socks—sleep with dry, warm socks.

■ Avoid socks and shoes that are too tight.

■ Do not add socks if your feet are cold. This causes more constriction inside your shoes. Move up to a larger shoe.

■ Rewarm gently; do not use a strong heat source.

■ Do not rub the skin; instead, use passive skin-to-skin contact.

■ Elevate the feet above the level of the heart.

■ Start an anti-inflammatory drug program.

■ Consider the use of an antiperspirant with aluminum hydroxide to reduce sweating—use this on your feet for a week before anticipated exposure.

■ Do not pop blisters, apply lotions or creams, or walk on injured feet.

Frostbite

Frostbite occurs when tissue actually freezes. Toes are particularly susceptible to this serious condition. Factors that contribute to frostbite include exposure to wind, wet skin (even from sweat), and tight socks and shoes that constrict blood flow.

Early signs of frostbite include numbness, a waxy or pale discoloration of the skin, and pain in the area. The tissue may also become firm to the touch. As frostbite progresses, the skin gets paler and the pain ceases. Often frostbite will thaw on its own as the person keeps moving or gets into a warm environment and out of the wind, wet, and cold. As the tissue warms, there can be redness, itching, and swelling.

In severe cases of frostbite, the skin becomes immobile as it freezes with underlying tissue. Blisters can form with clear or milky fluid. Blisters filled with blood indicate deeper damage. While the skin may change color, or even darken, do not assume that you will lose the toes. It may take weeks or months to know if amputation is required. Check with your physician as soon as possible to determine what care is necessary.

Be aware of moisture inside your shoes and socks in extreme cold conditions. Sweat and outside moisture can change to ice inside your socks, leading to frostbite.

Tips for Managing Frostbite

- Do not rub your toes to warm them—that causes even more tissue damage.
- Do not rub the frostbitten area.
- Unless absolutely necessary, don't walk on frostbitten feet or toes.
- Get into a warm environment as soon as possible.
- Immerse the affected area in lukewarm—not hot—water, or warm the affected area with the body heat from another person.
- Do not use a heating pad, heat lamp, or the heat of a stove, fireplace, or radiator for warming.
- Do not rewarm or thaw frostbite unless you are sure that you can keep the area warm. It is important to remember that thawing the tissue and then allowing it to refreeze can be devastating. Get professional medical help if possible.
- Dehydration will make you more susceptible to frostbite.

Snow & Ice

Hiking or running on snow and ice can be challenging. Traction is often severely compromised and unless one is careful, falls are common. Snow can cover a variety of rocks, roots, and other obstacles that can cause you to trip. Ice is a hard and unforgiving surface. The two most important factors in traveling over snow and ice are keeping your feet relatively warm and dry and obtaining traction.

Moisture-wicking socks are a must. Also consider wearing waterproof socks. You have two choices in these: the SealSkinz ChillBlocker socks, which have a fleece liner and will keep snow out; and the Seirus Hyperlite Stormsock, which are made from neoprene and designed to hold warmth. These socks are described in the "Socks" chapter.

Cole Hanley runs with hex screws in the soles of his shoes during the winter and has been pleased with the traction they provide. He adds that no screws have ever fallen out and no screws have ever poked the bottom of his feet.

An alternative is to use one of the traction devices that fit over the soles of shoes. Dot Helm, from Alaska, has tried many of these traction devices. She comments:

I should note that the 200 meters between my home and neighborhood mailbox is one of the most treacherous stretches of ice around on a small hill, maybe 15–20 feet high at a 10% slope. So traction devices get tested here. If the snow is soft enough for Yaktrax, I can usually snowshoe run. On the ice near me, the Yaktrax Pro doesn't have enough sharpness to provide traction on ice, like studded shoes do. They also keep my shoe off the ice, so I frequently have less traction than without them. I've also used ice joggers (studs like car tires) of one sort or another over the years to negotiate ice and they do fine, except when you have the rough ice and not enough of the studs contact ice.

Two cautions are necessary: If you use traction devices that fit around or over your shoes, be aware that they may fit differently on different shoes. Secondly, each traction device may work differently on different snow and ice surfaces.

TIP: Hex Screws for Ice & Snow

Sheet-metal hex screws can be used in the soles of your shoes to get better traction. This is a cheap and easy way to modify your shoes or boots to be safe in snow and ice. Use ⅜-inch screws in the lugs of your shoes' soles. Put 10–18 of them around the edges of your shoes' soles with several at the toes and heels. Be careful if your shoes have an air or gel insert. Use a ratchet screwdriver or a drill with a ¼-inch socket to make the job easier. Dipping the screws into epoxy before screwing them into the shoes will help them stay in place. For more detailed instructions, check out Matt Carpenter's (of Pike's Peak fame) screw shoe page at **www.skyrunner. com/screwshoe.htm.**

Ryan Wixom tried this with success: "It works great. I bought some small hex head screws and washers, and put about 13 into the bottom of an old pair of Montrail Vitesse. I used a couple of washers under each screw head to keep them from screwing in too deep." Doug Freese makes a good point when he adds, "Washers mean less screw in the shoe and are more likely to pull out so I would try to buy the right length." He also suggests using a hex head ratchet rather than a hand screwdriver. Doug even keeps an old pair of shoes with screws on hand for muddy races.

Shoe companies are introducing shoes that incorporate some form of spikes for traction. Be on the lookout for these and similar shoes. The Icebug is a shoe and boot line from a Swedish footwear company. With their BUGrip technology, their shoes have 15–16 smart studs that work independently to grip surfaces. The carbide-tip steel studs are set in the hefty rubber lugs on the shoe's sole. Four varieties of shoes and boots are offered: racing, training, active, and winter. Icebug shoes can be seen at **www.garmontusa.com/icebug.html.**

Tips for Managing Snow & Ice

- Consider wearing one of the newer Gore-Tex fabric shoes to repel some of the moisture that will lead to wet and cold feet.
- Use sheet-metal hex screws or one of the traction devices listed below.
- Use high gaiters to keep the snow out of your shoes or boots.
- Wear the best moisture-wicking sock available. Drymax or wool blend socks are a good choice.

WINTER TRACTION PRODUCTS

DUENORTH ALL PURPOSE TRACTION AID is designed for people who walk, run, or hike and want greater stability on ice and snow. It fits over your shoes and has bidirectional tread and six replaceable carbide spikes for maximum grip on ice and snow. It is made with a special compound rubber that retains elasticity in all temperatures. **www.surefoot.net**

KAHTOOLA MICROSPIKES, a flexible traction system, is designed to be used with any common footwear, from trail-running shoes or hiking boots to snow boots. Kahtoola's ten-point gripping system is made from the strongest aluminum alloy and weighs only 19 ounces per pair. Straps and quick-release buckles make it easy to put the system on any shoe. A unique LeafSpring extender bar and independent front and rear straps allow the system to flex naturally with any footwear. The extender bar is available in three different lengths and can be adjusted easily without tools. For serious ice conditions, consider their KTS crampons. **www.kahtoola.com**

KASTNER TRACKTION SOLES were designed by Sid Kastner, a world-class triathlete. The Tracktion Sole's outsole has patented carbide-metal studs that extend slightly from rubber protrusions on the sole. When used for running in adverse conditions, these studs remain extended on snow, ice, or trail surfaces. On hard (concrete or asphalt) surfaces they are absorbed into the sole, so that they perform like any other high-performance running shoe. The Tracktion Sole is available for license to shoe manufacturers. **www.kastnershoe.com**

STABILICER SPORTS are traction devices that have an aggressive cleat-and-tread combination held in place with their tension-fit binding. They are made with dual-density TPE elastomer construction with a traction tread outsole and replaceable cleats. **www.32north.com**

YAKTRAX PRO is a lightweight traction device, made of rubber tubing covered with stainless steel coils, that fits across the soles of your shoes. The Pro is made out of an injection-molded thermal plastic elastomer designed for easy on and off. The coils are protected against rusting and hand-wound to give you 360 degrees of traction on ice and snow. The Pro is equipped with a removable performance strap that fits across the top of the shoe for stability. Although Yaktrax makes a Walker model, the Pro is best suited for athletes. **www.yaktrax.com**

Heat

Heat can affect your feet when running on roads, as at the Death Valley Badwater Ultramarathon or in the desert. We can learn from athletes who have been there. Cathy Tibbetts-Witkes, who has raced at Death Valley, the hottest place in America, describes running in the extreme heat:

> Unless you train [in the desert heat], your feet just aren't going to get used to pavement that you can cook fajitas on. With temperatures best measured with a meat thermometer, runners attempting Badwater have to figure out how to make their feet last 135 miles (bad enough as it is) in almost that much heat. Not only will your feet sweat, but also your crew will be spraying you with water to cool you down. As dry as the desert is, your feet will be wet at Badwater.

Denise Jones, the Badwater Blister Queen, tells of doing a heat-training clinic in Death Valley:

> I did a PowerPoint presentation on blister prevention and care and went over all the aspects. I did one demo the first night on a callus that had blistered and opened on its own on the ball of the foot. . . . Her feet were a mess—callus everywhere, black toenails, and nails too long. [This person] has done some amazing things in running, and yet it was clear to me that she wasn't practicing preventive measures at all. This is all the more reason for pedicures.

Five-time Marathon des Sables finisher and 2002 Badwater finisher Blaise Supler was surprised at how few blisters she got at Badwater compared to the Marathon des Sables held in the desert of Morocco: "The pounding at Badwater killed me, especially on the downhill. Plus the skin on my feet turned white and soft, with creases—I guess from the feet being so wet. It made the soles of my feet seem like they were on fire." This fire sensation is caused by maceration of the feet, which happens when feet are wet over long periods. Blaise admits that she "never changed my shoes or socks past mile 72. I was afraid to see my feet; they were so painful. But it turned out that they were hardly blistered." Maceration is preventable by using moisture-wicking socks, changing them frequently, and allowing the feet to dry and the skin to return to normal.

Clive Saffery ran the extreme Badwater Ultramarathon from Death Valley to Mt. Whitney and came up with a creative method of protecting his feet from the heat. In the 1999 Badwater race, he added an extra precaution to his usual regimen of using petroleum jelly and powder. To reduce heat on his feet, he duct-taped a cut-up space blanket on all the nonwhite parts of his shoe uppers and lined the under side of his shoe insoles in the same way, using small pieces of duct tape to hold the silver blanket on the shoe and insole. Aside from one small heel blister at 122 miles, he was trouble free the whole race in spite of the temperatures. The space blanket under his shoe insoles fared worse, however—when it was removed after the climb out of Death Valley, it had been reduced to a transparent piece of cling film! Some hot-water heater blankets are thin enough to be used the same way.

Probably no one has had the opportunity to work in the heat as much as Denise Jones, the Badwater Blister Queen.

personal experience

"The heat of the desert has melted shoes. Imagine what it does to feet! Over the past ten years I have seen and worked on feet so unbelievably blistered from this event that it would make one think they have been boiled in oil. I have used a myriad of combinations to ensure that feet could handle the stresses of the Badwater Ultramarathon. Through this trial-and-error method, I have devised a system of foot taping that seems to work specifically for racing on pavement in temperatures exceeding 120°F. It has been my experience that if I can get a runner to pretape, it helps prevent a lot of wasted time as the race progresses. Blistering, if it does occur, is subsequently not as major and more treatable.

"Try this method in training first to see if it works for you. In the 2003 race Ben's feet did perfect. In the horrific heat, he had no blisters. I used a combo of my taping, the Injinji socks, and Hydropel, as well as powder, before placing his feet in the socks.

"I don't recommend duct tape. All tape should be breathable. This is very important in desert heat. We have found that duct tape doesn't breathe and causes the area that has been taped to become edematous, sometimes causing worse blisters underneath the tape."

—Denise Jones, the Badwater Blister Queen

Denise Jones's Tips for Controlling Foot Heat

- Pretape any potential problem areas on your feet. In the desert, a breathable tape such as Kinesio Tex is essential.
- Make sure the shoes aren't black, as they absorb heat.
- Wear moisture-wicking socks.
- For those prone to toe blisters, Injinji toe socks help protect each toe.
- Orthotics or extra insoles provide extra insulation from the heated pavement.
- Take several pair of shoes in larger sizes, so if your feet swell in the event, you can change to a larger size.
- You can also keep your shoes and socks cooler by placing them in zip-top bags in the coolers.

- It's also a good idea to keep the tape in a zip-top in your cooler too because the adhesive melts in the desert heat, even in the foot box. When it melts, it won't adhere to the foot.
- Have some substantial scissors available, so if need be, you can cut your shoes in areas where friction has blistered you.
- Have a foot care plan and the equipment to fix your feet.

Sand

It's all about the sand. Anyone who has traveled across sand knows how it gets into everything. Your goal is to keep it out of your shoes and socks. Take one race as an example: the Marathon des Sables (MdS), is a 150-mile race across the Sahara Desert of southern Morocco, which requires competitors to carry all their food and gear for the weeklong duration of the race.

Cathy Tibbetts-Witkes has done the MdS several times and has mastered the sand:

> With a little training, feet can get used to running long distances with a 15- to 20-pound pack. What your training at home can't replicate is the relentless sand, which commercially made gaiters don't sufficiently keep out. The trick to saving your feet at the MdS is to make your own gaiters, which completely cover your shoe and go up to your knee. I use 70- to 80-denier uncoated nylon and fasten them to my shoes with Velcro epoxied to the shoe.

Cathy's gaiters attach to the edge of the soles and end just below her knees. Check the "Gaiters" chapter for more information on using gaiters in the sand.

Whether or not you wear gaiters, try to use shoes that are not mesh (unless you use gaiters like those of Cathy Tibbetts-Witkes). The mesh allows sand to get inside your shoes where it gets under your insoles, into your socks, and onto your feet. The sand, along with the movement of your feet inside the shoes, can tear up the shoes' inner material, causing even more irritations to your feet.

Below, Jim Benike tells of what he learned about this event and the effects of the sand on his feet.

personal experience

"The Marathon des Sables is unique in that it lasts seven days, so one has to run every day. One thinks in terms of sand, but there is so much grit and dust that is smaller than the sand. The grit will get into everything. Every crack and crevice—nothing escapes the grit. It will get into the mesh of any shoe. With that preface one can begin to discuss foot care.

"I used double-layer CoolMax socks, which I have been very satisfied with, but they are the wrong sock for this race. The grit and sand gets trapped between the two layers, so after a day or two the socks turn into sandpaper. Hand washing will not remove the sand and grit. Plan on three pairs, which I think is the right number—one pair for the first three days, one for the long day, and one for the balance of the race.

"I wore gaiters every day. Aside from gaiters one needs to cover the mesh of the shoe for the dune day and the long day. I saw several versions of a full shoe gaiter, but they didn't seem to hold up. I tried duct tape on the toe box, but it fell off one shoe. I could have used more duct tape. I think nylon over the toe box might work—the grit would still get into the shoe, but at least heat could escape. Some people just used a large sock over the toe box.

"I wear size 12 shoes but ran in 13s with an extra shoe insole. I took the extra insole out after the second day because my feet were swelling as expected. I had sandals for after the race. My feet were almost too big. I saw several people who couldn't get their feet into shoes or sandals and walked around with shoe insoles duct-taped to their feet.

"The race is about blister prevention, then blister management. It is just a question of how soon the blisters start. I used New Skin on my blisters and potential blister areas. It made the skin tougher and didn't attract grit or sand. I also used duct tape over the ball of my feet, which is where I normally blister. Pretaping might have helped, but I didn't do it. I know of others, veterans of this event, who did pretape. The needle-and-thread method of draining blisters worked for me. I didn't have any infections. The air is so dry that your feet dry out after each day's run. They never stay 'punky.'

"The French take the skin right off the top of the blister. In my opinion this is a bad idea because you still have to run the next day. A visit to the medical tent was a sure sign of someone in deep trouble."

— Jim Benike on the Marathon des Sables

If you use a lubricant on your feet, watch for sand buildup on your toes and feet. The sand will stick to the lubricant and rub between your toes and feet, creating a coarse friction. When changing socks, wipe off any old lubricant and clean your feet before applying any new lube.

You may have noticed a theme in the advice from all these sand veterans: sand can ruin your feet, and you need to do everything possible to keep it out of your shoes and socks.

Tips for Managing Sand

- Avoid shoes with mesh materials.
- Avoid double-layer socks.
- Keep your feet as clean as possible.
- Wipe off any old lubricant before applying a new coat.
- Use gaiters that keep the sand out of your shoes and socks.
- Stop and check your feet regularly.

Jungle Rot

Jungle rot is a skin disorder induced by a tropical climate. In long adventure races or ultramarathons, particularly in foreign countries, feet are often exposed to all sorts of organisms and nasty creatures. The ELF Adventure is one such race. It has been held in the Philippines and Brazil, places where a racer can be exposed to unfriendly parasites.

It's easy to pick up a few bugs—protozoa or mites or who knows what—especially when going through streams, rivers, and damp caves. Many of these parasites enter the skin through open blisters, cracks between the toes, fissures on the skin, and scratches. Some may lead to a hemorrhagic appearance under the skin. They may ooze fluid, often yellow with pus, from infection. The feet may be painful and itch unrelentingly. There are some nasty creatures out there in adventure racing, that's for sure!

In most cases, a diagnosis will have to be made by a physician and oral antibiotics are prescribed. Some of these organisms will take weeks or months to be eliminated from your body. Many times the race organizations will be aware of the potential for this type of exposure and have medical recommendations for its control.

"H *personal experience*

aving experienced the worst foot problems I can imagine at the ELF, I can share what happened. What is it that allowed some teams to totally avoid foot problems while others had to quit? Should some of us spank our parents for bad genes or will enrolling in an Anthony Robbins fire-walking course do the trick? My team took no special precautions and might be a good control group to help generate some ideas to prevent these problems for racers in similar environments in the future.

"Although the race's website listed only three official withdrawals for sore feet, it's likely that feet played some part in many withdrawals. You could see many competitors hobbling. At one point my feet were swollen to twice their normal size with distention where there should have been arches. They had taken on a mottled white, blue, and pink coloring, and I'm told that I probably had a fever due to the infections raging within.

"The doctors have told us that we experienced a combination of fungus and hookworms on top of the general blistering and swelling we had expected. The race conditions were very wet, and so were competitors' feet, from a combination of creek crossings and rain. Wet feet and fine grit led to blisters, which in turn allowed penetration by the fungus under the skin, moving us from athlete's foot to Stay Puft marshmallow feet. Subcutaneous fungal infections were the largest cause of pain and severe swelling. The doctor said hookworms are generally acquired in sandy soil that enters shoes and carries the organisms, allowing them to burrow in. One teammate wore SealSkinz socks that kept the sand out and she didn't get hookworms. Those of us without SealSkinz were infected with the hookworms. I counted around 30 in my feet!

"Here is what little I learned. Betadine rocks. One of the French doctors suggested mixing Betadine with petroleum jelly, coating the feet, and wearing socks (and the obvious and ever so useless, 'Keep zee feet dry'). This really helped kill the external fungal infection as the stuff kills everything. Hookworms are easily treated by a single dosage of a prescription medicine that for me worked almost overnight.

"Hiking poles are a must for races this length, especially if there is any chance you may become foot impaired. I put 40% of my weight onto my Leki hiking poles for a good portion of the hiking sections and wouldn't have been capable of finishing without them."

—David Schmitt, who has raced in the ELF Adventure

Tips for Controlling Jungle Rot

- Do your utmost to keep your feet as dry as possible.
- Air your feet during rest breaks or food stops. If you can, expose them to sunlight when resting.
- Use a water-repelling ointment such as Hydropel or Desitin Maximum Strength Original Paste to keep moisture at bay.
- Change into dry clean socks as often as possible.
- When changing socks and shoes, check your feet for open skin and treat those areas with Betadine and an antiseptic ointment. Some

lubricants are made with antibacterial properties. The "Compounds for the Feet" chapter lists several of these lubricants (pages 120–121).

■ If you suspect a parasite, get medically checked as soon as possible.

Foot Care in Multiday Events

Multiday events are a challenge to even the experienced athlete. There may be changing weather conditions: water from rain, wind and cold, and heat and humidity. No two multiday events will be the same. You must be prepared for whatever is thrown at you. Proper pre-event planning with your shoes, socks, and foot care kit, along with your other gear, is crucial. Whether you are doing a 100-mile trail run that takes 40 hours, a six-day road race, a three-day adventure race, or a two-week backpack, you must take care of your feet from the start. Some suggestions are appropriate for road races but not for trail races or events that are a mix of road and trail. Modify the suggestions to fit your event.

Rob Byrne has participated in the Marathon des Sables in Morocco, the Gobi March in China, and the Sahara Race in Egypt, each a seven-day stage race about 150 miles in length. He uses petroleum jelly on his feet, and then a polypro liner sock and a cotton sock on top. Each day he gets a new pair of liner socks and replaces the cotton socks every other day. I cringe at his use of petroleum jelly and cotton socks, but they work for him. He had no blisters even with all the river crossings in the Gobi event. He does wear gaiters.

I love the last line of this quote from the Marathon des Sables website: "As to your feet, there is nothing better than training before the race to ensure the good condition of your feet during the race. They will carry you throughout the race if you take good care of them. During the race they will be subject to constant friction, and blister treatment at night is the daily routine of the medical team. Shoes two sizes larger and with a wider fitting at toe level will be more comfortable when your feet swell due to the heat . . . or plasters! All too few competitors go to the chiropodist to prepare their feet, a mistake that many regret afterwards."

Terri Schneider, an ultrarunner and adventure racer, talks about managing her feet in the seven-day Sahara Race in Egypt: "In a stage race, as long as you are draining blisters and airing your feet out each day after running, the blisters will start to heal by week's end (as long as you don't get more). I would take all tape off when I was done running each day, clean the feet (as much as possible without having showers), drain them, and let them dry out as much as possible. Using benzoin each day to keep the tape on was a problem, as over days it dried my skin out too much and they became irritated. I must say that the heat and pack weight didn't help our feet at all. Elevating my feet as much as possible post-running helped and I slept each night with my feet on my pack as well. By week's end my blisters started to heel—though I did lose a few toenails."

Adventure racer Ian Adamson gives three prerace tips for multiday events:

First, choose shoes that breathe and drain well. Water and moisture always get in, but you want to make sure they get out, and fast. Waterproof shoes have their place, but rarely on the feet of an ultra-endurance athlete because they have the propensity to turn your nicely conditioned feet to mush faster than you can say "hop, skip, and jump."

Second, look for adequate midsole cushioning. Racing flats are nice and light, but over a few days it will feel as if you are walking with bare feet over the rocks. Too much cushioning is also bad because it elevates your feet, sacrificing lateral stability.

Third, some form of stone bruise protection is essential. The Salomon adventure racing shoes all have superior stone protection in the form of an outersole Kevlar or plastic plate. Carrying extra weight in uneven, off-trail terrain can wreak havoc on the soft tissues of your feet with inadequate defense.

More Tips from Ian Adamson for Healthy Feet

Try a silicone-based lubricant, which helps drive moisture away from your skin and reduces friction between your feet and shoes. Sportslick and Hydropel are both good products.

Empty your socks of rocks and junk. The debris that accumulates as you thrash around in the forest can cause blisters, sores, abrasions, and cuts, all highly contraindicated for happy feet. Best of all, use a light gaiter to keep things out to start with.

Walk through very cold water whenever you can. Cold water is extremely useful to reduce swelling and has some lovely, if painful, therapeutic and preventive effects while racing on your dogs. Don't worry about the moisture; if you have fast-draining shoes and use a silicone lubricant, you will be fine. Otherwise, soak your feet in whatever cold water is available.

Dan Brannen, an experienced multiday ultrarunner, has several ideas for the problem of swollen feet in multiday races:

In the latter stages of multidays on tracks or road loops, my enlarging feet felt best with no socks and open-toe running shoes. The biggest cause of serious swelling during a multiday is, ironically, being off your feet. The best way to avoid really troublesome foot swelling is to stay on the track as much as possible. Any rest breaks longer than a few hours are just going to make your feet bigger. Forget icing, elevation, and rest during the race. Their effect will be inconsequential.

Dan also recommends wearing socks and sandals when traveling home after the event (especially when flying). Or wear your shoes loose and untied—even when walking through the airport.

Peter Bakwin, a veteran multiday trail runner, observed a multiday race and offered the following: "I noticed a lot of the multiday runners had the toes cut out of their shoes. We camped next to one runner, and she had several pairs like that and her shoes were probably two sizes bigger than you would normally use. She changed her shoes and socks frequently, rotating socks to get dry ones. I also noticed that a lot of the six-day guys were using very thin nylon stockings under their regular socks." Trauma shears make short work of cutting shoes and should be available at any race that has medical support.

Sharon and Chuck Chelin share a good suggestion for staying on top of foot care issues. Their suggestion can be used by anyone, from hikers to adventure racers:

> Except for urgent daytime events, evening is when feet are inspected and maintained. This includes cleaning, as best we can under the circumstances; inspection and repair of any blisters; sandpapering of any dry, rough, or cracked areas; trimming and smoothing of nails; and application of a favorite conditioner, such as lotion, salve, alcohol, powder, and so on. This is also the time shoes are inspected. Out come the insoles and inserts, so the dirt can be removed and an inspection can be made for nasty little sharp burrs and stickers that like to work their way through the fabric, padding, and linings.

Off with the Toes

If you choose to cut the toes out of your shoes, use EMT scissors or utility shears, not a knife. Plan ahead and have a pair in your medical kit. Using a knife can lead to injury when trying to cut through tough shoe uppers. Here are a few tips.

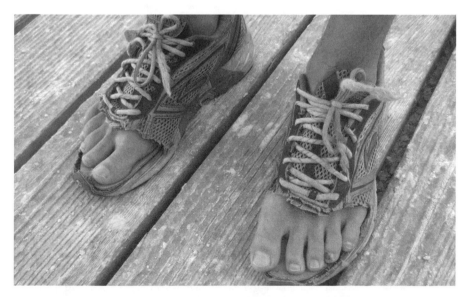

As odd as it may look, cutting the toes off shoes helps prevent common foot problems.

- Cut from just below the bottom pair of eyelets or the trim piece of fabric that the eyelets go through.

- Cut down to where the upper joins the sole, from one side around to the other side.

- Trim as much as necessary to clear the toes.

- If trimming the heels, keep the top part of the heel counter. Trim under this down to where the upper joins the sole.

- Use duct tape to cover any rough edges.

Ray Zirblis writes from the experience of 24-hour and multiday stage races. He knows first-hand that foot swelling can trouble racers: "After the Orlander Park 24-Hour, my feet are typically quite swollen for four or five days. Air and auto travel home is always excruciating. Once home, I keep a bucket of ice water by my bed and every couple of hours, when those 'dogs begin to bark,' I get up and soak them."

When I did a 72-hour road race, I learned that a quick 20-minute nap every six hours helped me stay sharp. From 12 hours on, I took these quick catnaps for the remaining 60 hours, and during each nap I slightly elevated my feet—with my shoes off.

Going into a multiday event without knowing the best way to care for your feet and how to fix blisters or a turned ankle can spell disaster. Practice before your event, and if you have a team or crew, or are on a team or crew, learn everything you can about how to take care of and fix your feet.

Tips for Multiday Events

- Use rest periods and food breaks to air your feet. This is crucial to let the skin dry and heal.

- Cut the toes out of your shoes (if the location and terrain allow). A piece of spandex or other stretch material can be glued over the hole to keep out trash.

- Frequently ice your feet or immerse them in ice water during occasional break periods.

- Elevate your feet when resting.

- Rotate your socks to keep your feet as dry as possible.

- Have extra shoes a size or two larger than normal, with interchangeable insoles.

- If you cannot change into larger shoes, start with shoes larger than normal and add a flat insole to help them fit from the start. Remove the insole as your foot swells.

■ Use different thicknesses of socks.

■ Use anti-inflammatory medications.

■ Change shoes and socks frequently.

■ Use very thin nylon stockings under regular socks.

■ Use Super Salve, Bag Balm, Brave Soldier Antiseptic Healing Ointment, or a similar ointment to keep your feet as healthy as possible.

Aching Feet

Wayne "Smiley" Herrick calls it thru-hiker foot pain: "It's that aching pain that many (most) long-distance hikers get on the bottom of their feet from overuse. It feels as if someone has repeatedly taken a hammer to the bottom of your feet."

Others can also feel the ache and pain of too much time on their feet. Sudden increases in mileage put undue pressure on the bones, tendons, ligaments, and muscles of the feet. If you are typically walking 3 miles a day and then suddenly walk 10 miles, you can expect your feet to feel sore, hot, and painful. Increasing your running miles from a 10K (6.2 miles) to a half-marathon (13.1 miles) will result in similar complaints. The same goes for other distances. Ultrarunners can feel this after a 100-mile, 24-hour, 48-hour, or 72-hour race. Adventure racers can feel it after a six- to ten-day expedition race. Typical causes are:

■ The day after day stresses of walking, running, or hiking long distances;

■ Trying to do many miles too fast;

■ Not properly conditioning your feet;

■ Pushing too hard in an event or race for which you are not fully trained;

■ Encountering conditions for which you are not prepared;

■ Wearing footwear—such as shoes, insoles, or socks—that is worn out; or

■ Having preexisting foot conditions, such as flat feet or plantar fasciitis, which contribute to the overall demise of your feet.

The rule of thumb for runners has always been to increase weekly miles by no more than 10% a week. This is good advice for all of us.

What Smiley learned can help anyone who experiences this same ache or pain. Read what he describes has worked for him and other hikers and apply it to your situation. For some, the ache and pain in their feet may take months or longer to resolve itself. He shares his experiences with aching feet and foot pain:

Do the bottoms of your feet still hurt or ache after changing to shoes? This is a common, almost universal, complaint of long-distance hikers, and I was no exception. The daily high mileage and long hours of hiking invited problems. At the beginning of each part of my two-part A.T. hike,

I endured intense foot pain of a variety I'd never experienced, even running marathons and ultras and being on multiweek climbing trips. I've since contacted a podiatrist and a sports trainer specializing in foot care. The only advice I got was, "Don't hike so much," and "Buy these $200 custom insoles."

Some of this is not scientific and only proven to work for me and other long-distance hikers. I was desperate and tried everything I heard and anything I could think of. First of all, reducing pack weight helps sore feet, and carrying a lighter pack to start with is a good preventive step. A solid training base is a strong preventive step. Changing to a new or different pair of shoes, especially a more supportive and/or cushioned model, could help. Taking a day off is an often overlooked, quite successful remedy. I've found that taking off my shoes and socks and elevating my feet and legs provide immediate, although somewhat temporary, relief. Elevating my feet and legs at night while sleeping was also helpful, as was getting a good night's sleep.

A self-foot massage and stretching the legs helps by increasing blood circulation to the feet. The variety provided by occasionally walking around barefoot at camp and in town helps. Avoiding pavement and particularly avoiding concrete in towns is a good thing and becomes more important while standing still. If you pay careful attention, especially while running, the difference in hardness among various surfaces is perceptible.

For some reason I can't explain, a huge meal provides immediate, complete, and lasting relief for my aching feet. It probably has something to do with a large part of the blood supply migrating to the stomach for digestion. Maintaining a very high level of hydration also helped. I noticed several of my days of more extreme foot pain on the A.T. were at times when I was not as well hydrated. I'd try to drink 8–10 liters/quarts of water on a hot day. Believe it or not, when my feet really hurt, sometimes I would just start running out of frustration. This increased blood flow, worked different muscles, and actually provided some relief. Soaking (numbing) my feet in a cold stream was very beneficial. While in a resupply town or after you get home, icing your feet is a good idea. I made use of snowfields along the Colorado Trail to ice my feet when they hurt.

I've found that the surest cure for aching feet is time. Three weeks of breaking my feet in using the above tricks and treatments brings an end to the pain for me. I've talked to others who just learned to accept their foot pain as a permanent part of their thru-hike.

16

Teamwork & Crew Support

There may be times when you are involved in a team sport or a sport that utilizes a crew. Adventure racing is typically done as a team. Backpacking and hiking, while not team sports per se, may be done as a group. Crew support is found in ultramarathon events, adventure racing, and team sports: football, soccer, and so on. Before your race or activity, develop a plan, draw up a list of supplies, and clarify all the responsibilities of each team or crew member. And be sure to discuss your group's notion of teamwork.

Teamwork

Any time you are with a group, teamwork is vital. You are only as strong as your weakest member and as fast as your slowest member. If you have a crew supporting you and you need foot care, can any crew member manage your feet—or only one? Do team members know how to care for each other's feet as well as their own?

For adventure racing, this is of particular importance. As you train and race, your team will learn from each other's strengths and build on each other's weaknesses. It may sound easy, but this aspect is rated as one of the most complex and difficult of all adventure-racing components. Each team member must have some degree of skill at all of the disciplines—including foot care. The same can be said for all members of a backpack or hike. The story of one team's experience during an adventure race will illustrate this point.

Patty Hintz, a member of Team R.E.A.R., participated in a two-day adventure race in the Shasta-Trinity Alps. She describes the race:

> The mileage for the running section was about 35 miles and one of my teammates had a problem with blisters. Being an experienced ultrarunner I brought along extra Spenco 2nd Skin. When she said blisters, I had no idea we were talking both heels, both forefeet, and multiple toes on each foot! We had three different types of tape to put over the 2nd Skin. I first tried moleskin—but a few miles later it was off. Next was cloth tape, but

it did not hold either. Finally, I remembered the duct tape in our team's mandatory gear. I don't know how she managed, but she said her feet felt 100% better. She was able to continue the race and the duct tape never came off.

This story is important in that Patty had anticipated foot problems and was prepared. She knew the value of 2nd Skin and knew how to tape the feet. She also knew how to improvise. If she had been on a team where no one knew how to properly drain blisters and tape over them, they may not have finished the two-day event. Patty describes some problems they encountered:

> Later we talked about what caused the blisters. [My teammate] had great running-type socks to reduce friction. Her shoes had plenty of break-in time and fit her feet properly. I personally think that it was not enough experience with time on her feet. I honestly feel that if your shoes fit properly and are the right type of shoe for the way you run, you wear appropriate socks, and you spend time breaking in a new pair of shoes before you race in them, blisters are still going to come until your feet have enough distance and time to toughen up. Until then, I'm a firm believer in duct tape and 2nd Skin. As far as my teammate's feet, I'm happy to say they healed very quickly—in about a week.

Planning for Foot Care

People participating in the same activity or on the same team would be wise to sit down before an event, particularly if it is your first or second event together, or your first multiday event, and talk about foot care. Who has the most foot care experience? What is the best way to prepare your feet—pre-event taping, toughening your skin, better socks, and/or better-fitting shoes? As Patty asks, "Does each member have enough time on their feet to toughen them for the distance?" What is the best method to use when fixing blisters? What about really big blisters? What is the minimum amount of foot care knowledge expected of each person? What foot care gear will you carry and how much of each item? Foot care kits are useless if only one person knows how to use the materials in

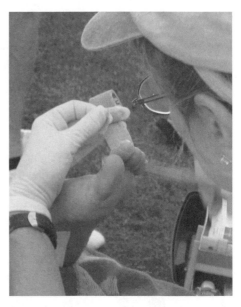

All team members need to be able to work on each other's feet. Here, a teammate wraps Coban over 2nd Skin on a toe blister.

them. Who then will fix that person's feet if problems develop? And who will manage the team's feet if that person is injured or has to be pulled from the race?

Planning should also include preparing a foot care kit. The chapter "Foot Care Kits" includes a list of what to include in your kit.

Team Responsibilities

You need to know how to use each item in your foot care kit. Each member of the team should know how to tape their feet to prevent and fix blisters. Each team member should work at finding what is best for his or her feet—lubricants or powders, two pairs or one pair of socks, double-layer or single-layer socks, the best way to lace shoes for specific foot problems, and the best-fitting shoes for his or her feet. It is the responsibility of the whole team to be sure each member is adequately trained in proper foot care. It can mean the difference between a good race and just finishing—or even not finishing.

Crew Support

If you will be participating in an event where you have crew support to help you at aid stations, be sure to discuss foot care issues with them before the event. Let them know if there will be shoe or sock changes at particular aid stations, and if so, what specific shoes or socks you will want. Let them know all of the following:

■ How to take your shoes and socks off to avoid making any foot problems worse,

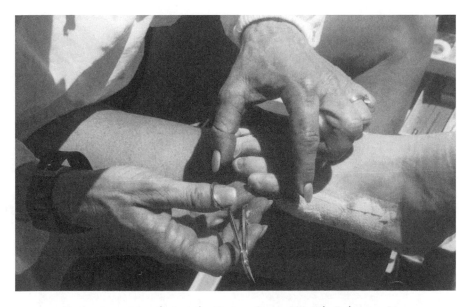

Denise Jones tapes feet at the Western States 100-Mile Endurance Run.

- How to put new shoes and socks back on,

- What powders and/or lubricants you use and where on your feet you use them,

- How tight you like your shoes tied and whether you use single or double knots, and

- How you want to deal with hot spots, blisters, toenails, or other unique problems.

Practice this with your crew at home, well in advance of the run. By trial and error find what works and what doesn't work. It is important to know the amount of time these activities will take.

When arriving in the aid station, let them know what you need for your feet. Advise them of any hot spots or blisters. Never let them pull shoes off your feet without proper unlacing. This action, however unintentional, can rupture a blister or cause increased pain to already hurting feet. A shoehorn can be a lifesaver—use it to easily slide the heel out of and into the back of the shoe without too much pressure on sore and tender heels.

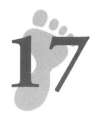

Providing Foot Care
for Athletes

Providing foot care for athletes is a huge responsibility. Their feet are what keep them going, and if you are known for providing foot care, the athletes will be appreciative of whatever you can do. If you are simply helping one runner, you might be a bit more casual. But if you will be part of a foot care team, you need to be prepared.

I have taught many people how to patch feet. Some of these, in turn, have taught others. Ordinary folks can patch feet as well as medical professionals can. Over the years, I have taught podiatrists, doctors, nurses, paramedics, emergency medical technicians, athletic trainers, and many other people who simply want to learn what to do. The skills to get an athlete back on the trail or road whose feet are badly blistered are not typically taught to medical professionals.

My goal when patching feet during an event is to get the athletes back in the race. That goal is the same regardless of the length of the race—a marathon, 50 miler, or multiday race. I need to be as prepared as possible to do whatever it takes to patch them up. That should be your goal too.

Being Part of a Foot Care Team

Whether working as a crew member or as part of a medical team doing foot care, it is imperative to have a solid understanding of all aspects of foot care. Blisters will be a large part of your routine, so knowing their types, and how to drain, patch, and tape them is vital. Whether taping over potential problem areas for an athlete before a run, over a patched blister during a run, or redoing a blister patch during a multiday event, taping skills are a huge part of providing quality foot care. Knowing how to drain a blister under a toenail is a good skill to learn. You need to learn what causes blisters, how to trim toenails, the problem with calluses, treating maceration, and more.

Make sure you study the following chapters in this book: "Taping for Blisters"; "Extreme Conditions & Multiday Events"; "Blisters"; "Strains & Sprains, Fractures & Dislocations"; "Tendon & Ligament Injuries"; "Heel Problems"; "Toe Problems"; "Forefoot Problems"; "Skin Disorders"; and "Cold & Heat Therapy."

In addition to having the practical skills, and just as important, one needs the ability to talk to the athletes you are treating and to listen to their concerns. When I am patching feet, I run my hands over the feet and ask what's going on. I always try to examine the whole foot, and both feet when possible. As I patch blisters, I try to educate the athlete about blisters, calluses, or whatever the issue is, and explain what I am doing and why. I believe strongly in helping athletes understand the ins and outs of foot care. While I'm patching their feet is a good time because they are a captive and interested audience.

If you are working with others who are also helping with foot care, be conscious of the degree of their skills. They may not know as much as you and will welcome you sharing your expertise.

This is no time for shortcuts. Not using compound tincture of benzoin will result in tape coming off and bunching up in the socks. Using the wrong tape, white athletic tape as an example, will result in the tape peeling off and causing further problems. Using a needle and not enlarging the hole will result in the hole sealing up and the blister refilling. Slapping on tape with folds and creases can cause discomfort to the athlete. You owe it to yourself and the athletes to do the best possible job.

Setting Up Your Station

A great tool to use for foot care is a chaise folding recliner. These adjustable chairs are perfect for patching feet because they provide full body support while the athlete reclines. The feet are lifted up for easy viewing. A chair for you to sit in while working will save your back. A massage table works well too. It is nice to have a table on which to spread out your materials. Plan ahead for events where you will be working at night. A good headlamp is at least 1 watt. Even with indoor lighting, a headlamp can help you see blisters more clearly.

Tips on Managing Blisters

Over the years I have worked aid stations at single-day and multiday events. I have patched thousands of feet of professional athletes, weekend athletes, and walkers who are not athletes. The one thing all these people had in common was their propensity to get blisters—often really bad blisters. Here are my tips on managing blisters.

PREPARATION
- Any blister should be drained. If the blister is causing discomfort to the athlete, drain it before it presents bigger problems.

- Use an alcohol wipe to clean the skin surrounding the blister.

- Cold and/or damp skin makes for difficult taping—try to dry and warm it.

DRAINING BLISTERS

- If using needles for draining blisters, move the needle side to side to enlarge the hole so it won't close up on itself.

- Λ #11 scalpel or pointed scissors can make a slit cut which will promote continued draining.

- Plan several drain cuts/holes in places where gravity and ongoing foot pressure will aid with continued draining.

BLOOD BLISTERS

- If draining a blood blister, warn the athlete about signs of infection.

- Usually it is better to drain and patch a blood blister in a controlled environment than to have it rupture out on the course.

- Add a dab of antibiotic ointment in or over the blister before patching.

MULTIDAY BLISTER TIPS

- Patch and tape feet after feet have been cleaned or washed. If the athlete has downtime during an event, encourage them to let their feet air out in order to dry the blisters.

- Use a syringe to inject a dab of zinc oxide in a blister to help the new skin dry and harden faster.

- Expect to redo blister patching and taping during the event.

PATCHING BLISTERS

- A dab of zinc oxide over a blister will prevent tape from sticking and works to dry out the skin.

- Spenco 2nd Skin patches are sufficient for short events but will lead to cold and damp skin on longer events, making further patching difficult.

- Blisters under toenails, if visible at the tip of the nail, can be drained there; otherwise, drilling the nail will be required.

- Tape can be applied directly over a blister as long as a dab of zinc oxide, antibiotic ointment, or blister patch prevents the tape from sticking to the roof of the blister.

TAPING

- Compound tincture of benzoin will help the tape stick better. Avoid getting it into open skin as it will sting.

- Round all corners of tape.

- Avoid folds and creases in the tape.

- If using Kinesio Tex tape, remember to rub the tape for about 30 seconds to warm and activate the adhesive for better bonding.

- Avoid tape that does not mold or shape to the contours of the foot.

Advising about Post-event Care

After spending time patching a blister, or several blisters, you want your patch job to hold. The best way to assure this is to advise the athlete to be careful as they put on and take off their socks. Tell them to bunch their socks up, top to toe, and then roll them onto the foot. This simple instruction can save your patch job and avoid having the tape come loose.

It is important for athletes to know how to manage their feet after the race or event. The most common issue is typically blisters, but sprained ankles and black toenails are two other common problems.

For blisters, advise athletes to expose the skin to air as much as possible by wearing sandals. Soaking feet several times a day in warm to hot water with a cup of Epsom salts helps dry out the blister. They should trim away any rough skin edges around the blister as they form. If there was blood in a blister, tell them to watch for signs of infection: redness and warmth at the blister site, red streaks going toward the heart, pus, tenderness, and/or pain.

Sprained ankles should be iced, wrapped with a compression wrap, and elevated above the heart. The ankle can be weight bearing as much as the athlete can tolerate.

Black toenails will benefit from Epsom salt soaks as well. Usually, black toenails will take months to resolve before the old nail falls off. If the nail is loose, wrapping a Band-Aid around the toe and nail will help keep it in place.

Your Tools

The final chapter in the book, "Foot Care Kits" on page 340, lists items that should be in a basic event foot care kit. When building a kit, add or subtract items based on your experience level. The quantity of supplies depends on the mileage, length of the event, the number of athletes you will be working with, and the number of days you'll working. My kit fits in a yellow toolbox.

At the 2010 Gore-Tex TransRockies Run, a six-day stage race in Colorado, I used two rolls of Kinesio Tex 1-inch tape, three rolls of 2-inch tape, and one roll of 3-inch tape. I also used several yards of HypaFix 2-inch tape and 60–70 compound tincture of benzoin swabs. Miscellaneous supplies included latex gloves, eight #11 scalpels, a tube each of zinc oxide and antibiotic ointment, several hundred alcohol wipes, a pack of 4x4 gauze, a container of hydrogen peroxide, a 10cc syringe and several 18-gauge needles, a bunch of ENGO Patches in different sizes, several scissors, tweezers, a Princeton Tec 1-watt headlamp, and several small bottles of hand sanitizer. There were 40 runners doing the three-day event and 220 doing the six-day event. In addition to me, two to three athletic trainers, who used supplies from their own trailer, were providing foot care daily.

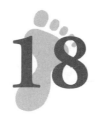

12 Mega-distance Athletes Talk about Foot Care

This is a unique chapter about 12 athletes who pushed the endurance envelope in an effort to accomplish something of significance. All 12 succeeded. Some ran while others walked. Six pursued their adventures predominately on trails; the others were mainly on pavement. The adventures range from walk or runs across America, the Pacific Crest and Appalachian trails, other long trails, and one run, amazingly, around the world.

I sent each of the 12 athletes the same set of nine questions about foot care and all graciously responded. The answers show how diverse the group was in how they managed their feet.

BOB BROWN Completed the Trans-America Race, the Trans-Australia run, and a 3,000 mile Trans-Europe run through eight countries. **www.bobbysrun.co.uk**

DEMETRI "COUP" COUPOUNAS Solo unsupported fast packs, not resupplied, of the Colorado Trail, Vermont's Long Trail, and California's John Muir Trail.

DAVID HORTON Completed the Trans-America Race, held the speed record on the Appalachian Trail for years, and in 2005 set the speed record on the 2,666-mile Pacific Crest Trail from Mexico to Canada in 66 days and seven hours. **www.extremeultrarunning.com**

BRUCE W. JOHNSON Ran across the U.S. from Oceanside, California, to Virginia Beach, Virginia, in 105 days. **www.unitedstatesrun.com**

TED "CAVE DOG" KEISER Fast packs and runs trails and mountain peaks. Completed a 50K hike in all 50 states in less than 100 days. **www.thedog team.com**

SUE NORWOOD Hiked the Appalachian Trail in 148 days. **www.runtrails.net**

JESPER OLSEN Ran 16,263 miles, circling the globe in his World Run starting January 1, 2004, and finishing on October 23, 2005. **www.worldrun.org**

ANDREW SKURKA In 2005 he made the first completion of the 7,700 mile Sea-to-Sea Route spanning the continent between the Atlantic and Pacific oceans in 339 days. **www.andrewskurka.com**

ANDREW "TRAILDOG" THOMPSON In 2005 he set a new speed record on the 2,174-mile Appalachian Trail in 47 days and 13 hours.

STEVE VAUGHT Calling himself "The Fat Man Walking," he walked 3,000 miles from San Diego to New York City to lose weight (he lost about 100 pounds) and regain his life. **www.thefatmanwalking.com**

JONATHAN WILLIAMS Ran across the U.S. in just over four months from Newport Beach, California, to Newport, Rhode Island, in 2005.

MATT WYBLE Ran across the U.S. from Atlantic City, New Jersey, to Lincoln, Oregon, in 2005 (with Brandon Newlin). **www.runacrosstheusa.com**

1 What shoes and socks did you use?

Bob Brown: I always wear Asics, usually whatever pair is on special offer. Because I don't get injured, I don't have to wear a specific type, but I always go for Asics. Socks: just cheap ankle socks.

Demetri "Coup" Coupounas: When I hike a day or two just for fun/training, I hike in crappy Walmart 88-cent cotton socks and put nothing on my feet. This trains my feet very well. When on big trails day after day, I wear either Wright Socks lightest version, two very thin pairs of CoolMax and just under the ankle high, or, if the trail is especially long and gritty/abusive to socks, I wear two pairs of dress socks—98% nylon, 2% Lycra, over the ankle, not stylish but very tough wearing. I like lightweight trail runners for almost everything—and very breathable uppers; the more mesh the better. Of course I change shoes when I get to the glacier/ice climbing, but I've gone to 18,000 feet twice in Salomon Tech Amphibians and loved them. When recovering, I wear Crocs, as the air is great for my feet.

David Horton: I used six pairs of Montrail Hardrocks and one pair of Montrail Leona Divides. I used about 15 pairs of Patagonia lightweight and silk-weight socks.

Bruce W. Johnson: I used New Balance 856. They quit making that shoe and I didn't research any other. When I only got 225 miles out of a pair before my joints started hurting, I ran out and had to experiment with other ones and that led to even worse problems. I finally found a pair of Nike Shox 2:45 and cut the sides open, and they are what I will wear next run. I bought 16 pairs in advance, a size larger than I wear.

Ted "Cave Dog" Keiser: Nike running shoes and Champion frictionless socks.

Sue Norwood: Four or five pairs of Montrail Hardrocks, one pair of Montrail Vitesse, and one pair of Montrail Highlines. The Hardrocks and Highlines have the same grippy soles and provided better traction on wet rocks, roots, and bog boards than the Vitesse. I replaced each pair after about 400 miles because the rocks chewed up the soles, but the uppers were all still in good shape. I was surprised to see so many hikers with backpacks wearing Hardrocks instead of hiking boots. I wore five pairs of Injinji socks the entire time and didn't get any holes in the socks or blisters on my toes. I wore very inexpensive thin socks over the Injinjis to reduce wear and friction. This system worked great!

Jesper Olsen: Due to sponsorship, I only used Asics Kayano and on occasion the Asics Gel 2000-series. I consider it optimal to switch between different brands and models during a training cycle of two to three weeks. But that was not possible during this run, and fortunately I didn't have any major problems on that account. I went through 28 pairs of shoes. For socks I used Asics's Kayano socks when available. Otherwise thin socks of whatever brand I could find. For instance, in Siberia there's not much choice. My favorite was without doubt the Kayano sock, mainly for comfort reasons.

Andrew Skurka: Socks: DeFeet Cush during the warmer months and DeFeet wool Blaze during the winter. Shoes: Montrail Masais and Highlines (I carried both and swapped off halfway through the day).

Andrew "Traildog" Thompson: I wore Flyrocs from Inov-8 along with their only variety of socks—MudSocks. In the north I used Fox River liners until I was confident in the resiliency of my feet.

Steve Vaught: SmartWool socks. I did not change my socks every time I stopped. I removed my socks, let them dry, and reused them. I used a cheap antiperspirant as a lubricant. I wear shoes that are one size too big for extra toe room but make sure that the box portion of the shoe is tight all the way from top to bottom.

Jonathan Williams: I wore New Balance 766s. Actually, New Balance gave me the shoes for the trip. I really liked the model and felt that they supported me well. As far as socks go, I wore cotton low-cut New Balance sports socks and I had a couple miscellaneous pairs with me.

Matt Wyble: We wore whatever shoes we could find cheap that were of decent quality. Brandon has a physical handicap that requires two different size shoes, so that also affected his choices. That being said, I think it really depends on the person. We bought shoes that we knew would work for us. As far as socks, we both wore Ultimax Ironman Triathlon half-crew socks almost exclusively. They are smooth and feel great. I get blisters pretty easily, and they really limited that and also dry very quickly.

2 How often did you change shoes and socks?

Bob Brown: I alternated socks every day. I usually have about ten pairs and change shoes every 500 miles.

Demetri "Coup" Coupounas: On long trips, I don't change shoes much at all. I find that I lose so much weight from both body and pack on alpine style thru-hikes that aren't resupplied that my feet don't grow appreciably—the weight loss offsets the mileage gain almost perfectly. I don't change socks much either. I almost always bring a backup pair (or pair of pairs if single socks) but have gone multiple weeks in the same socks day after day after day. I do take them off at night. I find that having the spare just in case or for the last few days works, as does rotating daily. On the very hottest of hot days, I'll take the shoes and socks off for an extended break in the heat of the day, but then I put the same ones back on.

David Horton: I changed shoes when I felt that they needed to be changed. I put on clean socks every day.

Ted "Cave Dog" Keiser: I change my shoes and socks according to the situation. If it is hot and my feet are sweaty, then I change them much more often than if they are cool and dry. I generally retire shoes after about 500 miles and socks when they have holes.

Sue Norwood: I never changed shoes or socks during the day. The longest I was on the trail each day was 14 hours. I usually averaged about 10–11 hours per day. My shoes and socks often got wet, but that doesn't cause me problems. Gritty and/or sandy trails are a problem for me (blisters), and I didn't run into those on the A.T.

Jesper Olsen: I did a maximum of 900K per pair of shoes with a minimum of 700–800K. I am almost certain that it makes a crucial difference in injury prevention. The strong Russian runner who started together with me in London had to give up in Siberia, approximately 9,800K into the run, due to severe injuries. He did around 3,000K per pair!

Andrew Skurka: Shoes: about every 500 miles per pair (1,000 miles total because I had two pairs with me). Socks: every ten days, or 250–300 miles.

Andrew "Traildog" Thompson: I changed both about once a day—whenever I thought the trail had dried out from dew. Sometimes I didn't change at all. I always had dry stuff at my disposal though.

Steve Vaught: Once a day.

Jonathan Williams: My trip was approximately 3,300 miles and I went through eight pairs of shoes. Unfortunately, I couldn't always get the pair right when I needed them because the pairs were mailed to me, and I had to be near a town with a post office I could get to in order for them to be mailed out. I also would carry with me two pairs of shoes at a time and alternate the pairs every couple of days. I would have two new pairs mailed out approximately every four weeks. I would change my socks every day. I brought about seven pairs with me and would always get a chance to wash them before I ran out.

Matt Wyble: We generally changed shoes and socks every day, switching back and forth between two pairs of shoes each day and rotating in a new pair as each pair got about 500 miles on them. If our feet got wet and later it was possible for them to dry out, we'd almost always switch.

3 Did you carry any foot care supplies? If so, what?

Bob Brown: Just carried Compeed in case of blisters and Vaseline. That's about it!

Demetri "Coup" Coupounas: I carry Hydropel and apply it liberally to both feet first thing every morning. Even after 50 miles and in and out of water all day, I find that the Hydropel is still there. I carry Dr. Scholl's foot powder and apply it every night. I think it cleans my feet pretty well, let alone dries them, and keeps athlete's foot at bay. I actually carry it in the original bottle because the delivery is so much better than in a film canister. I carry a very few other foot care items—a few Spenco 2nd Skin and the thin stretch cousin, a single moleskin and Molefoam patch, and a tiny bit of tape—but I find that I rarely (1 day in 50) use any of this stuff. I'm all about prevention.

David Horton: I used some moleskin and duct tape.

Ted "Cave Dog" Keiser: I do not carry any foot care supplies, but my support crew does: Vaseline, sticky spray, bandages, moleskin, tape, and so on.

Sue Norwood: In my Camelbak H.A.W.G. I carried a little bag with extra bandages (Blist-o-Ban, 2nd Skin Blister Pads, and Band-Aid Blister Block), an alcohol prep, a Wet Ones wipe, and a safety pin. I don't remember ever having to stop during the day to fix a hot spot or blister, just in the camper afterward.

Jesper Olsen: No. But I did have some scotch tape for worst cases, but fortunately I didn't need it.

Andrew Skurka: Just Sportslick.

Andrew "Traildog" Thompson: I carried nothing in terms of foot care supplies. In the truck I had cornstarch, waterproof tape, needles, clippers, and gauze.

Steve Vaught: I carried Hydropel Sports ointment and first-aid stuff.

Jonathan Williams: I had Dr. Scholl's moleskin. I didn't really use it, though. I did use Dr. Scholl's Blister Pads, which worked great, Band-Aids, and most important, orthotics.

Matt Wyble: We didn't really carry foot care supplies. I do own some, but I didn't even bring them with me. Beyond nail clippers and maybe an emery board, I don't think we had anything else. We always removed our shoes whenever possible, and I think that helped tremendously.

4 What problems did you have with your feet?

Bob Brown: I had one blister running across Australia but none across the U.S. and Europe. No problems at all. I cut the toe box out of my shoes, which prevents blisters.

Demetri "Coup" Coupounas: I rarely deviate from the above, so I rarely have problems. On the Triple Gem Alpine Style—the John Muir Trail, Long Trail, and the Colorado Trail—I had zero blisters in about 1,000 miles, for instance. I did get minor bruising on my heels on the Colorado Trail from trail runners that are too stiff for me—the Montrail Hardrocks.

David Horton: I got two blisters on my left foot, one under my second toe, and one between my little toe and next toe. These blisters started about the end of the second week and lasted for about five weeks.

Bruce W. Johnson: My feet were the biggest concern overall. Before this, I never took them into consideration. Now they are my main focus. Once swelling started and the pavement got hot—that led to more swelling.

Ted "Cave Dog" Keiser: If my feet are wet for a long period of time, they get wrinkled, much like a person's fingers when they are wet for a long time. There is a spot on the ball of both of my feet where the wrinkle is so deep that it feels like a knife piercing the skin with every step. Keep the feet dry, and it is fine.

Sue Norwood: Surprisingly few! The first three weeks I got 1) some fluid under a callous on the outside of my right big toe (minor bunion there) and 2) a blister on the outside of my other foot about halfway between the heel and little toe. I used the Blist-o-Ban bandages successfully on these two spots and they healed in a few days. I continued using the bandages for prevention for another couple weeks, then didn't need anything in those areas the rest of the trek. In New England, one of my little toenails became swollen and painful. I'm guessing it got infected in the swamps or mud I was running through. I drained it, soaked it a few times in Epsom salts, and bandaged it when I ran. Jim cut a slit on the side of three pairs of shoes I was alternating to take pressure off. My toe was OK in a few days.

Jesper Olsen: Usually I very, very seldom have problems with my feet. This is probably due to 22 years of marathon and competition running (I did my first marathon when I was 15). The same was the case during the 22 months of my 26,232K of my World Run—no feet problems. There was a beginning blister under the big toe on the left foot on day two in the Colac Six Day Race, which I did during the run (result 756K and first place overall). It was November and quite hot on the track. With immediate care before it got to be more than a sore red area, it didn't develop further.

Andrew Skurka: Bunion in left foot, which is partly hereditary and partly because of all the time I was spending on my feet.

Andrew "Traildog" Thompson: Problems: constant heel bump erosion/callousing, thickening of all foot calluses, splitting of the little toe ridge, blackening of the second and fourth toenails, and deep ridges on the bottoms of my feet due to moisture. Hot spots in the center of the bottom of the forefoot, soreness in all toes from kicking roots, and major soreness in the pinky toes due to swollen feet being crammed into shoes. My pinky toes doubled in size for the entire hike. Those little buggers were extremely beat up—all the time. I wore shoes that were a half size large for the whole trip, and every morning I was very glad I did.

Jonathan Williams: I had some blisters, although not as many as I thought I would have. I would put one of the blister pads and a Band-Aid on it and that would usually take care of the problem. I would also get aches and pains in my foot throughout the run but this was not unusual because I got aches and pains throughout my legs. Something hurt everyday. However, every time something hurt, the orthotics would be adjusted and the pain would go away from that spot.

Matt Wyble: We didn't have any serious problems with our feet. I probably had the worst of it. I lost most of the feeling in my toes early into the run from slapping on the pavement and general swelling, and the feeling didn't fully return until about a month after we finished the run. I also had a lot of foot blisters, but that was just something that I had to live with.

5 Did any foot issues compound themselves over time?

Demetri "Coup" Coupounas: The only problem [minor bruising on the heels] got worse over time but was never bad and never required treatment. Many years I go out much too fast and far much too early, get in really deep snow for eight to ten hours, get blisters, and take a few weeks off. So I know that what's working the rest of the time is doing the right things, not having some gift.

David Horton: The one blister under my second toe was very painful for a long time. I was afraid that it was going to get infected, but it never did. I would put a doughnut around it and then duct tape or some other kind of tape over that.

Bruce W. Johnson: Again, once the swelling started and the pavement got hot— that led to more swelling.

Sue Norwood: No, each problem healed pretty fast with the solutions I mentioned.

Jesper Olsen: No. I think it's important for athletes to train their abilities to sense injuries and blisters before they develop. It's trainable just like anything else!

Andrew "Traildog" Thompson: My heel bumps developed deep blisters under the calluses. I tore into one about halfway through the hike. It smelled like rotting flesh and it was immediately swarmed by 20–30 small flies that wallowed in the putrefied flesh and fluid—something was evidently dead in there. It was a gross concept.

Steve Vaught: No, if you maintain strict foot care routines, you will not have compounding issues.

Matt Wyble: I may have had a slight amount of compound issues with favoring a certain gait due to bad blisters. I had to focus to walk normally, even if it was less comfortable.

6 Did you have any overuse issues (for example, with tendons and so on)?

Bob Brown: I have had Achilles problems before, but I counter this now by cutting part of the heel tabs off. I feel they are too high on most trainers, which aggravates the Achilles.

Demetri "Coup" Coupounas: No—I'm not an overuse guy. I've always had the long run (walk) in mind and won't push myself beyond my limits. It's just so unproductive and miserable. No, thanks.

David Horton: I had no problems with tendons or ligaments. My knees did hurt quite a bit for the last 500 or so miles and they still hurt three months after finishing. I had cracks on my heels that developed. I had to make sure to put a lot of lotion on them to make sure that they didn't get any deeper or worse.

Bruce W. Johnson: My feet swelled up so badly that I didn't have to tie my shoes. The skin was splitting on the heels and bleeding. My feet are still the only thing that still had an arthritic feel to them.

Sue Norwood: Yes, about four to five weeks into the run. First one, then the other, outer side of my lower legs got swollen and tender just above the ankle joint. We went home three times during the adventure run. I saw my orthopedist when one of the legs was swollen. He determined the pain was at a nerve ending and diagnosed it as inflammation or herniation of soft tissue. Based on the location of the pain, he didn't believe it was a stress fracture. Both ankles/lower legs were fine after a few days of icing, elevation, and a different pain medication than I had been using. I didn't take any days off just for these injuries but ran through them.

Jesper Olsen: Yes, in the first five to eight weeks when my body struggled to adapt to the 50K a day I was averaging, and from pushing the baby stroller (with my gear). I had Achilles soreness, knee soreness, ITB [iliotibial band syndrome] soreness, and back and spine pain. After 5,000K into the run, I had no major issues.

Andrew Thompson: Even now, when I dorsiflex each foot, the tendons atop each foot are aching. Nothing really bothered me during the hike, however.

Steve Vaught: I pulled three tendons in my knee early on but nothing since.

Jonathan Williams: My Achilles was a big problem at one point. However, I was given a new orthotic with a heal lift in it and that alleviated the pressure on the Achilles. My knee, ankle, shin, hip . . . hurt at different points but were all helped by the orthotics.

Matt Wyble: My overuse injuries were mostly in my lower leg, nothing really in my foot.

7 What could have helped you better manage your feet?

Bob Brown: Nothing, as I haven't had any problems.

Demetri "Coup" Coupounas: I think they're pretty dialed.

David Horton: Stay out of the water and not run so many miles each day. Impossible!

Bruce W. Johnson: Wider and larger shoes.

Ted "Cave Dog" Keiser: Pay attention to your feet. They are your point of contact with the ground. An injury to your feet is more detrimental to your performance than an injury to most of the rest of your body.

Sue Norwood: Reducing the callus on my bunion more before I began the trek, putting a Blist-o-Ban on the side of the foot before it became a blister, and reducing my mileage (the latter was not acceptable, however).

Jesper Olsen: Dry socks and shoes. I had no injuries, as mentioned, but a lot of basic discomfort from running weeks in wet shoes and socks. The low intensity of the pace, around nine to ten minutes a mile, meant that it didn't develop into injuries to my feet.

Andrew Skurka: Nothing. I really had very few foot problems, or physical problems for that matter.

Andrew "Traildog" Thompson: Only time off would have improved my foot problems—unfortunately, the clock never stopped.

Steve Vaught: Only more experience.

Jonathan Williams: I don't really know anything about preventive care, so maybe if I knew something about that. It seems that with running this many miles, something is going to happen to the feet no matter what. I was just lucky that nothing really bad happened.

Matt Wyble: More Ultimax Ironman Triathlon socks, switching out shoes more often, probably some sort of powder to keep them dry.

8 Did you have a morning/night ritual for caring for your feet?

Bob Brown: In the early stages, Vaseline between the toes, but after about two weeks my feet are like leather, so I don't even bother with Vaseline after week two.

Demetri "Coup" Coupounas: I apply Hydropel to both feet first thing every morning. I squeeze one full index-finger's length onto each ball, and then work it in all over the sole, all over every toe, and just an inch or so up every side of my foot. I then put on my socks and shoes before heading out. All day I hike with the lightest load I can (less stress all over body including my feet), keep a moderate pace (which cuts down on klutzy moves among other things), and keep well fed and hydrated (better for every bodily function, including repetitive feet impacts and push offs). I use trekking poles on long trips, finding that the roughly 20% of force transferred to my upper body extends my comfortable range by about 25% (same work is done by feet and they are the limiting factor). I tend not to use poles on short training hikes to better train my feet. Light poles, such as REI's 12- or 13-ounce poles, are key, as the lighter they are, the easier it is for your hands to keep up with your feet. Each night, I take off my shoes and socks as soon as possible, powder with Dr. Scholl's, then hop in my sleeping bag. Eating, map work, and so on is all done from inside the sack to maximize my feet's warm and dry time. I find that they can take a lot of abuse each day if they get a full night's rest while warm and dry. I used to wash them but find the foot powder suffices for that function too.

David Horton: In the morning I would tape them up to try to prevent dirt from getting into the blisters. At night the first thing that I cleaned up was my feet. I tried to do that every night.

Bruce W. Johnson: Elevate your feet after running. I wore tight socks when elevating them. Ice them if you can. I slept with a pillow under the foot end of my mattress to keep feet elevated all night, even though it was harder to sleep. I found that this helped with the swelling.

Sue Norwood: In the morning I sometimes put Hydropel on my toes, but they seemed to do as well without it as with it. I put on new Blist-o-Ban bandages each morning when I needed them. I loved them, but they don't stay on well after a shower—expensive to use two new ones every day. In the afternoon I examined my feet carefully after I showered and determined what needed attention, looked for blisters or reddened areas (none after the first three to four weeks), cut the toenails or removed nails that were so soft they came right off, and filed down that callus every few days. By the end of the trek, the skin on the balls of my feet had thickened noticeably. I considered that a good thing; I never blistered there.

Jesper Olsen: For about the last 20 years I've done strength and mobility exercises for the feet, two to three times daily for five to ten minutes, unless impossible (seldom) and of course also during my World Run. For me it's my main strategy in preventing injuries—not only foot injuries. After all, the feet are the only body part that carries the full weight and impact during running. Therefore, I think it's essential to keep working on strength and flexibility of the feet, the toes individually, the whole foot, forefoot, and the ankle.

Andrew Skurka: Put on PossumDown socks from **www.backpackinglight.com.**

Andrew "Traildog" Thompson: I drenched my feet in straight cornstarch every morning, night, and between shoe and sock changes. At night I let my feet breathe as much as the cold would allow. I slept barefoot when I wasn't having night sweats. I would sweat nearly every night, though. Then I would wear a fresh pair of Inov-8 socks. My sponsor was generous enough to ensure that even late in the trip, I would find myself still pulling brand-new socks out of my bag—nothing better. Cornstarch was used as soon as I could get off my feet, get clean, and elevate my feet. Time was the major factor I was constantly up against.

Steve Vaught: I just wash them and give them a massage.

Jonathan Williams: Not really, except when I had a blister, and that just entailed putting a blister pad on it and a Band-Aid for padding.

Matt Wyble: Just taking off our shoes and socks and draining any blisters that had appeared using a safety pin.

9 What could others learn from your experience?

Bob Brown: You don't necessarily need tons of equipment and potions. Adapt your trainer shoes to suit your needs. If you do feel a blister coming in a long race, get it treated immediately. I have seen many people quit races because of blisters when they were otherwise in great shape.

Demetri "Coup" Coupounas: How to hike 1,000 miles without getting a single blister—though others should modify my methods some to suit their physiology and temperament. Also, doing all the right stuff works! And is big-time worth it. Finally, take it easy. Two miles an hour is gentle on your feet, and 15 hours a day is totally sustainable with a very light load—that's where consecutive 30-mile days come from, and once you've experienced them, you see how easy and enjoyable they are.

David Horton: If you can keep your feet dry, and you have the proper shoes and socks, blisters should not be a problem. In multiday adventures this is impossible.

Bruce W. Johnson: My advice is to monitor your feet closely and try to reduce swelling as fast as possible. Wear shoes that are wider and larger than you think you need.

Ted "Cave Dog" Keiser: Remember that it takes three factors to cause a blister: friction, moisture, and heat. Take any one of these factors out, and you will not be able to create a blister.

Sue Norwood: Run a lot of miles in training on the types of surfaces you'll be doing in an ultra or adventure run. It will toughen your feet and strengthen your muscular-skeletal system to help prevent blisters and injuries from occurring in the first place. Try wearing Injinji socks with a thin sock over them, use something such as Blist-o-Ban bandages on hot spots to prevent blisters from forming, and be sure that your shoes are large enough to prevent rubbing when your feet swell after hours and hours of running. I didn't know if my body would hold up over so many miles. I'm in my early 60s and have osteoarthritis in (probably) every joint. The two places I expected the most problems were my left ankle, where I had surgery a few years ago for two ruptured tendons, and my right second toe, where I had surgery six months before this trek (again, two ruptured tendons). Fortunately, neither site caused any problems. I didn't even tweak either ankle, despite all the rocks, roots, and other trail obstacles, because I wore ASO ankle supports on both ankles every day on the A. T.

Jesper Olsen: Listen to your body. A strong performance comes from a strong understanding and harmony of your body.

Andrew Skurka: It really helps to have tough feet to start with. I've been running competitively since high school so my feet are pretty tough. Wear non-waterproof running shoes. Carry a light pack. Coat your feet with a silicone-based ointment (such as Sportslick, Hydropel, or BodyGlide) when they get wet in order to water-proof them and to prevent cracking or blistering from them getting soft. If you are putting in long days, carry two pairs of shoes—the extra two pounds is a really good investment.

Andrew "Traildog" Thompson: I only want to stress my belief on always finding a way to deal with problems and continuing on. I never lost a mile on account of foot problems. Coming through Pennsylvania I thought that I had seriously messed up the inner workings of my right forefoot. It felt like I was walking on a golf ball—literally. We hemmed and hawed over the issue. I thought about going to a foot doctor. Instead I pushed a needle through the center of the bottom of my forefoot. A single drop of fluid was released and the pain was instantly alleviated. I ran hard the remainder of the day and never thought about it again. After my hike, the skin from the bottoms of my feet came off in sheets. In a few months, the numbness went away—again after I thought I had caused permanent nerve damage.

Steve Vaught: Listen to the advice of others, accept what sounds reasonable, but ultimately your body will tell you what you need.

Jonathan Williams: The orthotics were great. They really helped a lot, so if you are plagued with injury, it might be beneficial to give them a try. The blister pads worked well to help heal blisters. Blisters are painful, but we can run through them if we need to.

Matt Wyble: Do not let your feet stay wet for long periods of time. It causes blisters and can also lead to infection. Drain blisters with something sterilized only. Poke them open; don't cut them open. Make sure you get good insoles for your shoes if your own shoes don't have very good ones—it is extremely important and they are able to absorb a large amount of the impact from your foot striking the ground. If something with your shoe hurts during a short time wearing them, don't try to tough it out, as it is only going to get worse. Get professionally fitted for shoes, and do it at the end of a day when you've been walking quite a bit so that your feet are already swollen; otherwise, you may find that your shoes are too small. Blister problems? Get moisture-wicking socks!

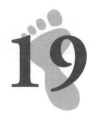

Preventing Blisters

Most athletes hold a common misconception about blisters—that blisters are simply a fact of life that one must learn to live with. Most athletes try tips that they have learned from others. If those don't work, they move on to another idea. Most try for a while, then give up and spend the rest of their life fixing their inevitable blisters. The fact is that there are many ways to prevent blisters.

Ultrarunner Mark Swanson writes about what he did for his feet at the 2005 Western States 100: "Here's what worked for me. I smeared BodyGlide over my feet and put on Injinji socks. Then I put Gold Bond powder in thin liner socks and put those on over the Injinji socks and wore gaiters. I ended the race with a couple of small starter blisters but nothing that gave me any trouble. Changed shoes and socks at Foresthill, though I wished I hadn't as the new shoes were a tad snug and I'll probably lose a couple of nails as a result—not to mention the minutes I lost!"

Mark applied something to his feet (BodyGlide), around his feet (socks), in combination (powder and another pair of socks), and then added a general item (gaiters). After one more story, we'll look at these types of things we can do to prevent blisters.

Adventure racer Dan O'Shea spent eight years learning what works for him in preventing blisters: "I have trained my feet for the stress of my sport, and they have a tough outer layer. For races, I use compound tincture of benzoin, followed by Sports Slick lubricant, and then a double-sock system." At the 1999 Beast of the East Adventure Race he raced with two first-timers whose feet were hardly conditioned to the rigors of a five-day race. After two days of racing Dan found that "both these individuals had blisters on top of blisters and could walk only with great pain." Dan and teammate Harold Zundel, both former Navy SEALs and experienced racers, had maybe one blister between the two of them. Over the years he has learned different blister prevention techniques that work best on his feet. But he also realizes that what works for him may change over time as he gets new or different shoes, as his feet change, and as he participates in different types of events under changing conditions. Dan has the right approach—keep on learning and always be open to new blister prevention ideas.

Understand that while the blister prevention techniques you currently use may work today, they may not work tomorrow. I have patched the feet of many ultramarathoners and adventure racers who claim to have never had problems before. Knowing what options are available will help you be prepared. The ideas that follow show the importance of learning what works for your feet.

Things You Can Do for Your Feet

Many athletes believe they that what they do to their feet helps prevent blisters. Here are the most effective:

- Pamper your feet with a pedicure.

- Give yourself foot massages whenever you can.

- Get rid of calluses and keep the skin on your feet soft.

- Keep your toenails clipped short and buff them to get rid of all the rough spots.

- Keep your feet dry by changing socks whenever possible.

- Try to keep your feet dry, air them out at breaks, and change from wet socks to dry ones.

- Toughen the skin on your feet by walking and running barefoot on grass, dirt, and sand.

Things You Apply to Your Feet

There are many things you can apply to your feet to help prevent blisters. Lubricants and tape are two of the most popular. Powders are a distant third. Remember that whatever you apply to your feet will react to what you put around your feet. When you apply a lubricant, your socks will pick up some of it, and more applications will be necessary. Tape works well, but tape applied poorly can be pulled loose as you pull on your socks. Here are the best ideas:

- Use a callus cream to soften calluses and prevent friction and resulting blisters.

- Use one of the popular lubricants to reduce friction. BodyGlide, Hydropel Sports Ointment, Bag Balm, BlisterShield Roll-On, Brave Soldier's Friction Zone, and Sports Slick are the most popular. Reapply each time you change your socks.

- Use powder—such as BlisterShield, Zeasorb, Odor-Eaters, or Gold Bond foot powder—to reduce friction.

- Use one of the popular blister patching products, such as Spenco 2nd Skin, Blist-O-Ban, or Bunheads Gel Toe Caps.

- Use one of the popular tapes—such as Kinesio Tex, Leukotape, Elastikon, or duct tape—to pretape known hot spots or problem areas before your event.

- Use Certain Dri Antiperspirant or Ban Roll-On on your feet to control perspiration.

- Use a slick energy gel wrapper between your sock and shoe to reduce friction.

- Avoid petroleum jelly—it's sticky, attracts grit, and hardens on socks.

- For wet conditions, coat your feet with Hydropel Sports Ointment, Desitin Maximum Strength, or Sudocrem twice a day during a big race. Primarily designed to prevent diaper rash, this antiseptic healing cream leaves an oily trace on your feet and lasts for ages.

- Put a patch of lamb's wool on a bruised, sore, or blistered area, and secure it to the foot with tape.

Things You Put Around Your Feet

What you put around your feet is one of the most important factors in blister prevention. The wrong type of socks or footwear that fits incorrectly can create pressure points and blisters. This is an area where trying different ideas can really pay off.

- Use an ENGO Patch inside your shoe or on your insole to reduce friction.

- Wear two pairs of thin socks, a liner sock under a heavier sock, or double-layer socks.

- Always use moisture-wicking socks—no cotton.

- Wear SealSkinz WaterBlocker socks for really wet conditions.

- Wear Injinji toe socks if you have frequent toe blisters.

- For bottom of the feet and heel blisters, try another insole.

- The heel is the first part of the sock to wear thin. Get new socks before they get too threadbare.

- Be sure to smooth the heels of your socks. Also, check the heels of your insoles and the inside of your heel counters for folds and either worn or torn material.

- Replace worn-out shoes.

- Use shoes that are tested for the event, distance, and the elements: cold versus hot, roads versus trails, and wet conditions.

- Try another pair of shoes—many shoes breathe better than others and are easier on your feet.

- To drain water, use a red-hot nail to burn drain holes on the sides of your shoes right at the sock liner height where the shoe bends.

- Well-made and well-fit orthotics will help prevent blisters.

- Wear gaiters to keep rocks, dust, and dirt out of your shoes.

Things You Do in Combination

Some blister prevention ideas work best in combination with other ideas: BodyGlide and wicking socks, compound tincture of benzoin to hold tape on the feet, and skin toughening agents and double-layer socks. The list goes on and on.

- Get a pedicure at least once a month to smooth out all calluses and rough spots, and put creams on your feet on a daily basis.

- Use one of the lubricants liberally on your feet and then pull on moisture-wicking socks.

- Use one of the tape adherents liberally on your feet; then apply powder to cut the stickiness, and then pull on moisture-wicking socks.

- Use one of the tape adherents liberally on your feet, and then tape your feet.

- Apply one of the moisture-controlling products (such as Hydropel Sports Ointment or Desitin Maximum Strength) to your feet the night before a race, and then the socks you will run in the next day. Reapply the ointment in the morning and use the same socks.

- Wear good shoes and socks that fit properly.

- Keep your feet dry and wear good clean moisture-wicking socks.

Things You Do in General

In addition to doing things to your feet, applying things to your feet, and being careful of what you put around your feet, there are other helpful ideas in preventing blisters. The ideas here run the gamut from lacing techniques, hydration, and proper footwear fit to regular changes of socks.

- Buy footwear only from sources where you can be fitted properly.

- Stay properly hydrated with electrolytes to maintain good sodium levels.

- Learn different lacing techniques to prevent your feet from slipping inside the shoes.

■ Change to a different insole that has a smoother surface or use a heat-molded insole shaped to your feet.

■ Inspect your feet at rest stops, breaks, and each evening to find hot spots and problem areas. At the same time, clean out your shoes and under the insoles, and change socks.

■ Get a pedicure to manage your toenails and skin.

■ Elevate your feet at breaks and at night to keep swelling down.

■ Avoid wearing damp socks.

■ Rotate between several pairs of shoes.

■ Allow your feet to dry out as often as possible, including taking shoes off during breaks when you're out for a long hike.

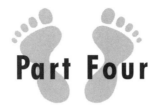

Part Four

Treatments

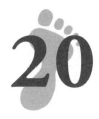

Treating Your Feet

The Fourth Law of Running Injuries:
Virtually all running injuries are curable. Only a minute fraction of true running injuries are not entirely curable by quite simple techniques.

—Tim Noakes, MD, **Lore of Running**[25]

No matter how hard we try to prevent problems with our feet, there may come a time when they need repairing. Then you become reactive. Many athletes are forced to be reactive in treating problems because they fail to take the time to find what their feet need and how they respond to the conditions they subject them to.

The following chapters explain how to fix typical foot problems. It is always best to know how to fix problems before they develop. Beginning a long trail run or a multiday hike without preparing for the possibility of blisters, a sprained ankle, or other potential injury is foolhardy. One or two unexpected blisters at the wrong time can spell the end to a long-anticipated event.

In 2000 I conducted a survey of runners, ultrarunners, triathletes, hikers, and adventure racers. While not a formal scientific survey, the 214 responses showed some interesting results:

■ Athlete's foot is more common in males.

■ Black toenails affect 71%.

■ Calluses affect 49%.

■ Ingrown toenails have affected 32%.

■ Morton's foot affects 30%.

■ Sprained ankles affect 11% now and have affected 36% in the past. Many participants have experienced this more than 15 times—the highest was 30 times!

■ Missing toenails have affected 57%.

■ Achilles tendinitis affects 11% now and has affected 25% in the past.

■ Plantar fasciitis affects 17% now and has affected 30% in the past.

■ Orthotics are worn by 36%.

As you can see from the results, most of us are not immune to injuries or problems with our feet. Of particular interest was that many of those surveyed had two or more problems with their feet at the same time. What the survey told me was that athletes need to know how to treat common foot ailments—not just what they now have, but what they might experience as a result of their activity.

The Marathon des Sables, an extreme six-day, self-supported race in the Moroccan desert, treats runners to 150 miles of sand, sand, and more sand; 200-foot sand dunes; rocky roads with small odd-shaped stones; heat that sucks the moisture out of skin, and winds and sandstorms that torment every inch of your being. Robert Nagle, a highly experienced Eco Challenge adventure racer, ran the race in 1997 and had only one blister. He commented, "Many of the participants have neither the experience nor knowledge of foot care for ultras—so they suffer mightily." The name of the game is to plan ahead to finish well and with healthy feet. If you don't, you are at a disadvantage right from the start.

In 1996 Dave Covey, an experienced ultrarunner, participated in a competitive and challenging 25-day 600K wilderness trek across Western Australia that stressed his feet beyond his wildest imagination. While working in a walking and backpacking shoe store, he studied the different types of boots and selected a nylon-and-leather boot with a Gore-Tex fabric interior. The combination of high temperatures, long pants, and wearing heavy-duty nylon gaiters to protect his legs from the spiny vegetation made his legs sweat constantly. With his feet always wet, and the terrain very uneven and rocky, his feet were subject to extreme punishment. Changing into dry wicking-style socks every two hours helped for the first two days. By the third day blisters had developed on the bottoms of his toes. Moleskin simply would not adhere to the wet skin. By the end of the eighth day he rested his feet for a few days to try to dry out the blisters. He then used Betadine and duct tape on the toes. By the 18th day, the skin finally began to callous over, and during the last six days of the trek, he did not have to use any tape. Dave gave his boots high marks for comfort, realizing the blisters were caused by other factors.

In the above two cases, Robert and Dave had done their homework. They knew what their feet needed to complete their extreme event. They planned and were prepared. Whether we are doing something similar or something much, much easier, we too need to have a basic understanding of treatments to fix our feet.

Some things are very basic. When your feet are tired, you have several ways to help them feel better. When changing socks, stopping for lunch, or whenever possible, take a few minutes and massage your feet and check for any hot spots. A short soak in an icy stream or in a bucket of cold water can revitalize tired feet. When you sit down to change socks or shoes after being on your feet for any great length of time, elevating your feet above the level of your heart will help reduce swelling of the feet. While hiking or on adventure races, try to wash your feet with soap and water at least once per day, preferably in the evening.

Other things are more detailed and complex and are included in the chapters that follow. The information includes descriptions of problems, ways to treat them, products that can help relieve or solve them, and, in some cases, exercises to strengthen the affected areas. Read the chapters that pertain to your injury history, and try the treatments and products to find those that will resolve your problems.

21

Blisters

An article in the August 2004 *Journal of Emergency Medicine*, "Event Medicine: Injury and Illness During an Expedition-Length Adventure Race," reported: ". . . blisters on the feet [represent] the single most common injury at 32.8% of all reported and treated cases." The article was written by David Townes, MD, an ER doctor who led the medical teams at the Primal Quest Adventure Races, and three other MDs.[26]

Blisters start out as hot spots. If caught in time and treated, hot spots can be controlled. Left to their own, they will develop into an irritating blister that can stop you in your tracks, end your athletic event, and sideline you for weeks. Blisters can be painful but can also cause you to change your gait to avoid putting pressure on the spot, thereby changing your stride, which can lead to injuries. Hot spots are simple to prevent and treat. Blisters are different. Many athletes think that there is one way to patch blisters. This chapter will show you many different ways to manage pesky blisters. Some are simple and quick. Others are complex and take more time—because they are meant to last during an ultramarathon or adventure race.

Part of caring for blisters is to also identify and eliminate the problem that caused them in the first place. One runner reported having developed the first blisters he had ever gotten while running, though he didn't notice them until afterward. After a 50-mile trial run he had two identical blisters, one on the tip of each little toe. Here is where detective work can get tricky. The blisters could have been caused by the seam welt over the little toes on the inside of the sock (a very common problem in a very common spot). It could have been the fit of the shoes—perhaps the shoes and/or the toe box were too short. The toenails could have been the culprits if they were too long, catching on the socks and making the socks bunch up at that point. Or the downhills could have been the culprit. Then too, the runner could have had a problem with his little toes—perhaps they were longer than normal or angled in such a way to be more prone to friction. Be aware of all the factors that go into the fit of your shoes and socks and how everything on and around your feet works as a unit. Simply patching a blister and continuing on is fixing only part of the problem.

Athletes talk about repeatedly getting blisters in the same place over and over and of getting blisters where they never had them before. Blisters can occur anywhere and at any time. When someone asks me about their specific blister problem, I always ask them, "What changed?" For more on this, read the section, "What Changed?" on page 12.

Treating blisters takes time and practice. Denise Jones tells of a runner at the Death Valley Badwater Ultramarathon:

> He had a combination of the wrong socks (all cotton), shoes that became too small once his feet swelled after 115 miles, and virtually no adequate tape with which to repair his throbbing feet. After nearly an hour and a half, I was able to drain and dress his blisters and cut the toes out of his shoes so that the swollen nubs—his toes—could become less crowded. I was pleased to learn that after that session of repair, he was able to complete the distance and finish the race. He thanked me over and over for helping him.

Hot Spots

Most runners experience hot spots in the areas where they are susceptible to blisters forming. The area will become sore and red—thus the name hot spot. You may also experience a stinging or burning sensation. Around the reddened area will be a paler area that enlarges inward to where the skin is being rubbed.[27] The area becomes elevated because the surface skin is lifted as it fills with fluid. The hot spot has then become a blister.

When you feel a hot spot develop, check your socks to be sure that they have not bunched up, retie your laces, and check inside your shoe to be sure that there is no debris that could be an irritant.

Treating Hot Spots

You must deal with these hot spots before they become blisters. By the time the hot spot has developed enough to be felt, protection is necessary. Take the time to deal with hot spots as you feel them develop. Continuing to run or hike on them will only make them worse. Untreated hot spots usually turn into blisters, which are harder to treat. Use your choice of one of the tapes or blister-care products described in this book to protect the area. If you have used lubricants or powders on your feet, clean the affected area with an alcohol wipe before applying tape, adhesive felt, or moleskin. In a pinch, when you are out in the middle of nowhere and develop a hot spot, use a dab of lip balm on the hot spot or put an energy gel wrapper or other slick paper over the hot spot between your sock and shoe.

Patty Gray, of the Muir Trail Ranch in the California High Sierra, learned of Dr. Scholl's lamb's wool years ago from a ballet dancer. Dancers use it in their toe shoes. She sees on average 1,000 backpackers through the ranch each year. Patty says, "I've suggested its use at the first sign of a hot spot, especially on/in the toe area to be wrapped around the digit. It stays in place nicely by itself and is also useful too in protection of the toes/toenails should they be bumping the end of the boot." The lamb's wool is a staple in their foot care box.

Hot spots typically develop from pressure caused by your footwear or socks. Examine your shoes or boots to determine whether you can modify them to remove the pressure point causing the problem. You may have to make a slit or cut out a small section in the side or toe of the shoe. Start with a small cut or hole and enlarge it as necessary. Be sure that your socks are not bunched up and creating pressure points. Run your hands inside the socks to remove any loose lint balls. After putting on your socks, use your hands to smooth the material around the shape of each foot.

Beyond Hot Spots: Blisters

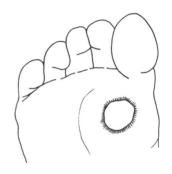

Basically, blisters are an injury. And as we all know, blisters can be painful. One blister in a sensitive place on the foot can easily ruin an otherwise good day. Blisters have often destroyed months of training and hundreds of dollars spent on a major event. Several blisters can drain your energy and reduce a runner to a walker or a hiker to a plodder, which in turn tends to create more blisters, which then slows forward motion even more. Too many athletes fail to educate themselves about blister prevention and how to do adequate blister care. Many runners and hikers think blisters are unavoidable and simply a part of the running or hiking process. Sometimes I think we should offer an award to the folks with the biggest blisters! Yet, somehow, when I remove a runner's shoe at the aid station and the skin falls off half of each foot, I realize the runner should not get an award but an education on good foot care.

An Experiment of One

Ultrarunner Mark Williams has learned that the blister issue is an individual one: "What works for one may not work for the other. You must experiment, experiment, and experiment. If something doesn't work, don't try to make it work. I've had some nasty blister issues. I tried taping, Bag Balm, Runner's Lube, Vaseline, wider shoes, and longer shoes. I think the blister issue is an individual one." Consider the following experiences of a few runners:

- "These Band-Aids on my toes will work fine."

- "I get a lot of blisters on my right foot and very few on the left."

- "I constantly get blisters when I run any longer distances of 25-plus miles and only on the side of the two toes next to the big toe on my left foot."

- "Wearing orthotics, I am prone to continual blisters on the inside of my right heel where the foot hits the orthotic."

- "The only blisters that I get are on my little or big toes, and then only during races."

- "I never had a blister until today."

Some athletes claim to have feet with skin as soft as a baby's bottom while others take pride in having thick calluses on the bottom of their feet. Both may claim to never blister and yet on another day, in a different race or activity with different conditions and variables, both may blister. We are each an experiment of one and our feet change. Other blister-causing factors also change race to race—weather conditions, a lack of foot conditioning through training, the body's hydration level, the length of the race, and running biomechanics as the runner reacts to a sore hamstring or tight quads, for example, all contribute to potential problems.

Blisters come in a variety of sizes. They start small, from a hot spot, and can continue to grow until they are treated. One blister may not seem like much, but suddenly you have two, and then, maybe three. Multiply the pain of one well-placed blister times three or four, like some people get, and you can imagine how severe a seemingly minor problem can become.

Ron Jansen consistently got big, silver-dollar-size blisters under the balls of his feet and in the middle of the foot. He shared, "I suspect that I have metatarsalgia because that same area goes numb and eventually gets very painful right in the same spot where the blisters form. Sometimes the blisters are the standard variety and sometimes they're blood blisters. I've found that if I use Hapad metatarsal pads (or even just a cotton ball duct-taped to the underside of my insole), that's enough to support the metatarsal and keep from going numb, and they also seem to help prevent the blisters. I still get them but not nearly as bad."

When ultrarunner A. J. Howie did the 1992 Trans-America, he described his blisters as "pepperoni pizza blisters," large enough to make the *Guinness Book of World Records*. Blisters can also become major nightmares. John Supler, participating in the Marathon des Sables, reported, "When I came in, my feet were shredded like noodles. And when I woke up, my foot was stuck to my silk sheet, with a pool of yellow pus underneath it, leaking out."

The time and conditions required for blisters to develop will vary from individual to individual. Runners and hikers tend to get either downhill blisters on the toes and forefoot caused by friction while going downhill, or uphill blisters on the heels and over the Achilles tendons caused by friction while going uphill. Blisters on the heel can also mean the heel cup is too wide. Blisters on the top or front of the toes or the outsides of the outer toes can indicate friction in the toe box. The chapter "The Best of 15 Years of Foot Care" includes a section on the little toe triangle where many athletes blister.

Kevin O'Neall has done dozens of marathons and ultras. He shares his attempts at preventing blisters:

I have never done a long race without getting blisters. I've tried it all: lubricants; double-layer socks; size D, E, 2E, and 4E New Balance shoes;

sandals; and military boots. I use a Dremel drill to sand calluses once or twice weekly, and a hacksaw and grinder to trim the soles near blister zones. I cut into my shoes for extra toe room, and then patch the hole with tape to keep dirt out. I've experimented with every kind of tape there is and used seven different brands of duct tape. Nothing works perfectly.

So what's the miracle? While surfing the Badwater website, I saw a mention of an ingenious toe product used by dancers. Bunheads (**www. bunheads.com**) makes flexible fabric toe socks with a gel lining. Sounds dumb, but I ordered some. The box has a photo of a dainty dancer's leg standing on its toes. So far I've got about 40 miles on one tube with no breakdown. The box says they're washable, but I've run without washing them to see how they'd stand up to sweat and grime.

Kevin attempted the Leadville 100 in 2002 and got hot spots on his right big toe even though I'd applied Elastikon. He rolled a piece of Bunheads Big Tips over the Elastikon and was able to continue until a fall strained a calf muscle and forced him to walk. He eventually missed a cutoff and was out of the run, but the Bunheads kept him in the race up to that point.

The bottom line is that finding what prevents blisters on your feet can take much time and experimentation. It may involve one or more of the prevention measures in the previous chapters. It may also involve using one of the treatments in this chapter.

Keeping Stuff Out of Your Shoes

If you have ever walked or run a trail, or hiked with a backpack, you have probably had stuff get in your shoes. You know the stuff—small rocks, sand, grit, leaves, twigs, thistles and stickers, cattails—that kind of stuff. The problem is, this stuff often leads to blisters forming.

What usually happens is that you feel the offending stuff—and make a choice. Stop and remove it or continue on. Sometimes we stand on one foot and kick the shoe against a rock to try and move the rock around inside the shoe. Other times we stop and take off the shoe and remove the offending piece. The sooner we remove the bad stuff, the better the chance that there will be no negative consequences.

It's when we ignore the stuff that we get into trouble. Small rocks, sand, and grit can cause a hot spot, which can develop into a blister. Other stuff can cause skin irritations and require an antibiotic ointment.

There is an easy way to keep junk out of your shoes. Gaiters. These can be homemade or store bought. In short, gaiters go around the top of your shoe and lower leg. They may zip, secure with Velcro, or pull on over your feet. They fit snugly at the top and keep stuff from getting inside your shoe. Styles fasten to the shoes differently. Some have a strap that goes under the shoe's arch while others fasten to the front and back of the shoe. Read more about gaiters beginning on page 150.

Blisters 101

A basic understanding of how blisters are formed is necessary to successfully treat them. Heat, friction, and moisture contribute to the formation of blisters. Studies have shown that the foot inside the shoe or boot is exposed to friction at many sites as it experiences motion from side to side, front to back, and up and down. These friction sites also change during the activity as the exercise intensity, movement of the sock, and flexibility of the shoe or boot changes.[28]

The outer epidermis layer of skin receives friction that causes it to rub against the inner dermis layer of skin. This friction between the layers of skin causes a blister to develop. As the outer layer of the epidermis is loosened from the deeper layers, the sac in between becomes filled with lymph fluid. A blister has then developed. If the blister is deep or traumatically stressed by continued running or hiking, the lymph fluid may contain blood. When the lymph fluid lifts the outer layer of epidermis, oxygen and nutrition to this layer is cut off and it becomes dead skin. This outer layer is easily burst. The fluid then drains and the skin loses its natural protective barrier. The underlying skin is raw and sensitive. At this point, the blister is most susceptible to infection.

The friction against whatever is touching the skin causes the friction between the layers of skin. As identified earlier, the majority of foot problems can be traced back to socks, powders, and lubricants—or the lack of them. In order to prevent blisters, friction must be reduced. Friction can be reduced in three main ways: wearing double-layer socks or one inner and one outer sock, keeping the feet dry by using powders, or using a lubricant to reduce chafing. It has been found that rubbing moist skin tends to produce higher friction than does rubbing skin that is either very dry or very wet.[29] Because the skin blisters more easily when soft and moist, it is important to understand the value of moisture-wicking socks coupled with knowing whether powders and/or lubricants are best for your feet and how to use them. Eliminating pressure points caused by poor-fitting insoles and/or ill-fitting shoes can also reduce friction.

Some athletes unknowingly clench their toes. This curling downward of the toes can lead to toe blisters or toenail trauma during the transition through the foot strike from mid-foot to push off with the toes.

Because your footwear causes blisters, the healing process truly begins when these are removed. If you have the option of a day's layover in camp without shoes and socks, this can speed the healing process and get you back on your feet faster

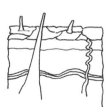

Normal skin

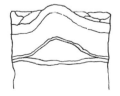

Blister forming

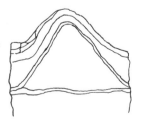

Large blister

and feeling better. Wearing sandals without socks exposes the blister to the air, which aids in healing.

Try to avoid getting blisters on top of existing blisters. When your skin is healing, protect or cushion the tender area.

Blisters Yesterday, Today, & Tomorrow

Most of us face it at one time or another: what worked for us in the past is no longer working. Ultrarunner Marv Skagerberg candidly warns, "Caveat pedis, or let the toes beware. I have completely solved the blister problem 12 times by perfecting various methods that allow me to run for 24 hours and up, blister free. However, the next time out with the exact same method, I have plenty of blisters." He has found that a combination of compound tincture of benzoin and silicone cream is by far the best for his feet (see the section "Extreme Blister Prevention & Patching," page 245, for his method). Yesterday's method may have worked for years. Today's method may work for years. But then again, as Marv warns, it may not.

"I *personal experience*

had hoped that 15 years as a long-distance runner and backpacker had eliminated the element of surprise in regard to foot problems and their treatment. I was wrong.

"The first day of my 17-day hike required an additional 11-mile climb to the trailhead atop Mt. Whitney's 14,500-foot summit. On the way up, both heels started to blister. A little early in the trip I thought, but not unexpected. I immediately applied my favorite remedy, 2nd Skin. This was to become a daily ritual. The 2nd Skin would ease the soreness and keep the wounds reasonably clean, but the Adhesive Knit that held it in place could not withstand the rigors of such a brutal, rocky trail, and the blisters worsened to more than an inch in diameter. Every step was painful, distracting me from the trail's beautiful surroundings. Soon, I ran out of Adhesive Knit and resorted to that trusty standby, duct tape. This kept the dressings in place longer, but after clambering up and over yet another 12,000-foot pass, it too would slip. Then I got a rash from the tape's adhesive and smaller blisters from the tape's edges.

"At my resupply point, nine days into the trip, I stocked up on 2nd Skin and duct tape and padded the heel cups of my two-year-old broken-in boots with moleskin and more duct tape. This stopped any future heel blistering but pushed my toes forward in the boots just enough to cause a whole new set of foot problems for the final leg of my trip. Some days it just isn't worth getting out of bed!"

—Tony Burke recalling the way he approached his 1996 backpack of the 211-mile John Muir Trail in California's Sierra Nevada

The late ultrarunner Dick Collins used to have problems with blisters. After trying recommendations from others, including tape, he formed his own conclusion. Dick learned, "Anything other than socks on my feet will over time become an irritant." He used only petroleum jelly on his feet and wore synthetic socks. Having completed 1,037 races, including 238 ultras, he found what worked for him and stuck to it. Like Dick, we each need to learn what works for us and be open to trying new ideas and products that could help keep our feet healthy.

We have no guarantee that what works one day will work another day. Ultrarunner Damon Lease experienced this frustration. By mile 20 of a 50-mile race he was feeling hot spots on his toes. By mile 38 he was reduced to a painful walking state. At the 42.2-mile aid station he made the difficult decision to stop. Damon noted, "I did nothing differently in this race than any other ultra." He had used the same shoe and sock combination in other ultras, but this course was steeper, with "more loose rocks and rough footing than the others." It happens. The trick is to play with all the variables in training to find what works best for your feet. Then be prepared with additional options in your gear bag.

Types of Blisters

There are many types of blisters. In my experience, toe and heel blisters are the most common, followed by ball of the foot and callus blisters.

Toe Blisters

Shoes with a toe box that is too short in length and/or height often cause toe blisters. The toes rub against the toe box and blisters result. Improperly trimmed toenails are also a common cause. Socks will catch on the toenails and push them back into the cuticles, causing blisters or fluid under the nails. Blisters between the toes are commonly caused by friction from skin on skin. Blisters on the bottom of the toes can be caused by friction from the insoles. Oftentimes the pinky toe curls under the neighboring toe, leading to blisters. Shoes with a good toe box and properly trimmed toenails are important to prevent toe blisters. Injinji toe socks can help those prone to toe blisters.

Ball of the Foot Blisters

Blisters on the ball of the foot are generally caused by friction. This may be from the surface of the insole or from socks. Often a lubricant or powder will help prevent these. Trying another pair of insoles can also help because your insole coverings may be rough. An ENGO Patch placed on your insole can effectively reduce friction.

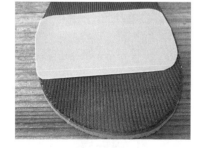

An ENGO Patch applied to an insole can reduce friction.

Heel Blisters

One of the more common blisters found on athletes' feet is on the heels. Is there a reason for this? Why do so many athletes blister there? The best answer is that heels move around a lot inside shoes, both up and down and side to side. Some shoes have plastic in the heel counters—a piece of plastic that is curved around the back of the shoe's heel counter. This plastic piece can sometimes be an irritant and rub on your foot, causing a hot spot that turns into a blister. Another irritant is the edge of the insole where it meets the inside of the shoe. Run your fingers around the inside of your shoe. Feel for seams or the hard plastic heel counter that can cause blisters. Feel the edge of the insole. Some insoles have a thick edge, while others are thinner. Another insole may fit better and not have the problem edge.

Bottom of the heel blisters can be caused by a rough surface of your insole or socks that are worn through or with a weave that has irritated the skin.

Steep downhills can lead to large blisters covering the entire bottom of the heel. These can be treated with an ENGO Patch on the insole under the heel and by draining the blister. Injecting zinc oxide into the blister will help dry the new skin and when taped, allows for walking or running.

Calluses and Blisters

An adventure racer told me, "My teammates who had calluses as protection from blisters had the worst blisters." I have seen this time and time again. Calluses can offer a bit of protection against blisters, but the trade-off is that when you do get blisters with calluses, the blisters are bad. Oftentimes they are larger and deeper because they are underneath the callused skin. And more important, these blisters are next to impossible to drain because the depth and exact location of the fluid pocket is hard to determine. You are better off reducing your calluses and getting to soft skin.

Blister Look-Alike

Sometimes you find a blister on one of your toes—but it's not a blister. A mucocutaneous cyst is a small nodular single mass that forms on the top of toes. These frequently form at the joint just behind the toenail. Caused by a weakening of the joint capsule, they are firm and rubbery and filled with a clear fluid. A silicone toe cap can help when it rubs. Treatments range from doing nothing to surgical excision.

General Blister Care

From the perspective of runners and hikers, the goal of blister treatments is to make the foot comfortable because often running or hiking must continue. Bryan P. Bergeron, MD, identifies four therapeutic goals of blister management.[30]

He recommends that all blister treatments be considered with these four goals in mind:

- Avoiding infection,

- Minimizing pain and discomfort,

- Stopping further blister enlargement, and

- Maximizing recovery.

Ultrarunner Gillian Robinson of **www.zombierunner.com** has learned to "pay a lot of attention to healing, so I don't run on wounded feet. Even the worst blisters heal in about five days if you use Neosporin, cover it during the day, and leave it uncovered to breathe at night (if it's not too gross). My feet seem to toughen up after blister trauma, so I trim off the dead skin and keep going."

For years, normal blister care was gauze, moleskin, and petroleum jelly. Anyone can slap on a piece of moleskin, slather on some petroleum jelly, and hope for the best. But to really fix a blister so you can continue running or hiking is an art. Observing the podiatrists at the finish line of a marathon or ultra, one finds most blister-care practices incorporate these three materials.

The time-honored method of blister care uses moleskin to protect the blister. If the blister is intact, cut a piece of moleskin about 0.5–0.75 inch larger around than the blister with a hole slightly larger than the blister in the center. Press it on the skin around the blister and put an antibiotic ointment, Bag Balm, or medicated petroleum jelly in the hole over the blister. The final step is to place a piece of tape over the moleskin. Do not use gauze because it is too rough and can irritate the skin.

Personally, I am not a fan of moleskin. It does not stick well, even with a tape adherent; it is too thick; and it does not conform to the curves of the foot.

Alternatives to moleskin are adhesive felt or one of the tapes identified in the "Taping" chapter. You can also use one of the tapes or Spenco Skin Knit in place of the gauze. When using tape or moleskin over a blister, apply it as smoothly as possible. Use finger pressure to smooth it evenly across the blister, and then repeat the smoothing process several more times after the initial application. Remember to cut the tape or moleskin large enough to extend well beyond the edges of the blister. The most common failure in using tape or moleskin is not allowing enough necessary for good adherence. The larger the blister, the more the tape or moleskin should extend past its edges.

Basic Blister Repair

If the above treatment does not help or if you must continue running or hiking, take time to repair a blister before it enlarges and ruptures. Dr. Bergeron recommends draining the blister prior to applying a dressing when it is in a weight-bearing area

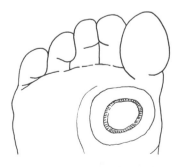

Moleskin with center hole cut out for blister

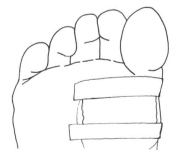

Gauze taped over moleskin to protect blister

and larger than 0.8 inch in diameter.[31] There are two basic ways to drain a blister: one using a needle and the other using small, sharp scissors or nail clippers. My recommendation is to drain any blisters that are in a pressure area (toes, arch, ball of the foot, and so on) or that are causing pain or discomfort. In my experience, it is easier to drain and manage them when they are small and before they become large and the roof tears off.

To drain a blister using the needle method, do the following:

1. Use an alcohol wipe to clean the skin around the blister.

2. Sterilize a pin or needle with a flame by heating with a match (avoid soot on the tip). Use it to lance two to four puncture holes. Move the needle side to side to make the opening larger so it will not seal up. Making a single large hole increases the possibility of the blister roof shearing off as you continue running or hiking.

3. Make the puncture holes on the side, top, and bottom of the blister where ongoing foot pressure and gravity will push out additional fluid, generally to the back of the foot and toward the outside.

4. Use pressure from your fingers to push out the fluid and blot the fluid away with a tissue.

5. Clean and dry the skin before doing further blister care. The outer layer of dead skin should not be removed.

It is important that the blister not be allowed to refill with fluid. Use one of the blister-care products in the next section to protect the blister. Occasionally recheck the blister and drain it if it has refilled with fluid.

If you are prone to getting hot spots and blisters, try dabbing on a bit of Anbesol or Cankaid on before patching. These products, sold in drugstores, are numbing medicines for your gums but will also work to numb the painful spots on your feet.

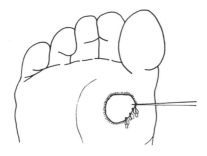

Use a sterilized needle to make several small holes on the outside edges of the blister.

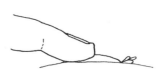

Gently push out the lymph fluid.

A better method for draining blisters is to use standard nail clippers or small pointed scissors and clip a hole at the edge of the most dependent spot and also 180 degrees from there. This lets both gravity and capillary action, along with muscular movement, fully empty the blister. The clippers make a V notch, rather than a simple hole. Podiatrist Dan Simpson reports, "I have never had a complication from this method and the clippers are easier to manipulate than scissors due to the shorter distance from your hand to the business end. The clipper also functions as a built-in depth gauge, preventing too deep an incision."

Another method helps blisters drain better when further hiking or running is required. Ray Zirblis picked up this tip while running the six-day Marathon des Sables in Morocco, and it would be appropriate for stage races or multidays where a runner needs to keep running. At the end of the day's run or other effort, if you find blisters, drain them and add another step: sterilize a needle and a few inches of thread with alcohol. Then thread the needle and run it and the thread through one side of the blister and out the other, leaving the thread in place with a 1-inch tail hanging on either end. The thread acts as a wick to further drain any moisture in the blister while one is running or sleeping. Ray reports, "I found that my blisters dried more thoroughly overnight than normal for me, and the inside was much less raw and less sensitive than usual."

However you lance blisters, the goal is to drain fluid so healing can start. This means making several holes where gravity and pressure will push out fluid. Picture a 1-inch blister on the side of a heel. I would make four holes—two on the bottom just inside the side edge and two on the top, also just inside the side edge.

In some cases, you should not attempt to drain blisters. *Do not drain a blister when it is blood-filled.* Doing so creates the risk of a serious infection, as bacteria is easily introduced into the dermis layer of skin and into the blood system. Pad around the blister with moleskin or adhesive felt. As the blister heals, the blood will turn from bright red to a reddish-brown.

Do not drain the blister if the fluid inside appears to be either cloudy or hazy. Normal blister fluid is clear and the change indicates that an infection has set in. If clear, the fluid can be drained, an antibiotic ointment applied, and a protective covering applied. Recheck the blister three times a day for signs of infection.

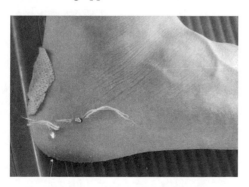

Thread through a side of heel blister

Each time you check, apply a new coating of antibiotic ointment and change the dressing. Early treatment can keep the infection from becoming more serious.

If the blister has ruptured, the degree of repair depends on the condition of the blister's outer covering. Clean around the blister as described below and apply one of the blister-care methods described in the next section. You can treat a ruptured blister—if the skin is generally intact.

If the outer layer of skin is torn off or only a flap of skin is left, carefully cut off the loose skin, clean the area, and cover the new skin with one of the blister-care methods described in the next section. As the blister heals, trim off any rough edges.

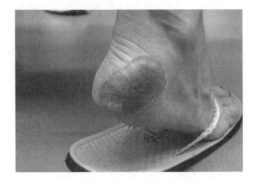

A heel blister filled with blood

Preventing Infection

Whether you get a blister or several blisters, whether you drain them or not, you need to watch them for signs of infection. If you pop a blister or you have a blister with its roof torn off, once you have the chance, apply an antibiotic ointment.

Did you catch the piece in the news about actress Hilary Swank's blister? News sources disclosed that Swank was nearly KO'd from the filming of *Million Dollar Baby* due to a foot infection—from a blister. It appears that she popped the blister on her own and continued with her workouts. When the pain increased, she found streaks going up her foot. Going to the doctor, she learned that the blister had become infected. There is a lesson here that we all need to learn. Just as Swank thought a blister was a simple thing, as they usually are, they can also become serious health issues. The lesson here is that blisters are an injury and must be watched for signs of infection. I'd wager that 99.9999% of all blisters heal just fine. But if that 0.0001% is on your foot, or on the foot of someone you know or love, you'd be more careful.

For open blisters, using soap and water and an antibiotic ointment or Betadine is important for avoiding infection. Though you may not use these on an open blister during a run or in the middle of the day while backpacking, at the end of the event or day, take the necessary time to properly treat the open skin. Applying an antibacterial topical ointment will help the open blister hcal up to 40% faster. Check your local drugstore for a broad-spectrum antibiotic ointment such as Neosporin or Polysporin that provides protection against both gram-positive and gram-negative pathogens. Brave Soldier Antiseptic Healing Ointment is an excellent all-purpose salve to have on hand for blister care.

Recheck blisters daily for signs of infection. An infected blister may be both seen and felt. An infection will be indicated by any of the following: redness, swelling, red streaks up the limb, pain, fever, or pus. Treat the blister as a wound. Clean it frequently and apply an antibiotic ointment. Frequent warm water or Epsom salt soaks can also help the healing process. Stay off the foot as much as possible and elevate it above the level of your heart. If the infection does not seem to subside over 24–48 hours, see a doctor.

Studies have shown that StaphAseptic (**www.staphaseptic.com**) kills more than 99.9% of staph and MRSA germs, preventing an infection without antibiotics. This pain-relieving wound treatment should be used as part of a complete staph prevention program to provide protection from skin infections. An alternative ointment is Bacitracin. A prescription ointment is Bactroban.

BASIC BLISTER-CARE PRODUCTS

ADHESIVE FELT is available in rolls in 0.125-inch and 0.25-inch thicknesses. This pink felt is extra thick and, compared to moleskin, provides extra cushioning and a stronger adhesive base. Check with your local drugstore, medical supply store, or podiatrist for availability.

BRAVE SOLDIER ANTISEPTIC HEALING OINTMENT was formulated for athletes and is popular among cyclists. Developed by a dermatologist to keep abrasion wounds moist and protected, Brave Soldier helps heal blisters, road rash, minor cuts, and burns. It's made with tea tree oil as a natural antiseptic, aloe gel for its natural healing properties, jojoba oil as a natural moisturizer, vitamin E to rebuild collagen and skin tissue, shark liver oil to reduce scarring, and comfrey to stimulate skin cell growth and wound resurfacing. **www.bravesoldier.com**

MOLESKIN is a soft, cotton padding that protects skin surfaces against friction and has an adhesive backing that adheres to the skin. Dr. Scholl's makes Moleskin Plus from thin cotton-flannel padding and Moleskin Foam from soft latex foam. Moleskin is available in a variety of sizes in most drugstores, and it can be cut to the size needed. Moleskin should not be applied directly over a blister because it can tear any loose skin when removed.

SPENCO PRESSURE PADS are made from closed-cell polyethylene foam that is soft, flexible, and thin. It is available in a six-pack of 3-by-5-inch sheets with two precut pads in ovals and circles and two uncut pads to be used over hot spots and blisters. **www.spenco.com**

Advanced Blister Patching

There are as many ways to patch blisters as there are products that can be used to patch them. Learn advanced techniques before a race. Experiment with different products and different taping techniques. Find what works for your feet and then perfect the method. Practice on your good feet so you will know how to make the patch or tape stick when your feet go bad. Learn how to patch intact blisters, drained blisters, and blisters with the skin torn off. The more you practice taping and patching blisters, the better you will become. Trial and error is a good way to learn.

Even though the time-honored blister-care products are still used by many, there are more efficient products to both prevent blisters and promote healing. The chapter "Taping for Blisters" contains information that can be used as treatments for blisters. By following the methods described, you can apply tape over a blister whether the blister roof is intact or not. Tape wherever necessary based on experience and circumstances. You can also apply tape over Spenco 2nd Skin or other blister-care products mentioned below. In fact, often the tape will help hold the patch in place, especially in an ultramarathon or multiday event.

My method of patching blisters has changed over the years. The care I administer depends on the type of event. In all instances, I drain the blister and apply a small dab of zinc oxide to the top of the blister, as a drying agent and to control moisture. Then, in a short race, up to a 50-mile distance or half-day event, I use Spenco 2nd Skin covered with Kinesio Tex tape. In longer events, I skip the Spenco 2nd Skin and apply the tape directly over the zinc oxide–covered blister. For longer events, I don't use 2nd Skin because of its tendency over time to lead to softened cold skin, not unlike maceration. In some cases, I will use one of the blister patches mentioned below. Kinesio Tex is my tape of choice. And I always keep a supply of ENGO Patches on hand to apply to the athlete's footwear.

For years the main product for patching blisters has been Spenco 2nd Skin. We have all seen the familiar blue squares of gel, either having them on our feet or applied to someone else's feet. The gel has helped many athletes make it to the finish line or get to the end of a hike or walk. Spenco 2nd Skin has two downsides, though. It requires a tape or dressing to hold it in place, and over long periods of time, the gel softens the skin—leading to a maceration appearance.

Several other products—Blist-O-Ban, Band-Aid Advance Healing Cushions, ENGO Patches, GlacierGel dressings, LiquiCell Blister Bands, Skin-on-Skin, and Spenco Sports Blister Pads—are designed to provide advance blister care and their information can be found in the advanced blister patching product list on pages 246–249. Blist-O-Ban, Band-Aid, GlacierGel, LiquiCell, and Spenco Sports Pads are all similar in that they have a pad inside with an adhesive strip around the outside. I like these style pads because they are easy to apply.

ENGO Patches are unique because they are applied to blister-prone areas of footwear, insoles, socks, and athletic equipment—not skin—for easier, longer-lasting, blister-free protection. Scientific and field tests show that ENGO's slippery blue surface significantly reduces the shearing effect of friction and rubbing, providing immediate relief. The ultrathin patches leave footwear volume virtually unaltered, a strong plus.

Compound tincture of benzoin applied to the area around a hot spot or blister will help blister products or tapes stick to the skin more effectively. Avoid getting tincture into a ruptured blister or other broken skin. After the tincture has dried and become tacky, apply one of the blister-care products on the following pages. Be sure to apply a light coating of powder or lubricant to counteract the still exposed benzoin to prevent socks or contaminants from sticking to the skin. Be forewarned that forgetting this step when using benzoin on the toes may result in blisters resulting from two toes being stuck together.

Be sure to carefully roll your socks on and off. This keeps the patch from catching on the socks and pulling off or bunching up. The use of a shoehorn will save patches applied to your heels.

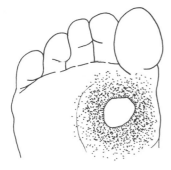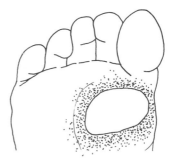

| Compound tincture of benzoin (or any tape adherent) applied around a blister helps protective layers to adhere. | Once the protective coating covers the blister, apply a light coating of powder or lubricant to exposed benzoin. |

There are several other types of blister patches. Spyroflex is adhesive but will stay in place better with tape over it. Xeroform is a yellowish petrolatum gauze dressing that can be cut and placed over a blister and then taped over. A small piece of 2nd Skin can be cut to fill an open blister and then covered with tape over the top. This allows a runner to continue with little pain. It's the fluid in the blister that causes the pain.

Kathy Hamilton has had success spraying her feet with several layers of New Skin before putting on her socks and shoes. She sprays her entire foot, especially between the toes. If she has a hot spot or blister, she uses a few extra coats.

U.S. Army Captain Dave Hamilton, a physician's assistant, learned a few tricks about how to treat torn blisters from Dutch Red Cross workers at the military Nijmegen 4-Day 140K March. Dave personally had this method used on his blistered feet after which he marched 25 and 26 miles respectively over two days with

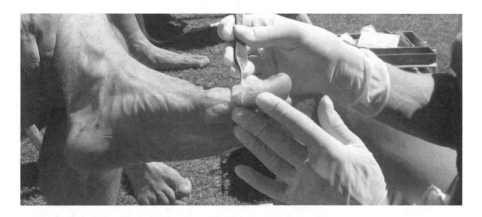

Applying 2nd Skin to blister

a 25- to 40-pound pack, wearing standard military boots. Here are their steps for dressing a torn blister:

1. Clean the blister area with an alcohol wipe.

2. If necessary, puncture the blister with a standard finger lancet, needle, or scissors.

3. Use the stick portion of a cotton swab in a rolling motion to force the fluid out of a blister.

4. Trim off any loose edges of the blister's roof skin.

5. If the blister is infected with pus, remove the roof of the blister and clean the blister cavity. Cut a piece of DuoDerm (or use 2nd Skin) in the shape and size of the open blister. Warm it in your gloved hands for five minutes to make it soft. Peel off the backing and place it inside the blister cavity. This forms an airtight dressing, soothes the wound, and fills the empty space inside the blister.

6. Tape over the patched blister.

If you have toe hot spots or blisters, you can use a gel toe cap to protect the whole toe. The caps are either solid gel or a fabric with gel inside. Bunga Toe Caps, Bunheads Jelly Toes, Hapad's Pedifix Visco-Gel Toe Caps, and Pro-Tec Toe Caps are examples of these caps. With care these caps can be washed and reused.

TIP: Integrity Check

When using any of the products listed on the following pages on your blisters, be sure to occasionally check them. They may peel off, shift their position, or ball up under the stresses of hiking and running. When doing hills, the constant uphill and downhill movements of the feet combined with the pressures of the running body or the weight of a backpack may compromise their integrity. If you sense a change in how they feel, stop and check it out.

Instead of putting something on your feet, you can put ENGO Patches inside your shoe or on your insoles. These thin fabric-film composite patches can greatly reduce friction in targeted locations within your footwear by giving a slick, slippery surface to the area of your footwear or insole where friction is a problem. They can also be used to patch over a worn spot inside the heel of the shoe.

Removing tape and blister patches can be tricky. If you pull the tape too quickly, you'll pull the skin too and risk pulling the top skin off the blister. Nik Weber has found that rubbing alcohol removes tape the best, but it will sting until it evaporates when applied to open wounds. But it still hurts less than lifting the blister skin up with the tape. He says, "I use a long cotton swab with a wood stick and soak the tape if it is porous like Elastikon, then use the soaked cotton swab to peel the edges of the tape loose. You sort of push at the tape-skin interface with the cotton swab until the tape releases."

Extreme Blister Prevention & Patching

Some athletes may choose to use extreme methods to initially prevent blisters or subsequently treat their blisters in order to continue on in a competitive event. These are aggressive methods. A competitive 100-mile, 24-hour, 48-hour, or six-day run may motivate a runner to want to try any means to keep running. Likewise, hikers may need to deal aggressively with blisters when in the middle of a multiday hike. The team participation rule in an adventure-racing event may force a team member to consider treating blisters in an extreme method.

The use of a light coating of zinc oxide can help to dry out the skin and repel moisture. Put a dab in the blister or under your blister patch. This can be especially helpful if you will be resting or sleeping for a spell.

There are two extreme methods of extreme blister prevention and care. Review the following methods to determine whether one may be useful for you in your running and hiking adventures.

The **first extreme method** uses one of several products to glue the blister's roof to the skin underneath. Dr. Trolan has participated in several Raid Gauloises and served as a medical consultant to adventure-racing teams in the Eco Challenge as well as to Naval Special Warfare. He describes two more extreme methods of treating blisters, warning that they are "not for the faint of heart."[32] These methods have helped many adventure racers finish their events. The methods should not be used if the blister is infected. Likewise the following technique with compound tincture of benzoin can lead to infections and should only be used if you accept the possible consequences. Permanent damage to the skin surfaces can occur.

At the 2010 six-day TransRockies race, many of the runners came to the medical station with huge blisters on the bottom of the heel. We felt that the cause was the repetitive daily running on the course's steep downhills, probably with moisture on the feet. These blisters spread across the whole bottom of the heel, and oftentimes the skin tore. I found that the best treatment was to inject zinc oxide directly into the blister cavity once it had been drained. I gently massaged the zinc oxide to fill the whole blister. Then I taped over the blister as described in the "Taping for Blisters" chapter. This dries the inside of the blister, and the tape anchors the skin against the foot. This method is described below and is my favorite. I used 18-gauge needles because that was what I had on hand. A blunt needle is safer and can be used if the skin is torn. If the blister's roof is intact, you will need to use a pointed needle. A 16- or 18-gauge needle is recommended because of the thickness of the zinc oxide.

After you have opened the blister and drained it thoroughly, and your feet are dry, use one of the following methods to seal down the blister roof.

- Use a syringe and a large-bore 18-gauge needle to inject zinc oxide into the blister. Because the zinc oxide is rather thick, warm it in the sun or

ADVANCED BLISTER PATCHING PRODUCTS

BAND-AID ADVANCED HEALING BLISTER CUSHIONS are made with an elastic polyure-thane film over a moisture absorbing and adhering layer, or gel, both covered with protective silicone papers that are removed for use. Functioning as a second layer of skin, these products cushion the area, virtually eliminating blis-ter pain, while protecting it from further damage caused by friction. Tapered edges help adherence to the skin without rolling. It is not meant to be cut and can be worn for several days. For larger blisters, put two pieces side by side. Be careful not to wrinkle the edges of the pads. The hydrocolloid construction creates optimum conditions for rapid healing, while embedded cellulose parti-cles absorb excess fluid and perspiration from the wound surfaces. Additionally, bacteria are sealed out, reducing the risk of infection. These pads can be left on until they come off on their own. There are large ovals and smaller cushions designed for toes and fingers. Look for Band-Aid products at drugstores and running and sports stores. **www.bandaid.com**

BAND-AID SINGLE-STEP LIQUID BANDAGE is a liquid wound protection in pre-moistened swab applicators. It forms an invisible yet flexible shield that is waterproof and doesn't sting. **www.bandaid.com**

BLIST-O-BAN BLISTER PATCHES from Sam Medical Products use patented technology called Bursatek, which externally reproduces the function of the body's internal bursal sacs. When force is applied to the area, the patch provides a gliding surface, reducing friction and shear forces. Blist-O-Ban patches are two layers of breathable plastic film bonded together, except for an area in the center. This creates a dome-type area, like a collapsed perforated bubble allowing the two plastic sheets to glide freely against each other—taking the pressure off the skin underneath. The patches are only 0.006-inch thick. Offered in three sizes, all ovals, the medical-grade adhesive skin contact layer is breathable, perforated, latex-free polyurethane. **www.blistoban.com**

BUNGA TOE PADS AND TOE CAPS are made from a medical-grade polymer material. **www.bungapads.com**

BUNHEADS GEL PRODUCTS are made of a nonsilicone polymer, formulated with medical-grade mineral oils to cushion and protect those areas of the foot prone to friction trauma. They are washable, supple, comforting, hypoallergenic, nontoxic, dermatologist tested, and cost effective. The gel doesn't migrate, so it won't bottom out. The Jelly Tips, Jelly Toes, the Big Tip, and the really Big Tip are designed specifically for toes. Available at local retailers. **www.bunheads.com**

COBAN is a self-adherent wrap that can be used around feet, ankles, and heels to hold blister products in place. Its elasticity and flexibility allows movement of the joints. Because it adheres to itself, it contains no adhesive. Because it is elastic, be careful not to apply it too tightly and cause constriction. Pharmacy or medical supply stores typically carry Coban or similar self-adherent wraps. Most are available in 2-, 3-, and 4-inch widths.

ADVANCED BLISTER PATCHING PRODUCTS

DR. SCHOLL'S BLISTER TREATMENT sterile pads prevent blisters and help protect existing sores from pressure and abrasion. Cushlin pads adhere directly to skin, forming a tight seal around blisters. Available at most drugstores.

DUODERM CGF FLEXIBLE STERILE DRESSING is a polymer wound dressing used in hospitals. Packaged in a 4-by-4-inch size, it can be cut to fill the space inside an open blister. Buy the borderless dressings. Available in medical supply stores.

ENGO PATCHES are low-friction patches uniquely applied to blister-prone areas of footwear, insoles, socks, and athletic equipment—not skin—for easier, longer-lasting, blister-free protection. Ultrathin patches leave footwear volume virtually unaltered. Strong, latex-free adhesive prevents migration and movement, even through moisture and sweat. Scientific and field tests show ENGO's slippery surface significantly reduces friction and rubbing, providing immediate relief. Several sizes are available: small ovals for toes; large ovals for the ball of foot, arch, and heel areas; and rectangles for custom trimming. **www.goengo.com**

FLEXI CARE TRANSPARENT BANDAGES are 0.01 millimeters thin. Four designs are offered: a small 0.75-by-0.75-inch spot film, a 1-by-1.5-inch film, a 1-by-1.5-inch film with a pad, and a larger 2-by-2.75-by-1.5-inch film. These very sticky, superthin bandages are waterproof and breathable and can be used as a covering for a hot spot or blister. **www.libatapeusa.com**

GLACIERGEL BLISTER AND BURN DRESSINGS contain 50% hydrogel to cushion, cool, and provide pain relief. They come in a kit with three large oval and three rectangle dressings and alcohol wipes. They are made to stay in place for three to four days, and they have an adhesive edge for easy application. **www. adventuremedicalkits.com**

LIQUICELL BLISTER BANDS use an advanced liquid technology to place liquid in a cell, which circulates and moves in all directions against friction and pressure. They come in one size, a large oval with a adhesive backing and are sold in packs of eight. **www.pro-tecathletics.com**

NEW-SKIN comes in two forms: a Liquid Bandage useful as a skin protectant or toughening agent and a Wound & Blister Dressing. The Liquid Bandage, in a spray or liquid, dries rapidly to form a tough protective cover that is antiseptic, flexible, and waterproof, and it lets the skin breathe. The Wound & Blister Dressing comes in 2-inch squares. Available at most drugstores.

Hapad offers **PEDIFIX VISCO-GEL TOE CAPS** that can be used over toe blisters. **www.hapad.com**

PRO-TEC'S TOE CAPS, made from custom-grade silicone, are soft and stretchable to fit all toes. Locate a reseller through their website. **www.pro-tecathletics.com**

SKIN-ON-SKIN from Medi-Dyne is a product similar to 2nd Skin. It comes in 1-inch squares, 3-inch circles, and 1.5-by-2-inch rectangles and is made with water, hydrogel, and vitamin E with a flexible adhesive knit that secures the hydrogel in place. **www.medi-dyne.com**

ADVANCED BLISTER PATCHING PRODUCTS CONTINUED

SPENCO ADHESIVE KNIT can be used to cover 2nd Skin pads or as a skin protector to prevent blisters. Spenco Adhesive Knit is a highly breathable woven fiber with the ability to stretch and conform, and it does not come off from sweat or bathing. It cuts to size and fits easily around toes and hard-to-tape areas. Adhesive Knit comes in 3-by-5-inch rectangles in a six pack. **www.spenco.com**

SPENCO 2ND SKIN BLISTER PADS should be applied directly over blisters. Made with the 2nd Skin hydrocolloid pad bordered with a thin adhesive film, the pads keep blisters from drying out, absorb moisture and perspiration, and promote a scab-free, naturally healed blister. **www.spenco.com**

SPENCO 2ND SKIN DRESSINGS are unique skinlike hydrogel pads that can be applied directly over closed or open blisters. The pads help reduce friction and the discomfort of blisters. They can also be used over abrasions, cuts, or similar wounds. Use one or more pads to cover the blister area. Remove the cellophane layer on one side of the pad, apply that gel side to the blister, and then remove the cellophane from the other side. The pads do not stick to the skin and require tape to hold them onto the skin. They should be kept moist and changed daily. Cover the 2nd Skin pads with either Spenco Adhesive Knit, one of the tapes mentioned, or a self-adhering wrap. These pads are available in a variety of sizes: 1-inch squares, 3-inch circles, and 3-by-6.5-inch rectangles. Be sure to keep your packet of pads moist or they will dry out. **www.spenco.com**

SPENCO'S SPORT BLISTER PADS come in three sizes—small, medium, and large ovals. The small is great for toes, while the large works well for heel blisters. Each pad contains a soft hydrocolloid pad covered by an ultrathin film dressing

roll it between your hands. This changes the viscosity to make it easier to inject. Inject enough to fill the blister evenly, using your fingers to spread the zinc throughout the inside of the blister. The zinc dries the skin and makes it possible to walk and run when the blister is taped. It does not adhere the blister's roof to the inner skin as do the following two methods, but there is no pain and the possibility of infection is low.

■ Use a syringe, without a needle, to inject compound tincture of benzoin directly into the blister. Immediately apply pressure across the top of the blister to evenly seal down the blister's outer layer to the underlying skin. This also pushes out any extra benzoin. Be forewarned that injecting the benzoin is momentarily painful. Dr. Trolan rates it as an eight on a one-to-ten pain scale where "childbirth and kidney stones are a ten and a paper cut is a one."

Others have expanded on this method with other products. These methods of gluing blisters should be used at your discretion and with a watchful eye toward later infection.

to promote faster healing. The hydrocolloid pads contain aloe vera. Moisture is absorbed to help prevent the blister from drying out until healed. The pads are made to stay on for up to five days. The film dressing is adhesive-backed to hold the pad in place. **www.spenco.com**

SPYROFLEX is an adhesive wound dressing. It consists of a thin two-layered polyurethane membrane that has an adhesive inner side that goes against the skin and an outer layer that is moisture-vapor–permeable and microporous. As an "intelligent" dressing, Syproflex is open-cell, designed for moisture management. It helps protect the blister from external moisture and bacteria while speeding the healing process. Moisture from the blister is absorbed by the porous membrane, passes through, and evaporates. The pad, cut to size, is applied directly over the blister and may be left on for up to seven days, yet it is easily removed without sticking or tearing. Spyroflex works extremely well on inflamed and infected blisters. For maximum adherence, use as much of the pad as possible on the skin around the blister and cover the pad with Spenco Adhesive Knit or a similar porous tape. Spyroflex is available in an Abrasion Dressing Kit with three 4-inch square pads. Pads may be cut to size. **www.outdoorrx.com**

XEROFORM PETROLATUM GAUZE DRESSING is a sterile, nonadherent fine mesh gauze wound dressing. This product can be used over blisters. Xeroform is packaged in a 1-by-8-inch strip, a 5-by-9-inch rectangle, or a 4–by-108-inch roll (for medical crews). It can be found in medical supply stores.

Lisa Bliss, MD, found, "Instant Krazy Glue works great, but I always seem to get into a battle with the bottle and end up gluing my fingertips together. I prefer to treat my own blisters, and I really don't want to have to put gloves on to do so, so I use either benzoin or Orajel (Orajel Maximum Strength Toothache Pain Relief Gel). In my opinion, benzoin works a bit better, smells better, and, yes, burns like hell for a few seconds. Orajel, on the other hand, is great for sticking down the roof of a blister after draining, and it has the added benefit of 20% benzocaine that helps soothe the burning. I've used Orajel both during and after runs to treat blisters. It's sticky enough to hold down the roof of a blister (just squirt a drop in the hole you've cut to drain), but I have always dressed the blister afterward because I'm not sure if it will hold if I have to continue to run. It's not as adhesive as benzoin and certainly not as much as Krazy Glue. It does help the sting somewhat, at least enough to get you running again. No problems with it. It doesn't glue fingers together, which is good for me!"

Instant Krazy Glue is now offered in an Advanced Formula and as an All-Purpose Brush-On. It is best used on small- to medium-size blisters. When you want to apply Krazy Glue to blisters, here are some tips.

- Make sure that the skin is dry and free of oils or powders.

- Use small, sharp scissors to trim the edges of skin to be as even as possible.

- Hold the edges of the blister's skin together.

- Apply light layers over the blister, allowing 20–30 seconds between layers.

- Cover the patch with your favorite tape, with a piece of tissue over the blister.

There are several alternatives to Instant Krazy Glue. Super Glue (**www.super gluecorp.com**), which has been around for years, and the newer Gorilla Glue (**www.gorillaglue.com**) are also good choices for sealing blisters.

At the 1996 Western States 100-Mile Endurance Run, Teresa Krall found out the hard way how painful tincture in a blister can be. The cotton ball used to apply the tincture was dropped into the dirt and one of her crew mistakenly decided to pour the tincture directly onto her blistered heel. As Brick Robbins, her pacer, recalls, "The benzoin was poured before I could object, followed by a blood-curdling scream. After a while (it seemed like forever), Teresa quit screaming." Teresa recalls the blister being about half-dollar size and the pain being intense. She would not do it again unless it was the only method left to let her run.

Using Syringes & Needles

You may see medical aid station people using syringes with needles to draw out the blister fluid and then to inject the tincture. Syringes with needles must be sterile in order to prevent infection. There is no safe way to dispose of the syringes and needles, or sharps, as they are called in the medical profession, except in a sharps container. If you use syringes and needles outside of a medical station, store the sharps in a hard-shelled container until they can be safely disposed.

In this time of hepatitis, HIV, and AIDS, we need to practice universal precautions—in this case, hand washing and switching to new gloves before treating each person. An open blister must be treated as an open wound, and the blister's fluid must be treated as a bodily fluid. Additionally, there is a danger that using a syringe, you might inject more tincture than is necessary to get a good seal or not enough to cover all inner surfaces. By making several small puncture holes in the blister, and using a syringe without a needle, excess tincture can be pushed out when pressure is applied to the roof of the blister. A good seal is then ensured.

Pushing a sharp needle into a drained blister must be done with care. The sharp point can easily penetrate the new, raw skin, which will be painful. Because needles have a beveled point, insert the needle with the tip toward the roof of the blister. An alternative is to use a blunt-end needle or a teat cannula, which is used on cow udders and can be found online.

Needles used to drain blisters can be any size. Needles are known by their gauge size. The larger the needle gauge number, the smaller the needle. A 25-gauge needle is very small and can used for normal draining; however, a larger gauge 20- or 22-gauge needle will make a bigger hole and make draining easier. Needles used to inject zinc oxide should be either 18- or 16-gauge because of the viscosity of the zinc. Compound tincture of benzoin can be injected through a 20- or 22-gauge needle.

The **second extreme method** of blister prevention uses compound tincture of benzoin, or a similar benzoin-based product, and a lubricant. Marv Skagerberg used a benzoin and silicone-cream combination that worked for him for the last 78 of 86 days of the 1985 cross-country Trans America race. Averaging 43 miles per day through 12 states, Marv did not get a single blister.

1. Clean the feet thoroughly, and dry them completely.

2. Coat the feet, heels, soles, and toes with compound tincture of benzoin.

3. Let the feet dry for three minutes, keeping the toes spread. The feet will still be quite sticky.

4. Apply your choice of lubricant (Hydropel is a good choice as it controls moisture).

5. Reapply the lubricant and change socks every four to six hours.

Bill Trolan, MD, uses Hydropel Sports Ointment over Cramer Tuf-Skin in the same manner as Marv described above. He recommends reapplying Tuf-Skin, or a similar benzoin product, and cream at every sock change. Many adventure racers swear by Hydropel because it repels moisture. Never underestimate the creative search for blister preventing ideas. Some athletes have found that Sno-Seal Original Beeswax Waterproofing is effective when applied over compound tincture of benzoin. Atsko's Pro-Tech-Skin is similar and

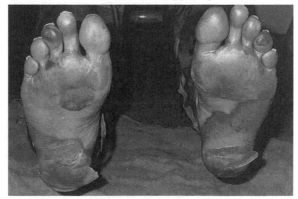

Under extreme conditions, entire feet can blister and whole skin layers can separate. It's best to do all you can to prevent such dire circumstances.

is made for use on skin. Remember that any of these products needs to be reapplied when changing socks or every four to six hours when on your feet.

The choice is yours. These types of blister sealing works to seal the blister's roof to the inner skin so running and hiking can continue. But there is definitely pain and always the risk of infection, and other treatments are available.

After sealing the blister, Dr. Trolan suggests several options. Apply a coating of benzoin to help the tape or moleskin better adhere to the skin. Or apply Instant Krazy Glue over the blister. This layer provides an extra layer of protection and helps your tape covering better adhere to the skin.

For severe cases, Dr. Trolan has used the tincture of benzoin injection, followed by a coating of tincture of benzoin on top of the blister, followed by a coating of New-Skin Liquid Bandage, followed by a layer of Krazy Glue, and finally followed by tape. He recommends using an emery board or fine nail file to smooth any rough spots on the blister coating before applying tape or moleskin.

Ultrarunner and Pacific Crest Trail record holder and former Appalachian Trail record holder David Horton recommends using the combination of anti-biotic and drying-agent zinc oxide on blisters when you have an overnight stop or a rest period for the zinc oxide to do its magic. He remembers using the zinc oxide method on blisters when running the Trans-America (across the United States). He advises that you "take a needle and drain the blister. Then using the same hole, inject zinc oxide back into the blister until it is full of zinc. Put a Band-Aid over that. Many times we would do that in the Trans-Am, and the next day the blister would be nearly dried up. It is still the best thing I have seen to do to a blister." David made this blister fix one time on ultrarunner Dusan Marjele, the eventual Trans-Am winner, and he came back several more times because it was so effective. For multiday events, this is a great method.

"L *personal experience*

eukotape rocks! This was the best tape. Unfortunately, [at the Primal Quest Race] we had only one roll and went through it quickly. The adhesive was far superior to any other we had available and the tape shaped well to toes and feet.

"For blisters that were open with macerated or infected tissue, we used Xeroform gauze. This is the petrolatum- and antiseptic-impregnated bandage that is often used for sucking chest wounds. It worked particularly well for blisters in between the toes. We cut the gauze pads to size and wrapped them around the toes and then taped over them. Unfortunately, we could not talk to the racers at the end to see how well this worked, but it seemed like a good idea.

"We used syringe needles (mostly 18-gauge) to drain the blisters. The larger-size needle allowed the fluid to drain easily through the needle, without risk of it closing back up. Some also used the bevel edge to cut a slightly larger opening. We drained any blisters, large or small, that had palpable fluid. To clip or not to clip blister was on a case-by-case basis. We never clipped intact blisters, but open or torn skin was often removed to prevent further tearing.

"If the area was tender, we taped it. Any reddened or sore area was either taped or covered with moleskin. If the racers had done this earlier, I think we would have seen fewer patients.

"A podiatrist showed us a trick to keep tape from curling at the edges. She takes a normal votive candle and, after taping, rubs it over the edges of the tape. The small amount of wax reduces friction and helps prevent curling. This is less messy than using Bag Balm or petroleum jelly.

"Two people had infected cuticles due to ingrown toenails. The doctor had to lift the cuticle and drain the pus. Obviously, these racers didn't read John's book on trimming your toenails!"

—adventure racer and paramedic Jane Moorhead,
relating how her medical crew managed feet in the
2003 Subaru Primal Quest Adventure Race

Deep Blisters

Deep blisters are blisters under a callus, which means they can be many layers of skin deep. Usually the only way to treat deep blisters is to use a syringe and needle to drain the fluid. The athlete knows that a blister is there—but it is almost impossible to drain because the fluid is difficult to see and finding the exact depth is hard. Pressing on the callus to try to expel the fluid by hand is too painful. Using a pin or scalpel won't work. The blister is so deep that nothing else can get in that deep. Only in the biggest races with a full medical staff will there likely be a doctor who has the Zylocaine and equipment to properly care for these blisters. If I am treating an athlete with deep blisters, I will only use my scalpel with their consent after I explain the problem.

Read the section on calluses below to understand how to soften these problem areas. It is true that many athletes value their toughened feet and calluses. For some, they help. For others, they mask hidden deep blisters.

"D *personal experience*

eep blisters are next to impossible to treat. I can think of one instance in which a runner used a combination of compound tincture of benzoin and Hydropel in combination to do a Badwater double. He got through the one way to the top of Mount Whitney, but his feet were a mess by the time he was ready to do the return trip. You see, he didn't want to bother with pretaping. I don't blame him; it's a time-consuming effort to do it. But he developed blisters so deep on his heels and the balls of his feet that he could not move forward. They became blood blisters. My husband, Ben Jones, who is a medical doctor, injected him with Zylocaine, so that the blisters could be drained and treated. Under normal race circumstances it's impossible to get an injection to drain blisters. Usually there isn't that resource in a race.

"That is why I recommend filing calluses down so that if one develops a blister on that area, it can be drained and treated. Otherwise, [the blister] just grows and it becomes impossible to move forward. Once the fluid is drained, the blister is treated with antibiotic ointment and 2nd Skin and taped. It's then possible to keep on moving quite comfortably."

—Denise Jones, the Blister Queen of Badwater

Beyond Blisters

There may be times when blisters develop and even with treatment, due to continued running or hiking, additional care is needed. Several things may happen. The skin may slough off and ball up in the sock, leaving raw exposed skin. The skin may stay in place but fall off when the sock is removed. The raw skin may bleed. When blisters have developed to this point, you have to make a choice. Continuing to run or hike may lead to infection and further damaged tissue. Ideally, stay off the feet as much as possible. If you must continue, treat the problem and recheck frequently.

Sterile wound-dressing products will help the healing process. Medical personnel should have several of these products in their kits to manage extreme blisters and cases where the skin has separated from the foot. These dressings are typically available only through medical supply stores and online.

- AmeriGel's Wound Dressings and Hydrogel Saturated Gauze Dressings
- Cramer's Nova Derm Sterile Wound Dressing
- DuoDerm CGF Flexible Sterile Dressing
- Ferris' PolyMem Wound Care Dressing
- Spenco's 2nd Skin Moist Burn Pads
- Spyroflex's Wound Care Blister Dressing pads

Use these products over the blister or raw skin and leave them on as the healing process begins from the inside. The nonadhesive dressings require a tape covering or self-adhering wrap to hold them in place. One of these carried on a multiday hike could easily save your feet.

Fixing Blisters, Their Way or Yours

You may find yourself entering in an event in which you do not have control over the blister treatments and how they are applied. Participate in a 100-mile trail event or an adventure race, and you will find medical aid stations manned by podiatrists, podiatry students, nurses, emergency medical technicians, and an assortment of individuals with various medical skills. These individuals will treat your blisters according to what they know and what materials they have available to them. How they treat your blisters may not be how you would like them treated. Most aid stations are stocked with moleskin, petroleum jelly, and gauze. They may or may not have 2nd Skin and compound tincture of benzoin. If you want your feet treated with a specific product, you will have to carry a few in your fanny pack. If you want a specific powder or lubricant, you will need to carry these in a small container. I am always happy to see athletes who are able themselves, or with their crews, to manage their own feet. It can be very taxing on a small medical staff and on their supplies to manage everyone's feet and special needs.

For example, the Marathon des Sables is unlike any other marathon or ultra-marathon. The six-day, self-supported race in the Moroccan desert has 150 miles of sand, sand, and more sand. Cathy Tibbetts-Witkes, a many-time Marathon des Sables finisher, calls it a blisterfest: "Even people who never get blisters get them." While the medical care is adequate and very good, it is not everyone's first choice of blister care. Cathy reports the usual procedure is to lance the blisters, cut the skin off, apply benzoin, and then apply a blister patch. While this is not my first choice of treatment, it does work. Runners report a low incident of infection despite the high level of open blisters. Remember: A lack of preparedness on your part means that you will be treated as the medical team has been taught.

Dr. Trolan stresses the importance of understanding how your feet change when you add things to them. Adding moleskin and gauze to your foot changes the way your foot fits inside your shoe or boot. The extra thickness of the blister patch changes pressures and angles of the foot inside the shoe. This in turn changes the shoe from its usually broken-in fit to that of a mismatch. New pressure points develop, turning first into new hot spots and then into blisters. The biomechanics of the foot, ankle, and leg are altered and the gait changes. Additional problems are likely to develop. Dr. Trolan recommends using as little and as thin a blister patch as possible. This has become my teaching too.

Do not hesitate to give medical personnel at these aid stations instruction on how you would like your feet patched. I remember the bulky gauze patch put on the bottom of my right foot in 1986 during the final stages of my first Western States 100-Mile Endurance Run. While it was a good patch job, it simply did not fit right and turned me from a runner into a walker. Be aware of how medical staff are treating your feet. If you prefer a specific method of blister patching, you need to tell them, and be prepared to describe it to them—or better yet, be prepared to do it yourself.

Post-event Blister Care

I have worked the finish line of many events. Runner after runner comes to have their blisters lanced and patched. Most times, their feet are dirty and sweaty. My rule is that I don't patch anyone at a finish line unless they have washed their feet, and preferably after they have showered. I don't want to apply dressing only to have them get it wet.

Many times, their blisters are small and not worth lancing. I recommend that at home or in their motel room, they soak their feet in hot water with Epsom or Pepsom salts several times a day, if possible. The salts help dry out the skin, and often the fluid will be reabsorbed into the tissues. Epsom salts are very cheap and I would encourage you to add a zip-top bag filled with the salts for your post-race supplies.

I never put tape on a foot at a finish line. I use only Coban or a similar self-adhering wrap. Rolls of the wrap in 1-, 2-, or 3-inch widths can be found in most drugstores. A tube of antibiotic ointment should also be packed for open blisters, scratches, and cuts.

As your blisters dry, if the skin has torn, it will harden. Keep this trimmed so it won't catch on socks. A nail file can be used to sand down any rough edges.

A simple post-event foot care kit can be carried in a large zip-top bag. Being prepared with Epsom salts, antibiotic ointment, a roll or two of Coban, small scissors, and a nail file is always a good idea.

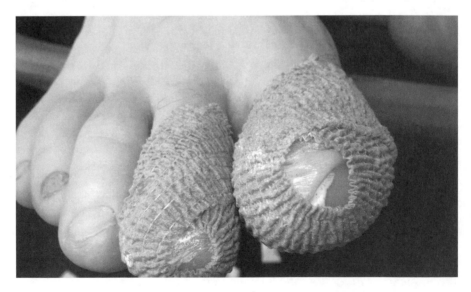

Wrap Coban around the toe and then around the tip.

22

Strains & Sprains, Fractures & Dislocations

nkle sprains and strains are common occurrences—some even with resulting fractures. Bones can break as a result of falls or twisting motions, and stress fractures can occur if athletes push themselves too fast and too soon, an unfortunately common tendency. A sudden fall with its resulting wrong landing can result in a dislocated ankle or toe. The cause may be rocks or tree roots hidden in leaves or grasses, unsteady footing while trail running at night, or twisting motions coming off a curb. Athletes need to be prepared to deal with these injuries quickly and appropriately, as late or inadequate treatment can worsen the injury, sidelining you longer and possibly setting you up for future injuries.

Strains & Sprains

A strain is the overstretching of a muscle or tendon—but without the significant tearing common to a sprain. There may be bleeding into the muscle area that can cause swelling, pain, stiffness, and muscle spasm followed by a bruise. Strains can come from overuse, repetitive movements, excessive muscle contractions, or prolonged positions.

A sprain is a stretching or tearing injury to the ligaments that stabilize bones together at a joint. Sprains are usually associated with traumas such as falling or twisting, and ankles are frequently the sprained or strained joint. During a fall or sudden twist, you may experience sudden pain or hear a pop. If you cannot walk after a few minutes of rest or if you heard the infamous pop, you can be fairly certain you have a sprain. After a sprain occurs, the fibrous joint capsule swells and becomes inflamed, discolored, and painful. An X-ray is in order. Delaying treatment for sprains or strains increases the risk of swelling and further injury.

One ankle sprain will make you more susceptible to repeated sprains, as the ligaments are left weakened, lengthened, and less flexible. Without proper care, you could get sprain after sprain and develop chronic ankle problems.

It is important to properly treat your sprained ankle. Swiss researchers analyzed health histories of 268 people and noted that 18% of those with osteoarthritis have suffered previous ankle injuries. David Weinstein, MD, head of the U.S. medical staff at the 2004 Olympics, states that when ankle ligaments are stretched, the ankle bones slide against each other and wear down the joint surface. This may, over time, increase your risk of osteoarthritis fivefold.

Ultrarunner Sue Norwood calls herself the "queen of ankle sprains." She shares this advice: "I have learned from my 22 years of experience as a patient with recurring ankle problems from trail running. My ankle sprains got progressively worse until I ruptured two peroneal tendons in one ankle and had to have surgery to reattach them. It's better to learn effective preventive techniques than to let yourself get this injured!"

The most common ankle sprain is an inversion sprain, in which the foot rolls to the outside and the ankle turns out. The injured area is the lateral ligament just below the ankle joint on the outside of the foot. An eversion sprain, in which the ankle is turned inward and the medial ligament injured, is less common. In a serious sprain, both the lateral and medial ligaments can be injured. An X-ray will reveal whether there is a bone fracture that would require immobilization of the joint.

There are three degrees of an ankle sprain. A grade I strain has minimal swelling, and the athlete can still put weight on the leg with the twisted ankle. The ankle's ligaments have been stretched and some are torn. A grade II sprain has moderate swelling and moderate pain when weight is put on the injured ankle. There is a partial tear of the ligament. A grade III sprain has a large amount of swelling, and weight placed on the ankle cannot be tolerated. Grades I and II will heal in about 4–6 weeks with full recovery in 10–12 weeks.

A grade III sprain requires medical attention. With a severe sprain there is the possibility of a related fracture. If there is a great deal of pain and swelling, and you are unable to bear weight on the foot, an emergency room visit and an X-ray are in order.

There are ways to minimize ankle sprains. Obvious but often forgotten, specific strengthening exercises can go a long way toward preventing strains and sprains (see "Strengthening Exercises," page 264). In addition, always be aware of how your feet land. If you sense your foot starting to roll over, quickly transfer your weight to your other foot. When on the trail, be attentive to changes in the terrain, especially on downhills and in the late afternoon and evenings, when shadows merge into darkness. On the road, be aware of curbs, manholes, and grates, as well as the slanted, concave surface roadway. On grassy areas, watch for hidden holes and roots. Any of these can trip you up and throw you off balance. Additionally, you are more susceptible to making wrong moves and being slower to respond to sudden terrain changes when you are tired.

Treating a Strain or Sprain

The initial treatment for a strain or sprain includes the classic RICE treatment:

■ R = rest

■ I = ice

■ C = compression

■ E = elevation

Ice your injury within 30 minutes if possible. The first 24 hours are the most critical for beginning treatment. The typical sprained ankle takes four to six weeks to fully heal. Severe ankle sprains can require a cast for complete immobilization.

Early treatment within the first 24 hours decreases swelling and lessens the risk of additional injury. Initial rest of the foot is also important. A lightly applied Ace wrap will provide compression to help keep swelling down while providing support. Apply the Ace wrap from the forefoot toward the ankle. Do not wear the Ace wrap at night. Apply ice for 20 minutes at a time at least four times daily. Six to eight times a day for the first few days is even better. The chapter "Cold & Heat Therapy" gives more information on making the most of icing techniques.

Elevate the injured area above the level of the heart as much as possible during the first 48 hours. This keeps blood away from the injured area and reduces pain and swelling. In bed at night, elevate the foot on a pillow. The treatment goal is to return the ankle to normal motion and to be weight bearing as soon as possible. The combination of rest, icing, compression, and elevation, especially in the first few days, will help the healing process and decrease the pain and swelling.

Heat increases blood flow to an injured area, which makes swelling worse. For this reason, the use of heat is not recommended for at least a week after an injury. Moist heat can be applied by using a moist heating pad, a warm towel, or a warm bath. Dry heat can be applied by using a heating pad for 20 minutes at a time.

The use of anti-inflammatory medications is usually warranted. Nonsteroidal anti-inflammatory drugs, commonly called NSAIDS, are used to control pain and swelling after an injury. The most common NSAIDS are aspirin, ibuprofen, and naproxen sodium (Aleve). These pain relievers should be taken according to their instructions and usually with food. Be careful if you continue training because the NSAIDS block pain signals that would warn you of further injury.

Natural science can also help. Traumeel is a natural pain reliever that works with your body to promote healing while reducing recovery time (**www.traumeel usa.com**). Homeopathic treatments use minute doses of natural substances to stimulate the body's self-healing response. For sprains and strains there are three recommended remedies: arnica montana, Bryonia alba, and rhus toxicodendron.

Depending on the severity of the injury, you might be able to walk on it. With minimal pain and swelling, self-treatment at home can often be sufficient. If the pain is severe with a large degree of swelling and there is discoloration of the injured area, prompt medical attention is mandatory.

Bryan Whitesides, a board-certified orthopedic clinical specialist, suggests the following two tips to help athletes more quickly and completely recover from an ankle sprain. "First, the use of crutches for even a few days can dramatically improve recovery time," he says. "Encourage walking using the crutches to reduce weight on the ankle instead of keeping the foot off the ground. Second, a compression wrap with the addition of a horseshoe-shaped felt pad greatly reduces the effects of swelling." To wrap an ankle sprain, Bryan cuts 0.25 inch of thick felt into a horseshoe shape and places it so the U cradles the malleolus (ankle bone). Then he uses an elastic wrap to firmly compress the entire horseshoe against the ankle. He adds, "The horseshoe and wrap should be used until the swelling is nearly gone." Bryan maintains the website **www.injuredrunner.com,** which offers a DVD about stretching, strengthening, and balance training—vital for athletes.

Wrapping an Ankle

Bryan Whitesides offers the following tips to wrapping an ankle. This technique provides compression and support following an ankle sprain. Two-inch-wide elastic wrap works best, and the tension should be firm but still allow normal circulation.

1. Start the wrap 3–4 inches above the outer side of your ankle. Pull the wrap straight down under your heel and around to the arch.

2. From your arch proceed around to the front of your ankle and then around to the back of your heel/Achilles.

3. From the Achilles, continue diagonally along the inner side of your heel; then wrap under your arch to the outer side of your ankle and up to the front of your foot.

4. Proceed around the inside of your ankle and pull the wrap behind your heel/Achilles. Continue around the outer ankle diagonally, coming under the foot again and around to the front of your ankle. This pattern can be repeated for additional support/compression.

5. With any additional wrap, spiral up the lower leg.

There are two schools of thought on how soon to start running, exercising, or bearing weight on an injured ankle. One says to get out on it as soon as possible and let pain be your guide. If the ankle is stiff and sore when you first start, keep going and see if it loosens up. If the pain increases, you should call it a day, go home, and ice. If it doesn't get worse or feels better, you are probably OK. The other says to work through the healing process at the ankle's speed. You must choose your course based on available information. Even if you can't bear weight on the injured ankle, starting range-of-motion exercises or using a Thera-Band resistance band can help jump-start the rehabilitation process (**www.thera-band.com**).

Certified athletic trainer Jay Hodde, MS, ATC/L, points out the following dangers of running too soon on an injured ankle:

Running with a severe sprain can cause more problems than just reinjuring it. Several things may happen. First, your gait will change as you guard the injury. Because your body is not used to these changes, overuse injuries may occur in other areas of the body. Second, the severity of the sprain may increase, prolonging recovery. Third, the ankle joint may develop the tendency to partially dislocate (subluxation). This is more common if the sprain is severe. Usually, there is some minor slipping of bone surfaces that can cause problems if the joint mechanics are thrown off by the sprain. Bruising of the bone surfaces can occur and can lead to complications later in life, such as an increased risk of arthritis.

When you can start to put weight on the ankle, begin with easy walking and slowly build back to the routine you had before the injury. Wear an ankle support if you cannot bear your full weight on the ankle. Walking even a little bit a few times a day will aid on the road to recovery. After each exercise period, ice as necessary. Following a few of the strengthening exercises described below will also help you gain back ankle strength and normal motion.

When Your Ankle Still Hurts

Lisa Bliss, MD, shares some solid wisdom: "Soft tissue injuries should heal up within eight weeks with appropriate diagnosis and rehabilitation. If there is recurrent pain or swelling eight months after the original injury, there is either a missed diagnosis, insufficient rehabilitation, or recurrent injury.

"After my sprain at Western States, I rested the ankle and did the usual rehabilitation protocol consisting of range of motion, proprioception, strengthening, and plyometrics. I returned to running pretty quickly with the ASO brace, but the ankle never fully recovered. There was continued pain deep in the joint, especially with downhill running (when the joint is least stable and relies on ligaments for added stability). I never had real pain (such as when I had my toenails permanently removed!), only a vague discomfort, and only when running. After several attempts at running longer distances without pain failed, I finally got an MRI. It showed that I had completely ruptured the lateral ligaments in my ankle—the anterior talofibular ligament (ATFL) and the calcaneofibular ligament (CFL), and by exam and stress X-rays, the ankle was very unstable (grade III ankle sprain). No wonder all the rehabilitation in the world couldn't get me back to pain-free running.

"I elected to have surgical repair of the ligaments and am now three weeks post-op. Prognosis (my own) is a full recovery and return to running in a few months.

"The point I want to emphasize is that you should not take your ankles for granted! They should be in tip-top shape for the trails—no less. They should not be painful or swollen after a 'short' 50K. An ankle that's not 100% after eight months means that something is wrong. It may be as simple as weak peroneal muscles or as traumatic as a bruised bone or a cartilage fracture, but even a weak muscle can be a problem for an ultrarunner.

"I always recommend against surgery if there are other treatment options available. As most of us know, proprioception is key to nonsurgical rehab, but many of us fail to strengthen the peroneal muscles on the outside of the leg (those whose ankles evert). If the lateral ligaments are stretched out, then the muscles must be very strong to help stabilize against recurrent sprains. The other thing that is very important is protecting the ankle from reinjury. Wearing a brace will not make the ankle weak; not doing the strengthening and proprioception exercises leaves the ankle weak. The brace may prevent a severe injury."

Ankle supports are an important part of treating an ankle sprain or strain. The support will allow you to be up and about faster and will provide comfort as the ankle continues healing. There are many types to choose from. The section "Ankle-support Products" (on pages 266–267) describes an assortment of available supports. But rather than becoming dependent on ankle supports, work on strengthening your ankles and sense of balance.

You can strengthen your ankles by focusing on proprioception, the neurological signals from your body to your brain that tell it where your body is relative to the space around it. Several exercises below focus on this aspect of ankle strengthening, which improves your ability to balance. Many athletes swear by proprioceptive reconditioning after an ankle injury. When you are able to make a mid-stride adjustment as your foot hits the ground, senses an uneven surface, and sends a signal to the brain, you are more likely to avoid a sprained ankle. The more we practice this on varying terrain, the quicker and stronger this process becomes. Proprioception can be enhanced by walking and running on soft and uneven ground at every opportunity. Practice proprioception at home, or the office when doing simple tasks by balancing on one foot. The use of a wobble or rocker board is also helpful. Because injuries often occur when we are fatigued, doing these exercises at the end of a workout when our muscles are already tired can be helpful. Proprioceptive exercises will help strengthen your knees too.

Proprioception

Steve Gurney, an adventure racer (**www.gurneygears.com**), gives a good explanation of this important term. "Proprioception is the feedback between sensory tissue, our brain, and muscle. By sensing the angles and forces in each movement of our feet, the brain can fire the appropriate muscles for stability and then movement. The more we practice this on varying terrain, the quicker and stronger this process becomes. Proprioception can be enhanced by running on soft and uneven ground at every opportunity. Try making a rule to stay off sealed surfaces. Run on grass verge, in creeks and riverbeds, in parks, beside rail tracks, and in subdivisions. If you have to run on roads, then run up and down the gutters playing coordination games. (for example, three steps in the gutter, two steps up on the curb).

"Balance practice is excellent, using such things as a wobble board or tightrope-style balance on gate chains, parking lot walls, or fences. Running as fast as you dare on walls is great.

"Coordination for rock running is also enhanced by practice. We can simulate specific and quicker foot-eye coordination on plenty of things near home. For instance, running up and down stairs at speed, sideways and backward. Running off trails in a forest is good. You can also practice proprioception at home—or the office when doing simple tasks such as talking on the phone, thinking, cooking, or watching TV—by balancing on one foot (for greater challenge, shut your eyes) or a wobble board."

Josh Gilbert, a chiropractor, thinks a wobble or rocker board is a good tool. He suggests the following: "First, I would do a very simple activity. Stand on the injured ankle and balance for as long as you can. If you can do this for 30 seconds or longer, start doing the same exercise with your eyes closed. This helps to get your brain neurologically connected again with your ankle and the injured tissue and receptors. Only do this exercise if the ankle can bear your weight without pain (or not too much). Each joint in your body has receptors that tell your brain where it is. You don't have to look at your leg to know that it is turned in, out, pointed up, or down. The receptors in the joint relay this information to the brain. When the joint is injured, sprained, or stretched, these receptors start relaying incorrect information. It they are not retrained properly, you will end up like many people and continue having recurrent ankle sprains."

Supplements for Quick Recovery

Because ligaments and tendons do not have their own direct blood supply, their healing is slow. Ultrarunner Karl King found that the nutritional supplements of 1 gram glycine, 1 gram lysine, 0.5 gram buffered vitamin C, and one Aleve tablet is helpful in the healing process. Take this combination at breakfast and at bedtime. The supplements provide the major building blocks for connective tissue, while the Aleve is an anti-inflammatory.

Two dietary supplements, glucosamine sulfate and chondroitin sulfate, have been found to reduce joint pain. In 2005 the American College of Rheumatology announced a National Institute of Health–funded study that showed using the supplements was effective at reducing moderate to severe knee pain due to osteoarthritis. Smaller European studies have made the same findings.

Glucosamine sulfate is a natural substance that helps build cartilage, the cushion at the ends of our bones, and maintain joint fluid thickness and elasticity. Chondroitin sulfate, also a natural substance, helps lubricate joints and gives tendons and ligaments their elasticity. Initial studies have found these over-the-counter supplements helpful in stimulating cartilage to grow and inhibiting the enzymes that break down cartilage. Many athletes have added this combination to their daily vitamin and supplement intake as a must-have. Drugstores, pharmacies, and health food stores typically offer these two supplements (often in one capsule) in an assortment of supplement formulas by different companies. Give these supplements time to work—a month or more.

Strengthening Exercises

Strengthening exercises for the foot and ankle can help prevent injuries and can speed recovery from an injury. Balancing exercises and the use of Thera-Bands are good to help strengthen the ankles. Thera-Bands can be used with many of the exercises. Stop any weight-bearing exercises if you experience pain. Here are some exercise options.

- Sit in a chair and write the alphabet with your toes to simulate ankle motion in all directions.

- Stand on one foot on a pillow or similar soft and unstable cushion and try to maintain your balance, first with one foot and then the other. As your ability to balance increases, move into short controlled up and down knee bends.

- Use a wobble board to work the injured ankle as well your good ankle.

- Move the ankle up and down in a pumping motion to help decrease swelling.

- Rotate your feet up to 50 repetitions in each direction. Do four to five sets every other day.

- Strengthen your ankles by balancing with one foot flat on the ground and the other leg bent back at the knee, as if you were in the normal support phase of a running stride. Start at 30 seconds at a time and practice until you can hold your balance for several minutes. When you have mastered this step, close your eyes and do the same thing. Repeatedly losing your balance and then recovering gradually strengthens the ankles even more. Doing this exercise with your eyes closed retrains you to quickly react to changes as your nerve endings detect a twist or turn when the foot hits the ground.

- Stand on one leg and slowly rise all the way up onto your toes and then slowly lower your heel to a flat foot. Balance yourself as necessary. Start with 25 repetitions and work up to 50 daily. This is another good proprioception exercise.

- Stand with your forefeet on a raised surface (such as a book, low step, or block of wood), and rise up onto your toes and then back down again. Hold each, at the top and at the bottom, for 10–15 seconds. Repeat until both calves are fatigued.

- An isometric exercise with the feet pushing against each other helps strengthen muscles without joint movement. When sitting on a chair, push down with one foot on top while pulling up with the other foot on the bottom. Then reverse feet. When sitting on the floor, you can also put your feet bottom to bottom, first pushing the big toes against each other and then the small toes against each other. Hold the motions for six to ten seconds and repeat several times a day.

- Hop on one foot and then change to the other foot. Practice forward and backward, and side to side movements.

Work Those Calves

Matt Mahoney, one of the proponents of barefoot running and running without socks, feels the most important ankle muscle is the calf: "This is what you use to take the weight off your heel and shift to the ball of your foot when your ankle starts to twist." He recommends the following calf exercises, emphasizing, "You will know you're doing these exercises right if your calves are sore for several days afterward."

- Run backward.

- Run barefoot in sand.

- Climb stairs, both up and down. Land on the ball of your foot as you descend.

- Do calf raises on a step, with weights, standing for the gastrocnemius and sitting for the soleus. Using machines is useful for these. Do the standing calf raises one foot at a time on a step with a weighted belt. Do the sitting raises on a machine with weight resting on a padded bar across the top of the legs.

Research at the University of North Carolina supports Matt's thoughts. The study found that training your calf muscles can protect your ankles from injury. The study followed 20 athletes and found those who rolled or sprained their ankles had less range of ankle motion than healthy athletes. The two calf muscles—the

ANKLE-SUPPORT PRODUCTS

The **ANKLE STABILIZING ORTHOSIS (ASO)** is made to prevent or treat ankle sprains. It features an elastic cuff closure to decrease the degree of potential inversion, figure-eight straps to replicate ankle taping, a low profile to allow it to fit in any type of shoe, and a lace-up closure. It is designed to keep the foot in a neutral position. A model is available with rigid side stays to increase stability. **www.medspec.com**

The convenient **ANKLEWRAP** differs from the typical Ace wrap. Made from a knitted blend of nylon and Lycra with a foam inner layer, it breathes to wick away perspiration, stays put with superior sticking power, and is fully adjustable. At 10 feet long by 1.5 inches wide, it is long enough to make a complete figure-eight wrap with three heel locks. **www.fabrifoam.com**

CHO-PAT'S ANKLE SUPPORT provides compression to the ankle with a removable Velcro fastener that wraps in a figure eight around the ankle, giving additional compression at specific locations of the ankle while providing stabilization. The support is made of neoprene. A Dynamic Ankle Compression Sleeve is also offered. **www.cho-pat.com**

CROPPER MEDICAL'S BIO SKIN is a compression support material made with four layers: a hypoallergenic Lycra knit outer layer, a SmartSkin membrane that absorbs moisture and wicks it from the skin, a Lycra knit/fleece inner layer, and a SkinLok layer against the skin. Bio Skin stretches with the body's movement, giving compression without bunching and binding, and it does not constrict the joints. Unlike neoprene, Bio Skin breathes. The three designs include a TriLok Ankle Control System, a Visco Ankle Skin that has visco polymer inserts around anklebones, and a Standard Ankle Skin. The visco and standard wraps have an optional figure-eight wrap. **www.bioskin.com**

The **KALLASSY ANKLE SUPPORT** is a proven design for rehabilitation of severe ankle sprains. The support is made of nylon-lined neoprene that provides warmth and compression. A strap that wraps around the ankle provides stability, and a

gastrocnemius and soleus—limit the ankle range of motion. Cathleen Brown, MA, the lead study author, advises calf raises with knees slightly bent to strengthen the soleus. To stretch the gastrocnemius, use the familiar stretch where you lean against a wall with one leg in front of the other. Repeating this with the back knee bent stretches the soleus.

Ankle-support Products

Weak ankles can be a problem, particularly on trails. After turning or spraining an ankle, an ankle support will provide the support and protection necessary for light training. Otherwise weak ankles can also benefit from an ankle support. Adhesive taping of the ankle can be helpful; however, for it to be effective, someone who is experienced must do the taping. While taping restricts extreme motion, the tape

A N K L E - S U P P O R T   P R O D U C T S

nonstretch lateral strapping system helps prevent inversion motions of the ankle. If you are prone to turned ankles, this support is one of the most stabilizing ankle supports available. It is often available in sporting goods stores or can be purchased online.

OPTP (ORTHOPEDIC PHYSICAL THERAPY PRODUCTS) has a wide range of devices for balance/proprioception, stretching, strength training, and more. **www. optp.com**

THE PERFORM 8 LATERAL ANKLE STABILIZER provides excellent external stabilization of the ankle's lateral (outer) ligaments, similar to ankle taping. While a lightweight elastic compression sock provides support to soft tissue, an elastic figure-eight strap wraps around the foot. Pads protect and relieve pressure on the Achilles tendon. This support is excellent for athletes prone to chronic ankle sprains. **www.brownmed.com**

PRO-TEC ANKLE WRAP stabilizes the ankle joint, preventing sudden twists or turns which may cause further injury. Made with a neoprene sleeve for warmth and compression and a figure-eight elastic wrap for support control and stabilization. **www.injurybegone.com**

STROMGREN makes several ankle supports that provide good stabilization to prevent turning an ankle or to support a previously sprained ankle. Their Double Strap Model offers a unique sock-style support with two elastic straps that wrap around the ankle to provide the benefit of taped ankle support without the tape. The Stirrup Lock Ankle Support has four straps that restrict inversion/eversion. **www.stromgren.com**

WOBBLE AND ROCKER BOARDS can be used to improve balance and strength, retrain injured muscles, improve muscle memory, and build core strength. You can get a wobble board for both feet or two smaller wobble boards, one for each foot. FitterFirst has the most comprehensive line of boards, as well as training charts and programs. **www.fitter1.com**

loses strength as it moves with the skin—40% of its strength can be lost within 20 minutes. Ankle supports are better at providing support.

Ankle supports are typically made from a compression-type sock. Some offer a figure-eight–style stretch wrap, which gives additional strength and support. Some ankle supports can be found in drugstores and sporting goods stores. Cramer, DonJoy, Futuro, Mueller, Pro-Tec, and Spenco all make basic ankle supports. Many are simply a one-piece pull-on neoprene or stretch device with a hole for the heel and toes. Ace wraps, or similar elastic wraps, are helpful after a sprain but provide little support against initially turning your ankle. Sue Norwood, who has an eversion problem, likes the ASO Ankle Stabilizer that her doctor told her to wear for the year after her surgery—it's supportive but lightweight and easy to use, and is one of the most popular.

All the ankle supports listed on the preceding pages are compact in size and fit easily into a fanny pack or backpack. Because the supports vary in fit and material, experiment wearing the support against the skin or over a sock to find the best fit on your foot. If you are prone to ankle injuries, consider carrying one as a preventive measure.

Fractures

Any bone in the foot can fracture; however, some are more prone to injury than others. The terms break and fracture are synonymous—both describe a structural break in the continuity of the bone. A fracture may occur from a fall, the twisting motion of a turned ankle, a blow from hitting your foot on a rock or tree root, or simply from a bad foot plant. The toes are the most likely bones to fracture in the foot—usually the first (big toe) and the fifth (small toe). The Jones fracture (breaking the fifth metatarsal on the outside of the foot) is common. This type of fracture is common with a fall or loss of balance where you put a sudden and undue amount of pressure on the outside of your foot. But there are many types of fractures.

Types of Fractures

AVULSION—the tearing away of a part of the bone attached to a ligament or tendon

BUTTERFLY—a bone fragment shaped like a butterfly and part of a comminuted fracture

COMMINUTED—more than two fragments; may be splintered

COMPLETE—the bone is completely broken through

DISPLACED—bone fragments are moved away from each other

IMPACTED—fragments are compressed by force into each other or into adjacent bone

INCOMPLETE—the continuity of the bone is destroyed on only one side

NONDISPLACED—the bone pieces are still together in the correct locations and angles

SEGMENTAL—several large fractures in the same bone

SPIRAL—the fracture line is spiral in shape

Fractures usually manifest themselves with a great deal of pain and tenderness directly above the fracture site. When a soft tissue injury has occurred, there will also be discoloration of the skin above the fracture. Fractures that are ignored can result in a malunion or nonunion of the pieces of bone as they heal. This could require surgery to correctly align the bone ends.

Emergency room physicians and sports specialists often use the Ottawa Ankle Rules[33] to determine the likelihood of an ankle fracture before an X-ray is taken (and to avoid unnecessary X-rays). The study takes two approaches:

- Pain in the malleolar (ankle bones) zone and either an inability to bear weight immediately and in the emergency room, or bone tenderness at the posterior (back) edge of either malleolus.

- Pain in the mid-foot zone and either an inability to bear weight immediately and in the emergency room, or bone tenderness at the navicular (the bone at the top front of the foot at the curve up the ankle) or fifth metatarsal (the mid-foot bone on the outside of the foot).

Treating Fractures

Treatment of fractures typically combines ice, immobilization, and elevation. Toe fractures are usually buddy taped, and the patient is advised to wear a firm-soled shoe or a wooden orthopedic shoe that restricts flexion of the foot. Buddy taping is done by lightly taping the injured toe to the toe next to it, with a piece of cotton between toes (never tape skin to skin). Buddy taping provides support and a limited degree of immobilization of the toe. A fracture of the big toe can warrant a full foot cast. A Jones fracture or any other fracture of the foot or ankle will require a cast and immobilization for four to six weeks.

Standard practice with fractures is to immobilize the joint above and the joint below the fracture. You may start with a non-weight-bearing cast, requiring the use of crutches, and later have it changed to a weight-bearing walking cast.

Refer to the chapter "Cold & Heat Therapy" for more information on making the most of icing techniques.

Stress Fractures

Stress fractures are a common sports injury. Sudden or repetitive stress, usually from overuse without proper conditioning, results in a small crack in the outer shell of the affected bone. Over time, if not treated, this crack will develop into a fracture of the bone. Often you will have no recollection of having injured the foot.

The most common foot bones to stress fracture are the second and third metatarsal bones in the forefoot—between the toes and the ankle. Some doctors will use an X-ray to make the diagnosis, but often a stress fracture does not show on an initial X-ray because the bone's callus formation has not yet taken place at the fracture site. A bone scan, which is different from an X-ray, is useful for a questionable diagnosis and will usually confirm whether you have a stress fracture. Some hospitals will use an MRI to make the diagnosis.

Other possible causes of stress fractures include wearing worn-out or poor-fitting shoes, or ill-fitting insoles; abnormal foot structure or mechanics (arch or pronation problems, or leg-length discrepancies); or tightness and inflexibility. Your medical specialist may recommend additional calcium in your diet and/or a DEXA scan bone-density test. Female athletes who have infrequent periods are most at risk for stress fractures.

At the point of the stress fracture, there is typically pain to the touch, often first felt as a dull ache or soreness. The pain usually becomes worse as the break grows. Swelling is common. Stress fractures are most common from overuse, over-training, or a change in running surfaces—from a softer to a harder surface. Stress fractures are also referred to as "march fractures."

Peter Fish's stress-fracture story is not so unusual. He remembers his first stress fracture (to the third metatarsal of the right foot), which happened in July 1995. His second fracture may have started as a stress fracture or may have simply been a fracture from the start:

> I had an unpleasant itchy sensation on the top of my foot for a month or so (I was ramping up mileage for the Portland Marathon), and during a training run, it turned into a sudden sharp pain. I limped home and went to my family doctor the same day. The fracture didn't show on the X-ray yet, but it appeared a couple of weeks later when I consulted my podiatrist. I didn't use the walking boot, but if I had to do a lot of walking, I found that a stiff-soled pair of medium-high work boots kept my foot from flexing painfully and enabled me to walk almost normally. I didn't run for six weeks, and then I started off cautiously, this time with the California International Marathon (early December) in mind.
>
> This time my training went quite well, with no protests from the injured foot, and I was able to get up to 40 miles a week with five or six long runs. I ran two races during the month or so before the marathon, one of 9 miles and the other a 20K, both at my projected marathon pace. A couple of weeks before the race, the top of my left foot felt sore. My podiatrist thought it was probably a neuroma from too-tight laces, as it was rather high up on the instep for a stress fracture. I ran the marathon, in some discomfort, although this didn't seem to get worse during the race, and I managed to attain my Boston qualifier by a couple of minutes with a time of 3:38.
>
> Immediately after the race, my foot became extremely painful, and I could hardly walk on it. It was a couple of weeks before I could run at all, and I had to run on the outside of that foot to do it. It didn't seem to be healing at all, so I went back to the podiatrist. An X-ray showed it to be fractured quite badly, nearly all the way through. The reason I could run on it was that the break was near the top of the third metatarsal, where there was less flexion. The doctor thought it seemed more like a break due to trauma than a normal stress fracture. During the 9-mile race I had run a couple of months previous, I got off the course once and had to jump a ditch to get back. I landed pretty heavily, and it seemed possible that this set up the fracture, which came on later, perhaps during the marathon. The regimen was the same as before: no running for six weeks, and as

before, I spent a lot of time in the pool, on my bike, and even did some cross-country skiing.

Treating Stress Fractures

After a confirming scan, a sports doctor, orthopedist, or podiatrist will usually recommend at least six weeks off. Follow their advice. To run or exercise heavily on a stress fracture is asking for more problems. Switch to more cushioned shoes and use this recovery time to focus on other non-weight-bearing exercises and cross-training: cycling, pool running, swimming, and weight training. Ask your doctor whether you can use a limited–weight-bearing exercise machine such as a stair climber or an elliptical trainer.

An Ace wrap or compression sock will help control swelling. An orthopedic or wooden shoe may be used to splint the foot. Anti-inflammatories are helpful. Elevation of the foot above the level of the heart will help reduce pain and swelling. Ice the area 20 minutes at a time three to four times a day and after any exercise. The "Cold & Heat Therapy" chapter gives more information on making the most of icing techniques. Difficult cases may require splinting, casting, or surgery.

Dislocations

A dislocation is a complete displacement of bone from its normal position at a joint's surface, which disrupts the articulation of two or three bones at that junction and alters alignment. The dislocation may be complete, where the joint surfaces are completely separated, or incomplete (subluxation), where the joint is only slightly displaced. The dislocation may be caused by a direct blow or injury, or by a ligament's tearing.

In the foot, the most common dislocations are the toes. Any of the toes can be dislocated, but the most typical are the big toe or the small toe. The ankle can be dislocated by any combination of fractures of the tibia (the big inner bone of the lower leg) or fibula (the small outer bone of the lower leg), resulting in a displaced talus. Ankle dislocations can be a major lower leg injury with severe consequences if the circulation to the foot is compromised.

Treating Dislocations

Dislocated toes are fairly simple to treat. Resetting dislocations is called reduction. With one hand, stabilize the ball of the foot with your thumb on the injured toe. With the other hand exert traction to the toe while pulling slowly and steadily on the displaced section of toe. Pull firmly enough that it clears the previous section of toe. The connecting ligament will then pull the toe back into place almost automatically. This reduces the dislocation. The toe then needs to be buddy taped to the toe or toes next to it for stabilization. A small piece of gauze, cotton, or tissue between the taped toes will prevent skin breakdown if the tape is on for any great length of time. A firm-soled shoe will help keep the toe in line and the foot-toe joint stable. If you are able, ice the toe before buddy taping. Frequent icing and elevation in the next 48 hours is recommended.

To temporarily correct and stabilize an ankle dislocation and related fracture, an orthopedic trauma surgeon recommends straightening the foot by exerting traction in a straight and steady motion—so that as much as possible it is in its natural position and angled to the lower leg. The foot, ankle, and lower leg then need to be stabilized with a splint. Use any available materials to keep the extremity stable. Check the toes frequently for normal skin color and warmth, which indicate good circulation. A dislocated ankle needs to be treated by an emergency room physician or orthopedic surgeon as soon as possible.

If either a toe or ankle dislocation is an open dislocation, where the bone has come through the skin, extra care must be taken. This open, or complex, dislocation is usually associated with a fracture, and the bone may still be outside of the skin or may have pulled back inside. First, clean the wound, and then proceed with the reduction. Then, leaving the wound open, apply a sterile dressing, and splint the extremity. Check the end(s) of the extremity farthest from the body to be sure there is adequate circulation, adjusting the extremity as necessary. When the open dislocation is stabilized, seek out immediate medical attention.

23

Tendon & Ligament Injuries

The primary function of tendons is to transmit muscle force to the moving joints with limited elongation. Tendons are ropelike structures that attach muscles to bones. Ligaments are similar structures that attach bones to other bones. When muscles and bones move, they exert stresses on the tendons and ligaments that are attached to them. The foot is a complicated but amazing engineering marvel. With 26 bones, 33 joints, 107 ligaments, 19 muscles, and tendons to hold the structure together and allow it to move in a variety of ways, it offers all kinds of opportunities for tendon and ligament injuries.

Troy Marsh, an orthopedic physical therapist, describes tendon disorders as "a major problem among competitive athletes, often interfering with training and competition. Tissue damage may result from a sudden traumatic episode such as an ankle sprain, or it may arise with no apparent cause but usually due to cumulative trauma or overuse."

The terms tendinitis, tendinosis, and tendinopathy all refer to tendon injuries. These terms are commonly confused and misused:

TENDINITIS—The suffix "itis" means inflammation. The term tendinitis should be reserved for tendon injuries that involve larger-scale acute injuries accompanied by inflammation. (*Tendinitis* is often spelled as *tendonitis*, but the preferred spelling used in most of the medical literature is *tendinitis*.)

TENDINOSIS—The suffix "osis" implies a pathology of chronic degeneration without inflammation. Tendinosis is an accumulation over time of small-scale injuries that don't heal properly; it is a chronic injury of failed healing.

When our muscles move in new ways or do more work than they can easily handle, our muscles and tendons can sustain damage. If the increase in demand is made gradually, muscle and tendon tissues will usually heal, build in strength, and adapt to new loads. It is this principle we use to build muscle and tendon strength.

Many athletes, however, participate in activities that injure a tendon on a microscopic scale and then do more injury before the tendon heals. If you continue the injurious activity, you will gradually accumulate these microinjuries. When enough injury accumulates, you'll feel pain. This kind of injury that comes on slowly with time and persists is a chronic injury; acute tendon injuries are sudden tears that cause immediate pain and obvious symptoms. Tendon injuries often require patience and careful rehabilitation because tendons heal more slowly than muscles.

Tendons are critical for converting the movement of muscle contraction to movement of the foot and/or ankle. The most common tendon injury is to the Achilles tendon, which connects the muscle of the posterior calf to the bottom of the calcaneus bone and mediates plantar flexion (toes down) function across the ankle. Injuries to other tendons that cross the ankle are usually the result of lacerations or direct trauma. Injuries to tendons can vary from mild (stretching) to moderate (tearing) to severe (rupture).

A common tendon problem affects the ankle flexors. These tendons are caught under the pressure of the shoe's tongue and laces across the front top of the foot. Walking or running steep hills can also cause this problem. Another common tendon injury is post-tibial tendinitis. This affects the posterior tibial tendon from the inside of the ankle and the foot. Major tendons and ligaments in the foot and ankle include the following:

- Achilles tendon,
- Anterior tibial tendon,
- Calcaneofibular ligament,
- Inferior talofibular ligament,
- Lisfranc ligament,
- Peroneal tendons,
- Posterior talofibular ligament,
- Sinus tarsi syndrome, and
- Tarsal canal ligaments.

Treating Tendon Injuries

There are multiple treatments for tendon injuries. Your podiatrist, sports podiatrist, or orthopedist is the best person to determine the treatment you need. In addition to the treatments below, sometimes a biomechanical assessment is needed. The list below is taken from **www.tendinosis.org,** a website devoted to tendon injuries (the following suggestions for tendinosis also work for tendinitis).

REST. By the time you feel pain from tendinosis, your injury has been gradually building for many weeks. Remember that tendons heal slowly.

PHYSICAL THERAPY EXERCISES can help heal tendinosis, as long as you are careful to progress gradually. Studies have shown that loading a tendon parallel to its length helps the collagen fibers grow with better parallel alignment and speeds the healing process. Find a physical therapist who has a lot of experience with tendinosis, and make sure he/she is willing to go as slowly as your body requires.

SONOCUR SHOCK WAVE THERAPY is a new treatment for tendinosis. The Sonocur machine is an extracorporeal ultrasound device that delivers sound waves to a very focused area of the tendon.

ICE is a common treatment for tendinosis. Many physical therapists suggest that you use ice following your exercises or whenever you need some pain reduction during the day. Don't use it just prior to your exercises. It's hard to say if ice has any long-term beneficial effect on tendinosis, but it can be an excellent form of pain control that has no negative side effects (as long as you take care not to get ice burn from too much ice).

SUPPORTS AND ORTHOTICS are often used for ankle injuries. Some people find that supports can add stability and support during activity. These should not be worn all the time because you can lose strength and flexibility.

NUTRITIONAL SUPPLEMENTS are somewhat of an unknown area. There has been little scientific research to investigate the effects of nutritional supplements on the healing of tendinosis. Glucosamine sulfate and chondroitin sulfate are not likely to help tendinosis. Other supplements that claim to help heal tendons and ligaments contain the amino acids glycine, lysine, and proline.

BODYWORK is done by physical therapists. Massage and other techniques can help loosen up. Many practitioners try to help you with your posture and body mechanics, and some do hands-on soft tissue work.

SURGERY should be a last resort for tendinosis. Some athletes have a positive outcome, while others a negative outcome. Educate yourself about the surgical procedure before you consider it for yourself, and give your injury plenty of time to heal on its own before you resort to surgery.

CORTISONE injections are not recommended by **www.tendinosis.org** because of the possibility of an adverse reaction on the tissue in the area of injection if repeated injections are given.

If pain and injury persists after a course of treatment, ask for an MRI. A partial or full tendon rupture can only be diagnosed with an MRI. Troy Marsh reports that "chronic Achilles tendinosis sufferers, most often seen among male recreational runners between 35 and 45 years old, responded favorably to a 12-week training program of high-load eccentric calf muscle training and returned to full running activity. A comparison group with the same diagnosis, treated conventionally with anti-inflammatory drugs, orthotics, rest, and therapy modalities, was not successful and each subject ultimately was treated surgically."

Tendon and fascia pain can be helped with a quick and simple minimally invasive medical treatment. The TOPAZ MicroDebrider utilizes patented Coblation technology to offer a quicker return to daily activities with a significant improvement in patient outcomes. This can effectively work on plantar fasciitis. Small punctures in key areas of the heel are made to allow the insertion of a pencil tip–size wand device, the MicroDebrider. Radio frequency energy is transmitted through the wand for short 500 millisecond intervals. The Coblation technology forms a plasma that gently and precisely dissolves soft tissue at relatively low temperatures and increases vascular blood supply. Check with your orthopedic surgeon or podiatrist for more information about this treatment.

How Tendons Heal

Tendons have limited blood supply, and nutrition is often supported via synovial fluid within the presence of a tendon sheath. In other words, tendons are designed to transmit tensile loads, have limited elastic properties, and heal slowly compared to other, more oxygenated tissue. This is important to know as one begins to understand the basis of optimal healing after injury and repair. It is very important to understand if prevention and performance is in mind.

Optimal healing consists of three phases: inflammation, repair, and remodeling. The first three days after acute tendon injury sees inflammation. During this time tendons are most sensitive to mechanical load and are chemically irritated. Relative rest is indicated. Interestingly, after about three weeks, inflammatory cells are not present and medications may lose the desired effect.

Repair of damaged tissue lasts about four to six weeks and consists of the deposition of new collagen. Early mobilization is a key factor for strengthening the repairing tendon and begins the process of organizing the new collagen along the lines of functional stress. Prolonged rest may not provide the controlled loading stimulus necessary for maturation of the healing tissue and may actually set up a degenerative process—a condition referred to as tendinosis.

Remodeling is the process of reorganizing the "contracted and disorganized" collagen fibers. Effective remodeling requires a progressive return to normal loads and activity to prevent contractures and to promote strength and flexibility. This process may take up to a year to mature and should include all three planes of functional motion. The three planes of motion at the foot and ankle can be appreciated when running trails as the surface becomes uneven or pitched, or when sharp turn angles are required.

Targeting tendon tissue for early treatment should focus on aerobic training and has been shown to increase tensile strength and endurance. This means high repetitions (100–200 per set) with low loads and introducing eccentric loading as soon as tolerable. Eccentric loading, unlike its concentric counterpart, is the lengthening of muscle under load. For example, a single leg heel raise using one's own body weight is concentric on the up phase and eccentric on the down phase. Standing toe raises are effective in strengthening tendons on the front of the ankle.

—Troy Marsh, an orthopedic physical therapist

Marsh suggests "remembering to keep the proximal muscle groups such as the hips and thighs strong and responsive in all planes of motion. Integrating functional and sport-specific strength and balance exercises, such as single leg heel raises, into your training will enhance performance and hopefully prevent any serious tendon disorders—and prepare you for the next athletic event."

Further information including reports on medical studies can be found at **www.tendinosis.org.**

Treatment Options: Trigger Point Therapy & ASTYM

If you receive treatment for tendon injuries and the pain, numbness, or other abnormal sensations continue, ask your health care practitioner about other treatment options. Two common options are trigger point therapy and ASTYM.

Trigger points are tiny contraction knots, a wad of muscle fibers staying in a hard contraction, never relaxing. A trigger point in a muscle could be painful or it could not manifest pain until touched. Often though, its pain is referred elsewhere. These muscle knots can send referred pain and numbness into the plantar fascia, Achilles tendon, toes, ankle, forefoot, heel, and arch. Referred pain from trigger points mimic the symptoms of many other common injuries—hence the relationship to tendons and ligaments. Massage or kneading of the trigger points is done to break up the knots.

Twyla Carolan, a kinesiologist and masseur, says of trigger points: "You might not even realize that you have such a knot until you apply direct pressure to it and the resulting pain has you leaping to your feet in panic. One of the odd things about trigger points is that they are notorious for hanging out in one spot while sending pain to another. This means that it can be quite difficult to actually locate the source of a pain problem, unless you find it by accident."

Nathan Wilson, an ultrarunner, wrote, "I found that by massaging trigger points on my lower legs and feet for a couple of weeks, I was able to gain flexibility in my ankles, which I have not had in years. *The Trigger Point Therapy Workbook* really complemented *Fixing Your Feet,* as it helped highlight the anatomical structure of the feet and the connections between parts of the body and the feet, which are also mentioned in your book."

Trigger points can be treated by a specialist or through self-treatment. If your health care specialist has experience with trigger points, the points are easy to locate and treat. If not, ask for a referral to a physical therapist or other specialist.

A couple of good sources of information about trigger point therapy include:

■ *The Trigger Point Therapy Workbook: Your Self-Treatment Guide for Pain Relief* by Clair Davies, New Harbinger Publications, Second edition, 2004.

■ Trigger Point Technologies Institute; **www.tptherapy.com.** It offers tips, charts, and products for trigger point pain relief.

ASTYM (A-stim) is a treatment process of soft-tissue injuries done by a physical therapist. Done properly, it can rejuvenate tendons, ligaments, and muscles by getting rid of scar tissue. An ASTYM treatment effectively stimulates scar tissue to be reabsorbed by the body and degenerated tendons to regenerate and heal. Following an ASTYM treatment, you will be given a stretching and strengthening regimen for the affected area. Compliance with these exercises is an important part of the treatment. On the feet, ASTYM can be used for plantar fasciitis, heel pain, Achilles tendinosis, and ankle sprains and strains. More information can be found at **www.astym.com.**

Achilles Tendinitis

The Achilles tendon connects the gastrocnemius and the soleus, the two major muscles of the calf, to the heel bone. It stabilizes the heel every time you take a step. The tendon makes it possible for you to rise up on your toes, run, and jump. Achilles tendinitis occurs when the sheath surrounding this cord becomes inflamed. There may be small tears in the tendon, or sudden and repeated stretching of the tendon causes an inflammation that is painful behind the heel, ankle, and lower calf while walking and running. The pain may be felt during the early part of your run or hike and then subside, only to worsen after stopping. This pain is your first warning, followed by swelling of the Achilles tendon and pain to the touch at the base of your heel.

A mild first-degree injury makes it difficult to rise up on your toes or walk on your heels. With proper treatment, you should be able to walk with little pain after about 48 hours. You should not resume normal athletic activity for several weeks. A second-degree injury is when there is partial tearing of the tendon from its attachment point. This injury will take six to eight weeks to heal, with an additional two to four weeks of stretching exercises before normal athletic activity can be resumed. In a third-degree injury, an extreme case, the Achilles tendon ruptures. This requires immediate

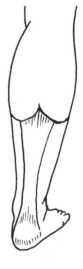

Achilles tendon

medical intervention, usually surgery, and a long healing and strengthening process. There is sudden calf pain and usually an audible snap if the tendon ruptures. The tendon will ball up in the calf with a related defect in the lower tendon. If the tendon is swollen, or you suspect a tear, usually a second- or third-degree injury, you should not risk running on it. You can further damage or rupture the tendon. If the pain is mild and goes away in five minutes with a warm-up, typically a first-degree injury, it is usually OK to continue.

Suddenly increasing your activity, increasing your mileage too quickly, or running steep hills can lead to an inflamed Achilles tendon. To prevent Achilles tendon problems, increase your activity, mileage, and hill training gradually. Strengthening your ankles, as well as lower leg and calf muscle stretching, can also help prevent problems. Overpronators, whose arches collapse when walking or running, are more prone than others to Achilles problems. Wearing shoes that do not fit or support the foot can also lead to an Achilles tendon injury.

Rich Schick, a physician's assistant, adds the following:

> The Achilles tendon is not a simple structure. It is more correctly termed the Achilles complex. If it were as simple as we perceive it, there would be a straight pull from the calf muscle to the heel, and the tendon would be very prominent instead of following the contour of the leg. In reality the tendon passes through a series of little tunnels of very tough tissue that hold it close to the leg.
>
> In severe cases of Achilles tendinitis, calcium deposits can form in and on the tendon, preventing it from passing through these little tunnels and resulting in a permanent disability or the need for surgery. This is called calcific tendinitis. If you grasp the tendon between your thumb and forefinger, move your foot up and down, and feel a grating or bubble-popping sensation, this is a sign of serious tendinitis. The finding is called crepitus and represents severe inflammation. If not treated appropriately, it can lead to calcific tendinitis. You must stop using the leg as much as possible. Some authorities recommend casting until this goes away. Ice and anti-inflammatory medication are also helpful.

Ignoring the signs of Achilles tendinitis and not seeking treatment can lead to a chronic inflammation or even tendon rupture. The pain may occur when warming up and then ease up. The athlete continues to train and the pain returns after the session has ended. Over time, the periods of pain-free training become shorter and shorter. Eventually, training may become impossible and treatment mandatory. This can lead to the formation of a cyst in the tendon. As the cyst expands, the tendon thins out and becomes more susceptible to rupture if overstressed.

Treating Achilles Tendinitis
The major causes of Achilles tendon problems are a lack of strength and flexibility in the calf muscles, a weakness in the tendon, or a weak ankle joint. Treatment may include any or all of the following: icing as described below, stretching and

flexibility exercises, wearing flexible shoes or boots with a well-padded heel counter, and avoiding the ups and downs of hills.

If you suspect you have Achilles tendinitis, stop running—do not run through the pain. Ignoring the symptoms may cause the tendon to rupture, which usually requires surgery. Call your orthopedist or podiatrist if the pain persists. The doctor may put your foot in either a flexible or immobilizing cast to reduce movement and weight bearing. Once the cast is removed, you will need to do stretching exercises to strengthen the tendon before resuming normal athletic activity.

The treatment for a mildly injured Achilles tendinitis is the same RICE treatment used for ankle sprains and strains: rest, ice, compression, and elevation, with the addition of a *P* (PRICE) for protection—usually a heel lift to reduce tension on the tendon. The first 24 hours are the most critical for beginning treatment. Early treatment decreases swelling and lessens the risk of additional injury. Initial rest of the foot is also important. A lightly wound Ace wrap will provide compression to help keep swelling down while providing support. Apply the Ace wrap from the forefoot upwards toward the calf. Do not wear the Ace wrap to bed at night. Apply ice for 20 minutes at a time up to six to eight times daily. Ice can be very helpful in the healing process. See the "Cold & Heat Therapy" chapter for more information on making the most of icing techniques. See also "Supplements for Quick Recovery" on page 263.

The injured area should be elevated above the level of the heart as much as possible during the first 48 hours. This keeps blood away from the injured area and reduces pain and swelling. The use of anti-inflammatory medications is usually warranted.

A small heel pad will alleviate the stresses on the tendon. For some individuals, wearing low-heeled shoes as often as possible will help keep the Achilles tendon stretched. An Achilles notch in shoes or mid- and low-top boots will accommodate the Achilles tendon in plantar flexion. The Achilles Tendon Strap made by Cho-Pat can provide relief from the discomfort of Achilles tendinitis.

Adding a small, thin, friction-reducing pad in the Achilles notch of the shoe's heel counter can reduce pressure on the inflamed tendon. Tamarack, the maker of the popular ENGO Patches, makes a thin Cushion Heel Wrap, which is perfect for protecting the tendon. If relief is needed during an event, you can cut a slit into the center of the shoe's Achilles notch in the heel counter.

A lightweight plastic night splint worn to bed can help to stretch the foot, limit contraction of soft tissues at night, and avoid morning stiffness. Night splints help avoid foot drop and accompanying muscle tightening. Night splints are proven as a treatment method for preventing the plantar fascia and Achilles tendon from contracting during the night. Many athletes swear by them. Check with your podiatrist, orthopedist, or medical supply store. Several night-splint models are available. If the pain persists, consult a medical specialist. He or she will need to rule out partial tears of the tendon, an inflammation of the tendon's sheath, or degenerative changes. Many physical therapists can apply a treatment called iontophoresis, which uses electrical current to apply a steroid medication over the inflamed tendon. Avoid cortisone injections into the area because they can cause tendon rupture.

Rupture of the tendon requires specialized care. If the rupture is fresh, within hours of the injury, surgical repair of the tendon is usually done. Older injuries may also be treated surgically, though many patients will improve by casting the leg. Diminished strength and re-rupture is more frequently seen in patients who are cast without surgery, so the preference is to surgically repair the rupture. Following surgical repair of Achilles tendon injuries, the patient is usually cast; then when the cast is removed, the patient receives extensive rehabilitation to regain strength and flexibility. Often a heel lift is required for six months to a year after the cast has been removed.

Scott Eilerts found relief from chronic tendinitis by wearing Earth shoes. They have a heel depression, rather than a heel lift, such that the foot is dorsiflexed when standing. The amount of dorsiflexion is similar to that with your heel on the ground and the ball of your foot resting on top of this book. It is so much easier to wear Earth shoes for everyday activities to keep your calves stretched than to have to wear a night split or adhere to a stretching regimen. One caveat: Earth shoes work best as a preventive for mild, chronic Achilles tendinitis, and for walking only. They should not be used for moderate/severe acute cases, given that rest and heel lifts are usually the best course of treatment.

Exercises to Stretch the Achilles Tendon

Stretching helps athletes improve flexibility and counter muscular imbalances that put them at a greater risk of injury. Proper stretching of the Achilles tendon can help prevent an Achilles injury.

One method of stretching is to stand far enough from a wall or heavy piece of furniture so that when you lean forward toward the wall or furniture, you can feel the tendons stretch in the back of your leg while keeping your feet flat on the floor. Lean forward and stretch only to the point of feeling the stretch, not to the point of feeling pain. Alternate a 20-second stretch with a 20-second rest standing straight; repeat 10–20 times. Continue this daily stretching until the Achilles stops hurting.

Les Appel, DPM, who designed the Powerstep Insole, recommends facing a wall with one foot flat on the floor and the other foot's heel on the floor and toes up on the wall 3–4 inches. Gently move your knee slowly toward the wall until you feel slight stretching on the bottom of your foot and the back of your leg. Hold this position for 30 seconds, and repeat five times per foot.

A Swedish study showed excellent results with a simple stretch. Stand on a step or ledge on the balls of your feet. Push yourself up with your good leg and slowly transfer your weight to the affected leg. Slowly lower yourself all the way down until the injured leg's heel is below the stair level and you feel the pull on the soleus calf muscle. Alternate this stretch with the injured leg's knee straight and then slightly bent. Repeat three sets of 15, twice a day. Additional strength can be gained by adding weight over time. Use dumbbells, a light barbell, or a weighted backpack.

The Prostretch is a popular tool to effectively stretch the plantar fascia as well as the Achilles tendon and the gastrocnemius and soleus musculature of the back of the

ACHILLES TENDINITIS PRODUCTS

The **ACHILLES HEALER** reduces stress on the Achilles tendon. The strap is made from ProWrap, a knitted blend of nylon and Lycra with patented foam lining. **www.fabrifoam.com**

The **ACHILLOTRAIN** is a lightweight, breathable sock that offers support for the Achilles tendon. It has silicone inserts in the back of the heel and under it. **www.bauerfeindusa.com**

CHO-PAT'S ACHILLES TENDON STRAP fits under the arch and around the ankle to relieve pressure on the Achilles tendon. Trials at the Mayo's Sports/Medicine Clinic have shown the strap effective as an addition to traditional treatments for Achilles tendinitis, particularly during the push-off phase of gait. The strap is available in four sizes based on ankle circumference at its widest point. **www.cho-pat.com**

THE CUSHION HEEL WRAP combines a thin layer of padding with a low-friction PTFE to ensure that painful rubbing and blisters don't occur and the Achilles tendon is protected. These wraps are designed to fit the curve of the shoe's heel counter with an easy peel-and-stick application. **www.goengo.com**

ENGO PATCHES are low-friction patches uniquely applied to footwear, insoles, socks, and athletic equipment—not skin—for easier, longer-lasting protection of the Achilles tendon. Ultrathin patches leave footwear volume virtually unaltered. Strong, latex-free adhesive prevents migration and movement, even through moisture and sweat. Scientific and field tests show ENGO's slippery surface significantly reduces rubbing, providing immediate relief. The back of the heel patches work well in the shoe's heel counter. Satisfaction guaranteed. **www.goengo.com**

HAPAD THREE-QUARTER-LENGTH HEEL WEDGES provide the necessary heel lift to help reduce the pain associated with Achilles tendinitis. They are available in

lower leg. Studies have shown that utilization of the Prostretch can more effectively increase ankle dorsiflexion (toe-up motion of the ankle) than the conventional and commonly used wall stretch technique mentioned on the preceding page. Its use is recommended as both a preventive measure and a treatment technique.

Ankle Tendons

The ankle is surrounded by tendons. The main ones that concern us here are the two peroneal tendons and the posterior tibial tendon.

Peroneal Tendons

The peroncus longus and peroneus brevis tendons run behind and around the lateral malleolus (the outside ankle bone). The peroneus longus flexes the ankle downward and out while the peroneus brevis tendon flexes the ankle up and inward. The

ACHILLES TENDINITIS PRODUCTS

three thicknesses. The coiled, springlike wool fibers provide firm and resilient support as they mold and shape to the foot. **www.hapad.com**

The **N'ICE STRETCH NIGHT SPLINT SUSPENSION SYSTEM** is made for both Achilles tendinitis and plantar fasciitis. This night splint uses bilateral suspension straps to provide continuous nighttime stretching of the Achilles tendon and plantar fasciitis. The straps allow for independent bi-plane dorsiflexion adjustment. A removable Sealed Ice pack provides cold therapy coupled with stretching of soft tissues. The unit is hinged to fold compactly. **www.brownmed.com**

The **PROSTRETCH** is a popular tool that effectively stretches the Achilles tendon, the plantar fascia, and the calf muscles. It builds lower extremity strength, balance, and flexibility benefits in three minutes of use prior to activity, thus reducing the risk of injury. The ProStretch can also be used for hamstring and anterior tibialis stretching. **www.prostretch.com**

The **SLANT BOARD** from Fitter adjusts to three levels and folds flat for travel. It comes in two widths. **www.fitter1.com**

The **STRETCH-EZ** from OPTP cradles the foot for a comfortable stretch of the foot, heel, Achilles tendon, hamstring, quadriceps, and inner/outer thigh and calf. Made of poly laminate and webbing. **www.stretch-ez.com**

The **TP MASSAGE FOOTBALLER, BALLER BLOCK, AND MASSAGE BALLS** were created to relieve plantar fasciitis, Achilles tendinitis, and heel pain. They work on the muscle of existing spasms and/or trigger points by applying pressure to the trigger point area. Also offered is a Performance Therapy for Foot & Lower Leg DVD, which shows a complete foot and lower leg exercise routine. **www.tpmassageball.com**

tendon, in a sheath, pass through a groove behind the lateral malleolus. The sheath forms a tunnel around the tendon and a band of tissue called a retinaculum reinforces it. When these are stretched beyond normal, as with a turned ankle, pain from the injury and inflammation will occur. A forceful stretch can cause a tear in the tendons. When the tendons momentarily slip out of the groove, it is called a subluxation.

Posterior Tibial Tendon
The posterior tibial tendon runs behind the medial malleolus (the inside ankle bone). It helps turn the foot inward when walking or running. Pain can be in the shin or down to the ankle and instep area.

Treating Ankle Tendon Injuries
A physical examination will help determine which tendons are involved and where they are inflamed, torn, or ruptured. An MRI may be ordered if a tear or rupture

is suspected. Icing, a combination of cold and heat therapy, and anti-inflammatory medications are in order. Wrapping the ankle for support will help. In some cases immobilization may be necessary. Start a program of stretching and strengthening of the ankle and lower leg—especially calf stretches. You may be referred to a physical therapist. Cortisone injections may be tried.

For a posterior tibial tendon injury, your podiatrist may prescribe an orthotic. Otherwise make sure you have good arch support in all your shoes and do not walk barefoot (Green Superfeet insoles are recommended).

Bursitis

Bursa are small fluid-filled sacs found between areas of high friction such as where muscles or tendons glide over bone. The bursa acts as a shock absorber, allowing movement between neighboring structures, usually in opposite directions. The body has more than 150 bursa sacs. Bursitis is the formation of an inflamed fluid-filled sac from trauma or overuse. On the feet, bursitis may develop beneath a callus or a bunion, under the metatarsal heads, or at the heel.

Typical causes of bursitis in the feet can be repetitive motions or an injury or sustained pressure to a joint. As the usually slippery bursa sac becomes inflamed, it loses its gliding capabilities and becomes gritty and rough. Inflamed bursas are painful and irritating. Bursitis in the heel can manifest itself with the same symptoms as plantar fasciitis, but the heel bursitis will persist with any weight-bearing activity, whereas with plantar fasciitis the symptoms are relieved after the fascia warms up.

Treating Bursitis

The first action is to stop or reduce the motion or action that is causing the bursitis. The use of NSAIDS will help reduce the inflammation. Heat will relax the joint and promote tissue repair. In severe cases, fluid may be drawn from the sac to relieve pressure. Gently warming up before strenuous exercise can help avoid bursitis. If you experience chronic bursitis, ask your doctor about medications and treatment options to relieve the pain and discomfort.

Plantar Fasciitis

The plantar fascia is a band of connective fibrous tissue that runs from the heel to the ball of the foot, forming the foot's arch. The band helps in support and stabilization of the foot during hiking and running. The arch flattens when standing. As you begin a step, the heel lifts up and also the plantar fascia tightens to form the curve of the arch and provides a strong push off with the toes. An inflammation of the fascia, called plantar fasciitis, occurs most often with overuse. The stretching and tearing of some of the fibers in the plantar fascia as it inserts into the heel bone causes the inflammation. If you have flat feet or high arches, or if you overpronate, the plantar fascia is strained, mainly at the heel. The stresses of impact sports, running, and hiking may flatten, lengthen, and eventually cause small tears in the plantar fascia. Tears near the heel bone often cause a heel spur to develop.

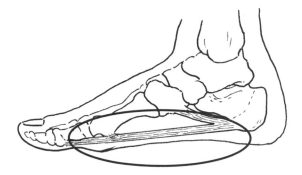

Plantar fascia

Athletes who are predisposed to plantar fasciitis injuries typically have increased their mileage too fast, increased the frequency and intensity of their workouts, increased the amount of hill work, and/or have a lack of flexibility and strength in their ankle and foot. They may also have a foot imbalance such as flat feet or high arches.

Plantar fascia pain is commonly felt in the morning or after long periods of sitting. The first steps at these times cause a sudden strain to the band of tissue that has started to heal itself during the night. The pain and stiffness is usually centered at the bottom of the heel, but symptoms may radiate into the arch. Although the pain may decrease somewhat with your initial activity, as the day progresses, it may return and be quite painful.

Consult your podiatrist or orthopedist if you are suffering from pain in the arch of your foot or suspect that you have plantar fasciitis. In some cases the fascia may involve a partial or full rupture, which will require more aggressive treatment. An aggressive multidisciplined medical approach using medical, biomechanical, and physical therapy treatments can help to return you to action as soon as possible. The Achilles tendon may also be involved, causing pain under the foot as it stretches.

Treating Plantar Fasciitis

Generally prescribed treatments for plantar fasciitis include rest, moist heat and stretching in the morning or before activity, icing massage after activity, heel cups, taping of the foot or an arch brace, orthotics, foot exercises, and shoe modifications. Ice your heels and the bottom of your foot after exercise (see the chapter "Cold & Heat Therapy" for information on making the most of icing techniques). By all means, replace your worn-out shoes and insoles. Usually you need either to provide more support to the arch or lessen the amount of overpronation. An arch support or arch pad can provide pain relief. Motion-control shoes can help if you overpronate. In extreme cases, oral anti-inflammatory medications, cortisone injections, physical therapy, cast immobilization, and even surgery may be necessary. Because the plantar fascia has low vascularity and a lack of good blood flow, it is slow to heal.

The first thing any doctor or physical therapist should tell you is to stop all impact activities for a period of weeks or months and to always wear shoes. Going barefoot is one of the worst things someone suffering from plantar fasciitis can do. Keep in mind that the tiny tears need to heal, and it makes sense to stop the activity that caused them in the first place. Have shoes by your bedside in case you have to get up at night. Avoid sandals unless they have an arch support.

You also need to regain flexibility and elasticity in the soleus muscle/sheath to prevent the condition from occurring again. Stretching is the way to do that, but you have to start out slow and easy, that is, writing the alphabet with your foot in warm bathwater. (See the section on stretching on pages 288–290 for various useful exercises for increasing flexibility.) Once you've started to heal, you can move on to the more demanding stretches. The most common comment by those who have conquered plantar fasciitis is how stretching helped more than anything else. A physical therapist or chiropractor can help adjust muscle imbalances.

A study by the American Orthopaedic Foot and Ankle Society looked at heel pain related to plantar fasciitis.[34] Dr. Glenn Pfeffer reported chronic heel pain as the most common foot problem, with up to 80% caused by proximal plantar fasciitis. The study compared a common polypropylene custom orthotic device, three over-the-counter heel pads (a ViscoHeel silicone heel cushion, a Tuli's Heel Cup, and a Hapad Comforthotic), and stretching alone. After comparing the results of five control groups, they found that stretching and off-the-shelf shoe inserts were just as effective as stretching and the more costly orthotics. Their recommendation: "For the initial treatment of heel pain, stretching and a simple, inexpensive, off-the-shelf device is the best way to go." When wearing heel pads, be sure to use them in all your shoes.

When Graham Wilson had severe plantar fasciitis, his podiatrist told him to throw away the inserts on new running shoes and replace them immediately. His preference is Superfeet Insoles. It is a good idea to check your insoles in all your shoes to see whether they provide good support.

In an interesting article, "Plantar Fasciitis—A New Perspective,"[35] Robert Nirschl, MD, makes a case for plantar fasciitis as a painful degenerative plantar tendinitis, not an inflammation problem. His research found no inflammatory cells in injured plantar fascia—meaning that anti-inflammatory medications and cortisone will not have curative potential. For plantar tendinitis Dr. Nirschl recommends stretching and strength training all areas of the leg to restore strength, endurance, and flexibility. Also recommended is the use of a night splint, arch bracing or a soft orthotic, and footwear with good mid-foot flexibility. In extreme cases, surgery may be indicated to remove painful tendinitis tissue. If your plantar fascia pain does not respond to prescribed treatment, consider asking your podiatrist or orthopedist to look into this study.

Cortisone Injections

While the inflammation for which corticosteroids are given can recur, corticosteroid injections can provide months to years of relief when used properly. These injections also can cure diseases (permanently resolve them) when the problem is tissue inflammation localized to a small area, such as bursitis and tendinitis. However, tendons can be weakened by corticosteroid injections in or near tendons. Tendon rupture as a result have been reported. Unique side effects of joint injections involve injury to the joint tissues, particularly with repeated injections. These injuries include thinning of the joint cartilage, weakening of the ligaments of the joint, increased inflammation in the joint (arthritis) due to a reaction to a corticosteroid that has crystallized, and introduction of infection into the joint. Source: **www.medicinenet.com**

Orthotics will often help relieve plantar fascia pain. AliMed Rehab and Aetrex make orthotics for plantar fasciitis. Gary Buffington recommends trying inexpensive orthotic shoe inserts before you have expensive orthotics made. Gary suggests you "wear them always until you are better—even in your bedroom slippers if you go to the bathroom at night. I think it would be best if you never took a step without them under your foot for a month." He also recommends contrast baths of two buckets of water, one at 68°F and the other at 103°F. He says, "Put your feet in for 5 minutes in hot, 2 in cold, 2 in hot, 2 in cold, and then 5 more in the hot for a total of 19 minutes twice a day or more." An alternative method is to ice the sole of the foot for ten minutes; then place the foot on a hot water bottle (as hot as you can stand it) for ten minutes. Repeat for three or more rounds, twice a day, for at least a week.

It is possible to tape the plantar fascia area under the foot for support, though doing so can be hard to manage. The tape, however, loses strength as it moves with the skin—40% of its strength can be lost within 20 minutes. Using one of the supports listed below will work better over time. An arch brace wraps around the arch to provide support and decrease the pull of the plantar fascia on the calcaneus heel bone. The Count'R-Force Arch Brace and the PSC wrap are two wraparound supports that provide relief from plantar fasciitis pain. The Hapad Longitudinal Metatarsal Arch Pads or 3-Way Heel/Arch/Metatarsal Insoles may also be used to relieve pain.

Lightweight plastic night splints are proven as a treatment for preventing the plantar fascia and Achilles tendon from contracting during the night. Many athletes swear by them. The splint helps stretch the foot, limit contraction of soft tissues at night, and avoid morning stiffness. Night splints also help avoid foot drop and accompanying muscle tightening. Check with your podiatrist, orthopedist, or medical supply store. Several night splint models are available. The Strassburg Sock is an alternative-style night splint that can be worn at night or while resting to lightly stretch the plantar fascia. Before getting out of bed, curl your toes downward eight to ten times to loosen the plantar fascia.

If the problem persists after trying some of these measures, make an appointment with a podiatrist or orthopedist. Advances in medical technology have resulted in the use of shock waves to reduce the troublesome inflammation and help jump-start blood flow, which in turn reduces pain and encourages healing. Common sense should tell you to try other conservative treatments before moving to the shock wave treatment or surgery.

Orthotripsy and extracorporeal shock wave therapies uses high-energy shock waves similar to those used for treating kidney stones. Shock wave therapy is indicated for use with patients suffering from chronic plantar fasciitis and heel-pain syndrome who fail to respond to the traditional and conservative treatments. The sound shocks cause microtears that heal with new blood vessel growth, allowing the plantar fascia to mend pain free. This noninvasive procedure is worth checking out before considering surgery. Recent studies show an 83% success rate after one treatment and 97% after two. Check with your podiatrist to find a specialist in your area who is trained in this new technology.

Endoscopic plantar fasciotomy is an invasive procedure in which a specialized camera is inserted into the heel area. Using the camera, the surgeon can see the plantar fascia through a very small incision, less than 0.5 inch, and release the extreme tension on the plantar fascia.

Plantar fasciitis pain can be helped with a quick and simple, minimally invasive medical treatment. The TOPAZ MicroDebrider utilizes patented Coblation technology to offer a quicker return to daily activities with a significant improvement in patient outcomes. Small punctures in key areas of the heel are made to allow the insertion of a pencil tip–size wand device, the MicroDebrider. Radio frequency energy is transmitted through the wand for short 500 millisecond intervals of treatments. The Coblation technology forms a plasma that gently and precisely dissolves soft tissue at relatively low temperatures and increases vascular blood supply. Check with your orthopedic surgeon or podiatrist for more information about this treatment.

Many athletes get so frustrated trying to resolve their plantar fasciitis that they try different things that others tell them about. Jayne Cassedy wrote, "Two things helped me recover from plantar fasciitis. The first is a homeopathic ointment called Traumeel. It's an anti-inflammatory and an analgesic from Germany. It works! I usually get it in health food stores. Second, lessons in Feldenkrais, a movement therapy. It helped me find my feet again! It's hard to find the lessons, though. I also used professionally made orthotics from a podiatrist. They helped, but Traumeel and Feldenkrais put me over the top."

Stretching Exercises for Plantar Fasciitis

Athletes can improve their flexibility and counter muscular imbalances that put them at a greater risk of injury by following a simple stretching program. The best results may come from a combination of plantar fascia and Achilles tendon stretching in multiple directions.

New Stretch Relieves Pain from Plantar Fasciitis

A new stretch is proving quite effective to help treat and potentially cure plantar fasciitis. In a study recently published in *Journal of Bone and Joint Surgery*, researchers found that patients suffering from the painful heel spur syndrome had a 75% chance of having no pain and returning to full activity within three to six months of performing the stretch. In addition, patients had about a 75% chance of needing no further treatment.

The study was a two-year follow-up on 82 patients with plantar fasciitis, all of whom were part of an original clinical trial of 101 patients in 2003. The patients were taught a new stretch, specifically targeting the plantar fascia, which was developed by Benedict DiGiovanni, MD, associate professor of orthopedic surgery at the University of Rochester and author of the study, and Deborah Nawoczenski, PT, PhD, professor of physical therapy at Ithaca College.

The stretch involves sitting in a chair with one leg crossed over the other knee. Then stretch the arch of the foot on the crossed leg by taking one hand and pulling the toes back toward the shin for a count of ten. The exercise must be repeated ten times, and performed at least three times a day, including before taking the first step in the morning and before standing after a prolonged period of sitting.[36]

Morning Stretches

■ Before getting out of bed, lie on your stomach, put your toes and forefoot against the mattress, and straighten your leg so your heel stretches your calf muscle. This can make your first steps less painful.

■ Also before getting out of bed, slowly stretch the toes upward toward the head at least three times, holding the stretch for at least 15 seconds.

■ Stretch the tendon by placing the ankle of the affected foot on the opposite knee. Then grab the toes and flex the ankle forward while gently pulling your toes toward your shin. Hold this stretch to a count of ten and repeat ten times, three times a day. Using a towel around your toes to pull them toward you is an alternative.

■ Another effective morning calf stretch is to stand facing a wall with your hands on the wall. Extend one foot behind you about 24 inches, while bending the other leg at the knee. Keep the heel of the back foot flat on the floor for two minutes and keep the knee straight—you will feel the calf muscle stretch. Repeat with the other foot.

Other Effective Stretches

■ Toe curls can strengthen your arch to prevent pronation. Sit down, take your shoes off, and curl your toes under as hard as you can and as many times as you can. In the beginning, you might get a cramp. Just walk around and try the curls again. Picking up marbles off the floor with your feet and dropping them into a bowl is another good toe exercise.

■ Les Appel, DPM, who designed the Powerstep Insole, recommends facing a wall with one foot flat on the floor and the other foot's heel on the floor and toes up on the wall 3–4 inches. Gently move your knee slowly toward the wall until you feel slight stretching on the bottom of your foot and the back of your leg. Curl your toes to raise the arch and transfer your weight to the outside of your foot. Uncurl your toes, hold for 30 seconds, and again curl your toes. Hold each position for 30 seconds, repeating five times per position per foot.

■ Rolling a tennis ball back and forth under the arch of the foot or simple self-massage across and along the arch can also help. Ice massage can be done using a small frozen juice can rolled under your arch.

■ Better than a tennis ball is the TP Massage FootBaller. Apply pressure with the FootBaller by using the floor, a table, or any hard surface to allow slight movement of your foot on the device. As pressure is applied, the material will slightly change shape in about five to seven seconds. As the materials change shape, roll the FootBaller to and fro, covering the entire affected area of the foot so that the trigger point or spasm is relieved.

■ The Prostretch is a popular tool to effectively stretch the plantar fascia, as well as the Achilles tendon and the gastrocnemius and soleus musculature of the back of the lower leg. Studies have shown that utilization of the Prostretch can more effectively increase ankle dorsiflexion (toe-up motion of the ankle) than the conventional and commonly used wall stretch technique mentioned above.[37] Its use is recommended as both a preventive measure as well as a treatment technique.

PLANTAR FASCIITIS PRODUCTS

ACCOMMODATOR ORTHOTICS provide relief from heel pain and plantar fasciitis. The High-Impact Accommodator offers the benefit of an Impact Plus energy-absorbing poromeric polymer pad in the heel. The Viscoelastic Accommodator combines accommodator and three-quarter–length design with the proven attributes of a pure, supple, viscoelastic polymer. Each offers a shaped longitudinal arch to relieve fatigue while supporting the arch, and a mild metatarsal arch, which supports and reduces unnecessary pressure from the metatarsal heads. **www.alimed.com**

BUNGA GEL HEEL CUPS are made from a medical-grade polymer material. **www.bungapads.com**

The **COUNT'R-FORCE ARCH BRACE,** an alternative to taping, is ideal for running and hiking. Designed by Robert Nirschl, MD, an orthopedic surgeon/sports

PLANTAR FASCIITIS PRODUCTS

medicine specialist, it has a curved shape that allow a wide distribution of the abusive forces causing the heel and plantar fasciitis pain. Two tension straps allow for personal adjustment. **www.countrforce.com**

CRAMER HEEL CUPS offer a basic heel cup that is made with Provosane II bonded to a layer of soft polyurethane foam. **www.cramersportsmed.com**

HAPAD ARCH PADS can relieve the discomfort of plantar fasciitis. The Longitudinal Metatarsal Arch Pads provide a corrective action that strengthens the longitudinal and metatarsal arches without restricting the natural flexibility of the foot. These pads may also help flat feet. The 3-Way Heel/Arch/Metatarsal Insoles is an all-in-one Longitudinal Metatarsal Arch Cushion and heel cushion that relieves plantar fasciitis and foot fatigue by supporting the arch, cushioning the heel, and distributing pressure across the ball of the foot. The Comforthotic Three-Quarter–Length Insole is a contoured one-piece arch, metatarsal, and heel cushion that helps support flat feet. **www.hapad.com**

HAPAD HEEL PADS AND CUSHIONS are useful in treating heel pain associated with stone bruises, heel spurs, leg-length discrepancies, and Achilles tendinitis. The Horseshoe Heel Pads relieve heel pain, and the Medial/Lateral Heel Wedges help correct misalignment of the heel and ankle. The Comforthotic Three-Quarter–Length Insole is a contoured one-piece arch, metatarsal, and heel cushion that relieves heel spur pain. The coiled, springlike wool fibers provide firm and resilient support as they mold and shape to the foot. **www. hapad.com**

The **LYNCO BIOMECHANICAL ORTHOTIC SYSTEM** is a ready-made triple-density orthotic system that comes in enough variations to accommodate 90% of foot disorders, including plantar fasciitis. Each model has either a neutral-cupped heel or a medial posted heel, and comes with or without a metatarsal pad. Additional Reflex self-adhesive pads can be added to the orthotics to relieve pain from Morton's toe, sesamoiditis, and leg-length discrepancy. **www.aetrex.com**

The **N'ICE STRETCH NIGHT SPLINT SUSPENSION SYSTEM** is made for plantar fasciitis and Achilles tendinitis. It uses bilateral suspension straps to provide continuous nighttime stretching of the plantar fasciitis and Achilles tendon. The straps allow for independent bi-plane dorsiflexion adjustment. A removable Sealed Ice pack provides cold therapy. The unit is hinged to fold compactly. **www. brownmed.com**

The **PF NIGHT SPLINT** comes in three models to relieve the pain of plantar fasciitis. The Original PF Night Splint is a lightweight plastic splint designed to lessen morning pain caused by contractures and muscle tightening while sleeping. The Freedom PF Night Splint II is a low-profile lighter weight splint, and the Soft PF Night Splint is made for sleeping but allows ambulation. All splints fit both right and left feet and include a liner and straps to protect the leg and instep from pressure. An extra-wide model of the PF Night Splint is offered for those individuals with larger calves and ankles. **www.alimed.com**

PLANTAR FASCIITIS PRODUCTS CONTINUED

POWERSTEP INSOLES BY DR. LES APPEL offer a unique four-phase design to relieve heel and arch pain. Made with a strong prescription-like arch support, it has a strong heel cradle that prevents the foot from pronating (rolling inward) and the arch from flattening—eliminating strain on the plantar fascia. **www.powersteps.com**

The **PROSTRETCH** effectively stretches the plantar fascia, the Achilles tendon, and the calf muscles. It builds lower-extremity strength, balance, and flexibility in three minutes of use prior to activity, thus reducing the risk of injury. It can also be used for hamstring and anterior tibialis stretching. **www.medi-dyne.com**

The **PSC–PRONATION/SPRING CONTROL STRAP** is designed to treat plantar fasciitis, chronic heel pain, heel spur syndrome, and shin splints. This reusable strapping device is made from ProWrap, a knitted blend of nylon and Lycra with patented foam lining. It wraps around the arch to provide superior support to the plantar fascia while also wrapping around the heel to reduce the force of heel strike and biomechanically move the foot's midline to a more neutral position. **www.fabrifoam.com**

SPENCO CUSHIONS are made from a noncompressible, viscoelastic material to relieve heel pain associated with heel spurs, thinning heel pads, and plantar fasciitis. Products include ViscoSpot and ViscoHeel cushions; Ipos Shock Absorber Heel cushions and SoftBase Insoles; and ViscoPed insoles. They reduce shock to the joints and evenly distribute pressure throughout the cushion. Available at sporting goods stores and some drugstores.

The **STRASSBURG SOCK** is easy to use at night or during extended periods of rest. A good alternative to the typical night splint, this system can be easily used and carried while backpacking. A standard over-the-calf tube sock uses two adjustable straps: one around the calf just below the knee; the other attached to the toe of the sock and passed through a D ring on the upper strap. Tension on the toe strap keeps the plantar fascia in a neutral to slightly stretched position, reducing or eliminating pain under the heel during initial weight bearing in the morning. **www.thesock.com**

THERMOSKIN PLANTAR FXT is a low-profile alternative to cumbersome night splints. The Thermoskin material helps increase skin temperature several degrees for the optimal level of heat therapy. Made with soft materials, it maintains the plantar fascia in a comfortable and flexed position during sleep. **www.swedeo.com**

The **TP MASSAGE FOOTBALLER, BALLER BLOCK, AND MASSAGE BALLS** were created to relieve plantar fasciitis, Achilles tendinitis, and heel pain. They work on the muscle of existing spasms and/or trigger points by applying pressure to the trigger point area. Also offered is a Performance Therapy for Foot & Lower Leg DVD, which shows a complete foot and lower leg exercise routine. **www.tpmassageball.com**

VISCOPED S INSOLES are made from a noncompressible viscoelastic material with a bar of softer silicone in the metatarsal and heel areas that is designed to relieve plantar fascia pain. The insole reduces shock throughout the entire length of the insole and distributes pressure evenly. **www.bauerfeindusa.com**

Plantar Fibromas

Occasionally a plantar fibroma (fibrous nodule) may form in the plantar fascia. These will usually not go away without treatment. There may be pain from the insole pushing against the nodule. Steroid injections may help and an orthotics can be made, but often surgical removal will be necessary.

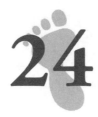

Heel Problems

The heel bone, called the calcaneus, is the largest bone in the foot and absorbs most of the shock and pressure from walking and running. The most common cause of heel pain is incorrect movement of the foot during running, hiking, or walking. With every heel strike, pressure up to four times the body's weight is placed on the heel, flattening the heel's fat pads and sending shock and stress to the bones of the foot and the arch. Some of the shock and stress travels on up the leg. As we age, the thickness of the heel's fat pads and the fat pads under the balls of our feet decreases; our natural shock absorption is reduced, pressure is increased, and we become more susceptible to injury. Heel pain may be caused by heel-pain syndrome, heel spurs, plantar fasciitis, or Haglund's deformity.

Heel pain can also be caused by dry and cracked skin at the back and bottom of the heel. This skin is often built up into a callus, and the fissures in the skin can be painful. Treat this problem the same as any callus (see page 327).

Heel-Pain Syndrome

Heel-pain syndrome is usually caused by overuse of and repetitive stress on the foot's heel. This can be caused by a sudden increase in athletic activity, by shoes with heels that are too low or that have lost their cushioning, or by the thinning of the fat pad on the bottom of the heels. This can be resolved by increasing activity level slowly, by wearing shoes with good cushioning, or by using a heel pad or cup.

Heel Spurs

Heel pain may also be caused by heel spurs or plantar fasciitis, which arise from the heel bone and attached soft tissues being stressed. Achilles tendinitis may also be a cause of heel pain. This type of heel pain is often the worst in the morning after getting out of bed and putting your feet on the floor—sometimes it improves after a few minutes. The section on plantar fasciitis in the preceding chapter should be considered mandatory reading for any athlete experiencing heel pain. Heel spurs and plantar fasciitis are closely related, and those with heel pain can benefit from many of the same treatments, stretches, and products. After reading about treatments for these injuries, make sure that you also read "Treatment Options: Trigger Point Therapy & ASTYM" in the preceding chapter.

Heel spurs are small points of calcium buildup sticking out and downward from the calcaneus heel bone, touching and irritating your plantar fascia. (Painful protrusions on the back of the heel are called Haglund's deformity; see page 296.) Stresses to the plantar fascia where it inserts into the calcaneus causes heel spurs to develop. A heel spur can usually be seen on an X-ray. A heel bruise or stone bruise is pain felt directly under the calcaneus. This pain is usually tenderness at a small site just forward of the heel's pad on the bottom of the heel.

Achilles tendinitis, flat feet, and excessively high arches are common conditions that make one prone to heel spurs.

Treating Heel Spurs

Proper conditioning of the feet and gradually working up to longer distances can help minimize heel pain. Many stretches can help prevent and also treat heel spurs, as well as plantar fasciitis (see section on stretching on pages 288–290).

Resting your feet and using ice is helpful when you first experience pain—ice 20 minutes up to six to eight times a day for several days. The "Cold & Heat Therapy" chapter gives more information on making the most of icing techniques. As pain subsides over time, warm soaks can help.

Tom Noll found his solution to heel pain by experimenting with different running shoes and using arch supports. By participating in discussions on an e-mail listserv, Tom began to see similarities as some people mentioned that they too had problems with the same model shoe he was wearing. He changed shoes and determined that he needed the arch support in all his shoes.

One very basic but important recommendation is to never walk in bare feet until you are pain free—especially in the morning getting out of bed. Keep a pair of shoes with an arch support at your bedside. Use sandals only if they have an arch support.

The use of orthotics in resolving heel pain has been proven. The biggest issue with custom orthotics is their cost. Many athletes first try an inexpensive over-the-counter orthotic. If that does not work, the more expensive custom-made orthotic may be necessary (see the "Orthotics" chapter, page 143, for detailed information on common types of orthotics).

The products listed on the following pages are quite varied. Some heel cups have a waffle design or special-density material on the bottom of the cup; others have a U-shape cutout at the bottom of the heel. Most heel cups simply cup the heel, while others are incorporated into a sock design. The new viscoelastic materials in some heel pads provide excellent cushioning. Heel pads are small and fit easily into a shoe to provide cushioning. Try several to find a design that works best for your pain or injury. Heel cups and pads are small and can easily be carried as preventive measures if you are prone to heel pain. The Count'R-Force Arch Brace and the PSC strap are alternatives to heel cups and pads.

PRODUCTS FOR HEEL SPURS

ACCOMMODATOR ORTHOTICS provide relief from heel pain and plantar fasciitis. The High-Impact Accommodator offers the benefit of an Impact Plus energy-absorbing poromeric polymer pad in the heel. The Viscoelastic Accommodator combines Accommodator and three-quarter–length design with the proven attributes of a pure, supple, viscoelastic polymer. Each offers a shaped longitudinal arch to relieve fatigue while supporting the arch, and a mild metatarsal arch, which supports and reduces unnecessary pressure from the metatarsal heads. **www.alimed.com**

BUNGA GEL HEEL CUPS are made from a medical-grade polymer material. **www.bungapads.com**

CRAMER HEEL CUPS offer a basic heel cup that is made with Provosane II bonded to a layer of soft polyurethane foam. **www.cramersportsmed.com**

HAPAD ARCH PADS can relieve the discomfort of plantar fasciitis. The Longitudinal Metatarsal Arch Pads provide a corrective action that strengthens the longitudinal and metatarsal arches without restricting the natural flexibility of the foot. These pads may also help flat feet. The 3-Way Heel/Arch/Metatarsal Insoles is an all-in-one Longitudinal Metatarsal Arch Cushion and heel cushion that relieves plantar fasciitis and foot fatigue by supporting the arch, cushioning the heel, and distributing pressure across the ball of the foot. The Comf-Orthotic Three-Quarter–Length Insole is a contoured one-piece arch, metatarsal, and heel cushion that helps support flat feet. **www.hapad.com**

HAPAD HEEL PADS AND CUSHIONS are useful in treating heel pain associated with stone bruises, heel spurs, leg-length discrepancies, and Achilles tendinitis. The Horseshoe Heel Pads relieve heel pain, and the Medial/Lateral Heel Wedges helps correct misalignment of the heel and ankle. The Comf-Orthotic Three-Quarter–Length Insole is a contoured one-piece arch, metatarsal, and heel cushion that relieves heel spur pain. The coiled, springlike wool fibers provide firm and resilient support as they mold and shape to the foot. **www.hapad.com**

The **HEEL HUGGER** is designed to treat heel pain and inflammatory problems of the heel. The neoprene sock surrounds the foot from the heel to the mid-foot, providing support, stabilization, and compression to control edema. Therapeutic Gel pads with Sealed Ice provide additional stabilization and cold therapy on either side of the calcaneus heel bone. The Heel Hugger provides relief from heel spurs, plantar fasciitis, Achilles tendinitis, heel contusions, narrow heels, and rear-foot instability. **www.brownmed.com**

Haglund's Deformity

Haglund's deformity is a bump in the form of an enlargement of the back of the heel bone (calcaneus) at the area of the insertion of the Achilles tendon. Sometimes it has the appearance of a square, shelflike bump. When the bump is irritated by wearing shoes, it becomes red, swollen, and painful. The enlarged bone may also irritate the Achilles tendon, resulting in pain with motion of the ankle joint and foot. Shoes with a rigid heel counter rub up and down on the heel bone. A bursa

POWERSTEP INSOLES BY DR. LES APPEL offer a unique four-phase design to relieve heel and arch pain. Made with a strong prescription-like arch support, it has a strong heel cradle that prevents the foot from pronating (rolling inward) and the arch from flattening—eliminating strain on the plantar fascia. **www. powersteps.com**

The **PSC–PRONATION/SPRING CONTROL STRAP** is designed to treat plantar fasciitis, chronic heel pain, heel spur syndrome, and shin splints. This reusable strapping device is made from ProWrap, a knitted blend of nylon and Lycra with patented foam lining. It wraps around the arch to provide superior support to the plantar fascia while also wrapping around the heel to reduce the force of heel strike and biomechanically move the foot's midline to a more neutral position. **www.fabrifoam.com**

SPENCO CUSHIONS are made from a noncompressible, viscoelastic material to relieve heel pain associated with heel spurs, thinning heel pads, and plantar fasciitis. Products include ViscoSpot and ViscoHeel cushions; Ipos Shock Absorber Heel cushions and SoftBase Insoles; and ViscoPed insoles. They reduce shock to the joints and evenly distribute pressure throughout the cushion. Available at sporting goods stores and some drugstores.

The **TP MASSAGE FOOTBALLER, BALLER BLOCK, AND MASSAGE BALLS** were created to relieve plantar fasciitis, Achilles tendinitis, and heel pain. They work on the muscle of existing spasms and/or trigger points by applying pressure to the trigger point area. Also offered is a Performance Therapy for Foot & Lower Leg DVD, which shows a complete foot and lower leg exercise routine. **www. tpmassageball.com**

TULI'S makes different versions of heel cups with a waffle design. The standard design is single-ribbed, the Pro Heel Cup has a double-ribbed waffle design, and the Gel Heel Cup is double-ribbed with gel polymer. For those with weak ankles, the CheetahWrap Fit ankle support incorporates a standard heel cup with a neoprene ankle sock-type support. **www.medi-dyne.com**

VISCOPED S INSOLES are made from a noncompressible viscoelastic material with a bar of softer silicone in the metatarsal and heel areas that is designed to relieve plantar fascia pain. The insole reduces shock throughout the entire length of the insole and distributes pressure evenly. **www.bauerfeindusa.com**

sac between the Achilles tendon and the heel bone becomes irritated, and over time bursitis may develop.

Haglund's deformity is also called pump bump or retrocalcaneal bursitis. It may be a bone deformity present from birth, or it may be acquired by injury over an athlete's lifetime. It is most often present in women and those who wear hardshelled ski or cross-country boots with rigid heels or heel counters. Individuals with a prominent protrusion of the heel bone are also susceptible to an inflammation in the heel area.

John Gale wrote, "I have been diagnosed with Haglund's deformity on my right foot. For the most part, street shoes and running shoes do not bother it. Hiking and mountaineering boots do (likely related to the stiffness), particularly on steep uphills. In particular, plastic mountaineering boots are a problem due to the stiffness of the boot. Unless I am very careful with fit and proper padding, boots will irritate it, remove the top layer of skin, and leave me limping about for a few days. I have had some success creating a doughnut out of Molefoam, which pads the bump and distributes the pressure from the heel cup around the whole heel rather than just the bump."

The primary symptom of Haglund's deformity is pain at the back of the heel. The tissues also may thicken over the bone bump forming a callus. The callus can grow quite thick and become inflamed while you are wearing shoes.

Treating Haglund's Deformity

The focus of treatment should start with reducing the painful pressure on the bump. In mild cases, a change of shoes will solve the problem and allow the irritation to heal. Changing to shoes with a lower or softer heel counter or a heel counter that is notched for the Achilles tendon can help. A heel pad can lift the heel up above the part of the heel counter that is rubbing on the bump. Pads around the bump may help. Moleskin, or Molefoam, as John mentions above, is not very thick and compresses with wear. A better choice is a pad made from the familiar Spenco green insole foam. These are flat insoles and you can easily cut them to make a pad with a hole in the center. Hold this pad on with a layer of tape. Be careful when applying the pad that this does not make the shoes/boots tighter and cause other problems. An ENGO Patch or ENGO's Cushion Heel Wrap, which adheres to the heel counter, will also reduce friction to the area. Icing the painful area, followed by warm water soaks, can help. Anti-inflammatories can be taken to reduce the pain. If this condition becomes unbearable during an event, cutting a notch or slice into the heel counter can relieve some of the pressure off the bump.

Surgery to remove the excess bone may be necessary in extreme cases. Cortisone injections are not recommended due to the area's proximity to the Achilles tendon.

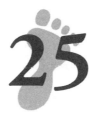

Toe Problems

"While we all have toes, some are better than others," says Herb Hedgecock, humorously relating the anatomy of his feet.

"I have ugly feet. My mother and father stuck me with an 'ugly foot gene,' which was a cruel thing to do. Sometimes I look at the perfect feet that others were blessed with and wonder what the hell I did to deserve Morton's toe and double-wides. The first place I get blisters is on my short fourth toe that curls under the long third monster. And the right foot does this even more. The second place is on the big toe and this seems to happen because the second toe is so damned long and the big toe curves in causing them to rub. Because the second and fourth toes are so out of proportion, this seems to cause toes one, three, and five to also get in on the act. Ergo, toe blisters near the toenails, but who needs ten toenails?"

Just as varied as the many shapes and types of toes are problems associated with them. This chapter will cover the whole gamut of common toe ailments, but first, a word about strengthening your toes.

Strengthening Toes

Strengthening exercises can help keep toes flexible. Practice picking up marbles off a carpeted floor with your toes. Release and repeat 20 times. Put a large, sturdy rubber band around all five toes. Spread your toes outward and hold for five seconds, then release. Repeat ten times. To work on toe flexibility, pull on each toe, gently twisting it to the right and then the left. Then push each toe up and down, while doing the opposite to the next toe. Healthy Toes, from **www.healthytoes. com,** are made from gel and fit over all five toes with spaces to separate each toe. The gentle stretching may help relieve pain from many foot conditions.

The Basics: Toenail Trimming

I mentioned earlier that I have three absolutes. The first is wearing **moisture-wicking socks,** the second is wearing **gaiters for trails,** and the third is **properly trimming**

toenails. How hard can it be to trim your toenails? I guess for a lot of folks, it's a huge deal and something they have a hard time doing. In all the years I have been patching feet, I have observed that untrimmed toenails are the number one cause of problems leading to toe blisters and black nails. Socks will catch on nails that are too long or that have rough edges. This puts pressure on the nail bed, leading to blisters under the toenails or at the tips of the toes or painful toenails, as they are pushed back into the cuticle. Nails that are too long are also prone to pressure from a toe box that is too short or too low.

Ultrarunner Joe Kallo wrote, "I followed your directions regarding using an emery board on the edges of my nails to smooth them, and it worked like a dream! This was the first ultra I've run that I've finished with no loose or painful toenails! And it was 100 miles!"

TIP: The True Meaning of Buff

Elisabeth Archambault has a great toenail tip: "Consider getting a nail buffer (available for a couple of bucks in drugstore cosmetic departments) and buffing them to a shine. Smoothing out the natural ridges is one more way to reduce friction. I'm convinced this helps socks to last longer too."

Toenails should be trimmed regularly, straight across the nail—never rounded at the corners. Leave an extra bit of nail on the outside corner of the big toe to avoid an ingrown toenail. After trimming toenails, use a nail file to smooth the top of the nail down toward the front of the toe and remove any rough edges. If you draw your finger from the skin in front of the toe up across the nail and can feel a rough edge, the nail can be filed smoother or trimmed a bit shorter. Remember though, the shorter you trim your nails, the greater the likelihood that you will experience an ingrown toenail. Conversely, nails that are too long can rub against the front of your shoes and catch on your socks, which can lead to a black toenail, wear holes in your socks, cut into other toes, and crack the nail when you run downhill. Shoes that are too tight in the forefoot or too short can cause the nail to press into the sides of the toe.

Use an emery board nail file from your drugstore. Better yet, invest a few bucks in a nice metal file that will last a long time and serve you well. To trim your nails, there are regular nail clippers, nippers, and scissors made exclusively for thicker toenails. If your local drugstore or pharmacy doesn't have them, check out **www. footsmart.com** for a great selection.

A little bit of care in toenail trimming goes a long ways in preventing toe blisters and black toenails, and in making your socks last longer.

Black Toenails

The technical name for the runner's black toenail, subungual hematoma, describes simply a blood-filled swelling under the nail. This common occurrence is caused by the trauma of the toe or toes repetitively bumping against the front of the shoe. Blood pools in the space between the nail plate and nail bed as they separate or compress from repeated trauma. Individuals with Morton's toe are most susceptible to experiencing black toenails. The nail becomes discolored and usually has associated pain. Most often the nail bed turns dark, almost black or blue because of the blood.

Some athletes tell of losing their nails after the nail bed has turned a whitish color. Vince Gerber wrote, "After finishing the Javelina Hundred my big toenail was floating on a giant blister. This was the first time I ever had white toenails, as opposed to the many black toenails I've experienced. The blister had no blood, just clear fluid. The first couple of days I used a safety pin to puncture and drain the blisters, which would seal and fill back up within a few hours. For the next few days, I would puncture and drain the blister once every day or two. Again, the blisters would slowly fill up again. After about ten days the blisters were totally deflated and the skin dried and started to peel off. Catching an edge of the nail while putting on a sock is what tore the first one halfway off. Then it was a matter of just pulling it off . . . no pain involved at that point. Caught the next one on a bed sheet, then snipped off the remaining side."

Vince makes a good point. Unless you want to tear the nails off, make sure to wrap a Band-Aid around the toe, covering the edges of the nail. Tearing a nail off before it is ready to fall off can be quite painful.

Many runners are simply prone to black toenails. The best means of preventing black toenails is to wear shoes with a generous toe box and with the proper length for your feet. Some runners cut slits in their shoe's toe box or cut out a portion of the toe box to gain relief. Jim Winne, who has perpetually black toenails, says, "When I have any toenails at all, I use moleskin." His strategy is to cut a piece of moleskin slightly larger than the nail area, put it on the nail, and round the edges. Use an alcohol wipe on the nail before applying and be sure the moleskin does not rub on adjoining toes. Kinesio Tex and Micropore tapes would also work.

Ultrarunner Nancy Shura-Dervin tells how she has resolved blood blisters under toenails: "Beginning about three months before the big race, I use an emery board to file down the thickness of the nails (I do all ten). You just sand the entire toenail surface . . . slowly. I perform this as a nightly ritual! This should be done gradually and gently, taking several weeks to get the entire nail paper thin! As new nail grows out, just sand it down. I also gently file over the end of each nail to take off any new growth. I came upon this idea based on the fact that several runners have had their toenails surgically removed. The thinner the nail bed, the more pliable it is to pressure. The end result is that my toes feel nailless to the touch. I stop sanding about three days before the event just to be sure the nail is not tender. As the nails get thinner, at first they can be a little tender (just like immediately after losing a nail) but the sensation soon diminishes." This greatly reduces the occurrence of toenail blisters caused by toe box pressure against a rigid toenail.

Black toenails can come from toenail trauma caused by clenching your toes. This curling downward of the toes can also lead to toe blisters. A small pad under the ball of the foot can help relax the toes, but many athletes have to mentally will themselves to uncurl their toes.

Peter Fish wrote, "I was quite interested in the material about toes that curl under, as I have a similar problem and have also considered surgery. In my case, it's mostly the little toes that get squeezed under the others, and taping them only contributes to the problem by increasing the pressure. I wear soft orthotics, and I have gotten a degree of relief by just making a cutout on the edge of the orthotic to make a depression for my little toe to fit into. These toes develop a sharp callus on the side of the toe, which I treat frequently, then sand it down with a callus file. The next toes in get blisters on the bottom, also from curling under, and these I tape, using one strip of duct tape over the end and another wrapped around perpendicular. As I've been doing longer races, I've felt that these solutions were not quite adequate."

Nancy offers a good tip to help manage these curling or overlapping toes. A good preventive measure is to cut the little toe out of the insole. This measure allows the little toe to ride on the shoe bottom while the foot and other four toes ride higher up on the shoe insole. It effectively prevents one toe from riding on top of another toe. This measure can be used for any of the five toes and can also be used for more than one toe as well. Here's how:

- Remove the insole and stand barefoot on the insole.

- Use a narrow marker pen to outline the space between the fourth and little toe then mark a bit toward the little toe where the toe meets the foot.

- With scissors, cut the little toe part out of the insole, making the cut smaller than the marks at first.

- Put the insole back in the shoe and try it on, noting that your little toe should ride on the bottom of the shoe.

- Continue removing the insole and trimming as needed to make the toe opening comfortable; you shouldn't feel the cuts at all.

Treating Black Toenails

If there is no pain from the black toenail, no action may be necessary. If the pain and pressure increases, the pressure must be relieved. To relieve pressure from a black toenail, use one of the following methods, depending on the look of the toenail. The treatment may have to be repeated several times. Although the two methods below might sound painful, they are usually not. The blood has separated the nail from the nail bed and is a barrier between the nail and the live skin underneath.

- If the discoloration does not extend to the end of the toenail, swab the nail with an alcohol wipe, and use a small nail drill, drill bit, or hypodermic needle to gently drill a hole in the nail with light pressure and rolling the needle/bit back and forth between your thumb and fingers. The blood will ooze through the hole. Keep slight pressure on the nail bed to help expel the built-up blood. Stopping too soon will cause the blood to clot in the hole and the problem will reoccur. I purchased a small nail drill through eBay and like its ease of use.

■ An alternative method is to use a match to heat a paper clip and gently penetrate the nail with the heated point. The heat in this method can cauterize the blood and stop the flow of blood out from under the nail. Press on the nail to expel the blood.

If the discoloration extends to the end of the toenail, use a sterile pin or needle to penetrate the skin under the nail and release the pressure. Holding slight pressure on the nail bed will help expel the blood.

Care must be taken to prevent a secondary bacterial infection through the hole in the nail or at the end of the nail by using an antibiotic ointment and covering the site with a Band-Aid. If the hole seals up, use the drill, needle, or paper clip to open it up again. Loss of the nail usually follows in the months ahead. The new nail will begin growing, pushing up the old nail, and may come in looking odd. David Hannaford, DPM, a podiatrist, tells of patients who come to see him thinking they "have cancer because their nails are growing in funny looking." Do not be concerned about the process unless an infection develops. Remember, it can take six to nine months for a new nail to grow in completely.

Judit Zubovits, MD, likes her toenails short. "I keep my nails ultrashort," she says. "I seem to have no problems trimming my big toenail quite short (less than 1 centimeter); the rest of my nails on my foot are literally just a few *millimeters* in length. I never get black toenails, no matter how long I run and no matter what terrain."

You may find relief by wearing a metatarsal pad, a small circular pad that pushes up the ball of the foot and drops the toes down, which takes pressure off the toenails. Contact Hapad (**www.hapad.com**) for information on these pads.

Once your toenail has come off, a new nail will grow in. Sometimes though, the new nail may grow in odd or wavy looking, thicker, or any other unusual appearance. Richard Schick suggests applying petroleum jelly or an ointment of your choosing to the nail bed a couple of times a day to keep it from becoming dry and stiff. Second, as Nancy suggests, use a nail file to keep the newly emerging nail as thin as possible until it is fully regrown. This keeps the nail flexible and without the structural strength to cause problems.

Athletes who have frequent problems with black toenails often choose

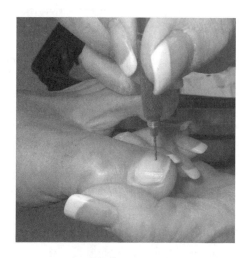

A nail drill makes a clean hole to relieve pressure.

to have them surgically removed. Tim Jantz, a podiatrist, describes the process of removing a toenail:

> After the toe is numbed, the nail is removed and the growth plate is treated with 89% phenol (some use sodium hydroxide) to destroy the growth plate. The area is then rinsed with alcohol and dressed with an antibiotic and a dressing. The usual post-operation care is daily soaks and dressing with a topical antibiotic and a Band-Aid for approximately four weeks, sometimes longer. The toe has endured a chemical burn and so heals by draining. It can have a raw feeling for a week or so, and I wouldn't want to stub it or have anyone step on it for a few weeks. You may also want to wear roomy shoes or sandals for a week. The procedure is about 95% successful. An option is to find a doctor who uses a laser, and the only difference is higher cost.

Kevin O'Neall wrote, "I was plagued with ingrown nail pain for most of my life. By the time of high school I had learned to grit my teeth and dig them out using an X-acto blade and tweezers. Ten years ago I submitted to surgery. As I watched, the podiatrist removed the ingrown nails and then treated the toes so they wouldn't regrow. The surgery was painless, took 15 minutes, and cost around $200. The toes were sore for less than a week, feeling as if I'd stubbed my toes walking barefoot into a heavy chair. I've never had a recurrence of the ingrown nails."

If you are prone to black toenails and have tried all the options to prevent them, consult a podiatrist about nail removal.

Big Toe Problems

Big toes are susceptible to problems in their joints. Hallux limitus is a decreased range of motion in the joint located at the base of the big toe. This condition can progress into hallus rigidus, wherein the joint becomes rigid. There can be pain in the big toe when it is pushed upward, as happens when we walk, run, or stand on our toes. The joint can become inflamed and swell. As the condition progresses, the pain can become more constant. There can be crepitus, or a grinding feeling in the joint with movement, and sometimes a bump can be felt on the top of the joint. Because the inflammation is on the top of the joint, it should not be confused with a bunion, which is on the side.

A premature wearing down and tearing of the joint's cartilage causes hallux limitus and rigidus. Without the cartilage, the bones rub together, and new bone growth occurs, often leading to bone spurs. The deterioration of the cartilage can be caused by repetitive injuries, age-related changes, and hereditary defects.

Treating Big Toe Problems

Early treatment is best to avoid long-term problems. Make sure your shoes are wide enough and long enough to prevent pressure on the toe. A shoe with as rigid a sole as possible is preferred. Use a soft-gel pad to cushion the ball of the foot and reduce pressure on the big toe joint. Resting the foot, warm water soaks, and gentle massage with topical pain relievers can help. Custom-made orthotics will help stabilize the foot.

Hammertoes, Claw Toes, & Mallet Toes

Hammertoes are toes that are contracted at the toe's middle joint, making the toe bend upward at its center and forcing the tip of the toe downward. The ligaments and tendons have tightened and are forcing the toes to curl. This can lead to severe pressure and pain. Blisters or corns may form at the top bend in the toe and calluses at the ends of the toes. Hammertoes can occur in any toe, except the big toe. There are two types of hammertoes: rigid and flexible. A rigid toe has no ability to move, but in a flexible toe, the joint can be moved. Hammertoes are typically the result of a muscle imbalance that causes the ligaments and tendons to tighten. Individuals with flat feet, high arches, and Morton's toe are prone to hammertoes.

Al Czecholinski relates his experience with surgery for hammertoes:

> I had hammertoe surgery on two toes on my right foot about four years ago. I'm very happy with the result. Prior to the surgery the foot was always swollen and sore where the toe joints were being rammed back into the foot. The podiatrist said that eventually these joints would be very damaged and arthritic, making even walking difficult. That being said, do not take the surgery lightly and try all conservative measures before getting the surgery. I lived with a sore foot for years and got a second opinion before I had the surgery. The surgery involved sawing out a section of bone to make the toe shorter so the tendon would become relatively longer. The sawed bones plus the pins that were inserted to hold the bones while healing hurt quite a lot. I spent about six to seven weeks in a big rigid foot immobilizer. Then it took a few more weeks to be able to walk fairly normally. If the hammertoes are only causing blisters due to rubbing and there's no swelling or joint damage, the surgery is probably not worth it. First try orthotics and modifying your shoe's toe box.

Claw toes are similar to hammertoes except they are contracted down at the middle joint and up at the joint at the ball of the foot. Mallet toes are contracted at the end joint only. Causes and treatments are the same as for hammertoes.

Treating Hammertoes, Claw Toes, & Mallet Toes

Be sure your footwear has a high and broad toe box. This usually allows the other toes additional room so there is less friction against the individual toes. For toes that are flexible, toe crests or splints that straighten the toe can sometimes be used. Gel caps or toe shields that slide over the toes can protect the toes from friction.

Strengthening exercises can help keep toes flexible. Refer to the "Strengthening Toes" section earlier in this chapter.

Pamela Adams, a chiropractor, offers another alternative:

Chiropractors who specialize in sports rehab and extremity adjusting may be able to help. Even yoga for feet or a course of Rolfing (which eliminates scar tissue) may help. Tendons can shorten; tendons can lengthen. Why not try conservative approaches while saving up for surgery? You may be pleasantly surprised. I've had patients with bunions; hammertoes; and overlapping, curly, or otherwise misaligned toes. Unless the problem is congenital, or due to an injury such as a fracture, most toe problems come from faulty alignment and biomechanics, poor shoes, and poor form during activity. I always suggest surgery as a last, not first, choice. Meanwhile, go barefoot at home and wear shoes that allow your toes to spread out when you toe off.

Adventure racer Steve Daniel's three outer toes on each foot curl up under the others—toward the big toe. When he did the Primal Quest 2003, he decided to go with what he thought was the best combination for his feet—Injinji toe socks and pretaping each toe at the joints and around any blister-prone areas with Leukotape. Even with these measures, his little toe felt as if it had been beaten with a hammer. That's obviously because it was pounded the whole time under the other toes. Steve talked to his podiatrist and was told surgery was his best option.

My wife had a problem toe that turned into a hammertoe. To help her, I used a thin strip of Kinesio Tex tape. I applied the tape to the underside of the toe, then up and over the tip, stretching it as I applied it to the top of the toe under tension. That helped straighten the toe and worked for her until she finally had surgery.

Corrective surgery may be the best option, but as Steve found out, it is expensive. There are often three surgical choices: cut the tendons on the bottom of the toes; cut the tendons, fuse the joints, and put titanium pins through the toes; or cut the tendons and then add some tendons on the top side of the toe to draw the toe up and out. Each has its pros and cons. Your orthopedic surgeon is the best person to explain each procedure and help you make an intelligent choice.

PRODUCTS FOR HAMMERTOES, CLAW TOES, & MALLET TOES

Assorted products are available in your local drugstore and pharmacy, among them Dr. Scholl's Hammertoe Pads and Gel Toe Shields or Toe Caps for cushioning the toes. Other products include the following.

FOOTSMART carries the Silicone Toe Crest that fits over one toe and nestles under the hammertoe for support while relieving pressure and friction. The Toe Straightener properly aligns hammertoes (also available in a double toe model). The Gel Toe Separator and Spreader may also provide relief. **www. footsmart.com**

HAPAD offers Pedifix Visco-Gel Toe Caps, Hammertoe Cushions, Toe Cushions, and a Toe Spreader. **www.hapad.com**

Ingrown Toenails

Ingrown toenails, most common to the big toe, may cause infection and require medical attention. One or both sides of your toenail may grow into the flesh of the toe. The result is a reddened, irritated, and swollen toe that is sensitive to any degree of pressure. These are usually very painful and require immediate attention. Increased redness, pain, and tenderness to the touch can indicate an infection. Toes are typically in a warm and moist environment, and bacteria can quickly take hold. The most common cause of an ingrown toenail is improper nail trimming (see "The Basics: Toenail Trimming" above).

Sometimes trauma from a stubbed toe or someone stepping on your toe can cause the nail to be jammed into the skin. Repeated trauma, such as the pounding to which athletes typically subject their feet, also can lead to ingrown toenails. The medical term for an ingrown toenail is onychocryptosis.

Treating Ingrown Toenails

Soak your foot in warm water or Epsom salts two to three times a day to reduce the infection. Do not poke at the ingrown nail. If you cannot trim the nail yourself, check with your orthopedist or podiatrist. An ignored ingrown toenail can become seriously infected. Apply a layer of antibiotic cream to help reduce inflammation and cover with a Band-Aid.

Rich Schick, a physician's assistant, recommends the following method to care for an ingrown nail:

> File the entire top surface of the nail from near the cuticle to the tip until you get it as thin as possible. A regular nail file will work, but a medium-grade metal file is much quicker. This weakens the nail. Then soak the foot in hot water for about 30 minutes to soften the nail, further weakening the nail. Then use a cuticle trimmer (available in most drugstore beauty departments) to free the ingrown portion. Do not attempt to work from the tip toward the base. Come from the side, and a little toward the base of the toe and use the "wings" of the instrument to lift and free the ingrown segment. As you continue forward, the trimmer will often cut the piece off. If not, snip it with a nail clipper. I prefer a small pair of wire cutters for the task.

Assorted products are available in your local drugstore and pharmacy. In addition to ingrown toenail files and toenail softening cream, here are a few specialty products:

- The Barrel Nipper, long-handled nail clippers made for thick, tough, curved nails;

- Dr. Scholl's Ingrown Toenail Relief Strips; and

- Toe Caps and Jelly Tips from Hapad (**www.hapad.com**) or Bunheads (**www.bunheads.com**) to cover and protect the nail.

Morton's Toe

Morton's toe, often called Morton's foot, is a common problem in which the second toe (next to the big toe) is longer than the big toe. In the 1930s, podiatrist Dr. Dudley Morton discovered that many people had a short first metatarsal bone. He concluded that this condition impacted their gait, causing their foot to hyperpronate—a dysfunction of the foot causing your ankles to roll in when you stand, walk, and run. Estimates for Morton's toe range from 15% of the population to as high as 50–60%.

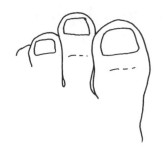

Those with Morton's Toe have a second toe that extends beyond the big toe.

The first metatarsal (of the big toe) is shorter than normal, and this makes the second toe appear longer than it actually is. This is usually a hereditary condition. The constant pressure placed on the longer second toe while walking or standing can lead to callus formation under the second metatarsal head due to this excessive pressure. The repeated pressure of the longer second toe against the front of the shoe or boot may traumatize the nail. If a hematoma develops under the nail, the nail will change color and may fall off. Because of the excessive pressure on the second metatarsal head in the forefoot, Morton's toe is often associated with metatarsalgia.

Morton's toe makes buying shoes harder. It is important to fit shoes to this longest toe. Your toes need space and breathing room and your longer toe is no exception. In addition, make sure you trim your nails and file them smooth. Good toenail care, especially of this long toe, will prevent the nail from hitting on the front of the shoe—jamming the nail back into the nail bed. If you are bothered by toe pain, gel caps could help. These are a gel substance that cover the toe, and many are reusable.

Treating Morton's Toe

To get a good fit, look for shoes or boots with a high and wide toe box. It may be necessary to use a shoe or boot a half size to a size larger than normal in order to have space for the longer first toe. The use of orthotics can align the foot by providing arch support. A metatarsal pad under the metatarsal heads of the forefoot can relieve pressure on the second metatarsal head. (A good source of metatarsal pads is **www. hapad.com**.) The use of a nonslippery insole will keep the foot from sliding forward. Look for an insole with a good heel cup, an arch that fits your foot, and a surface material that grips the foot and sock. Some runners will cut a slit over or on either side of the toe to relieve pressure. Another option is to cut out a small piece of the toe box over the toe. Orthotics may also provide relief. Surgery is usually a last resort.

If you find a blister or corn starting at the top of the toe, use a gel cap or tape to protect the area. If you begin to experience pain at the base of the toe, a pad might help. Use a U-shaped pad and position the cutout area at the site of the pain. To find the right position, first make a mark at the sore area with a marking pen. Then slide your foot inside your shoe and step down to transfer the ink onto the insole. Stick the pad to the insole with the opening toward the toes.

FOOTSMART carries Silicone Gel Caps and Digi-Cushions to cushion the toe, and Felt and Silicone Callus Cushions for the base of the toe pain. **www. footsmart.com**

Overlapping Toes

Sometimes toes will overlap other toes. This can occur with any of your toes and cause extreme irritation. Overlapping toes typically involve one toe lying on top of an adjacent toe. The fifth toe is the most affected digit with overlapping toes. Underlapping toes usually involve the fourth and fifth toes. The cause of overlapping and underlapping toes is unknown. Many experts suspect that they are caused by an imbalance in the small muscles of the foot.

Treating Overlapping Toes

Custom-made orthotics may help align the toes. Off-the-shelf orthotics commonly found in drugstores and sports stores will generally not help this condition. A podiatrist can make the correct type of orthotic. Shoes with a high and wide toe box can give toes the space they need. Gel toe straighteners, toe caps, and toe combs can be used on and between toes. A strip of 0.5-inch tape applied to the inside of the pinky toe and then over the tip, and applied to the side of the foot under tension, can straighten it a bit. Pamela Adams, a chiropractor, offers an option worth considering in the section on hammertoes. Chiropractic toe adjustments may be of help as well. If the condition is painful and causes problems when participating in sports, consult with your podiatrist to determine your options.

Surgical correction sometimes involves releasing the tendon and the soft tissues around the joint at the base of the fifth toe. In severe cases, a pin may need to be surgically inserted to hold the toe in a straight position. The pin, which exits the tip of the toe, may be left in place for up to three weeks.

FOOTSMART carries the Gel Toe Separators and Spreader. **www.footsmart.com**

Stubbed Toes

Occasionally we stub our toes badly, and this can result in a hematoma, a bruise, or even a fracture. Stubbed toes are more common in running shoes than in hiking boots. Stubbing a toe on a rock or tree root can be very painful. Check the toe for discoloration that can indicate a deep bruise or a fracture. There may be a laceration into the nail bed or into the toe itself.

Treating Stubbed Toes

Treatment includes buddy taping, icing the toe (a cold stream will also work), elevating the foot, and wearing a firm-soled shoe or boot. Buddy taping provides support and a limited degree of immobilization to the toe. It involves lightly taping the injured toe to the toe next to it after placing a piece of cotton between toes (never tape skin to skin). See the chapter "Cold & Heat Therapy" for information on making the most of icing techniques. For elevation to be effective, the injured toe should be above the level of the heart and iced. A firm-soled shoe will keep the toe from bending, providing additional immobilization.

If it heals in a few days, it is probably not fractured. On the other hand, if the injury does not respond to treatment, medical treatment and an X-ray may be necessary (see the section on fractures, page 268). A doctor may have you wear an orthopedic shoe, a wooden-soled shoe that does not allow the foot to bend. If the toe is fractured, expect a healing time of four to six weeks.

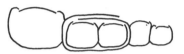

Buddy taping as seen from the front

If you stub your toe and the nail is bent backward, it's important to prevent the toenail from catching on your sock and tearing off. Wrap either a Band-Aid or tape around the toe to hold the toenail in place. The use of an antibiotic ointment under the nail will help prevent infection. Trimming off any loose parts of the nail will help prevent the nail from lifting off further.

Toenail Fungus

Toenail fungus is a major problem affecting many athletes. As I have patched feet over the past year, I have mentioned toenail fungus to many athletes and find most are in denial about this medical problem. John Mozena, DPM, podiatrist and marathon runner, says, "Because nail fungus can seriously impact your running as well as your general foot health, we urge runners to practice prevention and seek medical care at the first sign of the problem."

Nail fungus, also known as ony-chomycosis, is a persistent fungal infection of the nails that occurs when fungi called dermatophytes invade the nail bed. The fungus lives within the nail bed, making it difficult to reach and treat. Toenails infected with a fungus usually become thick and deformed. The infection may cause the nail to have a brown, white,

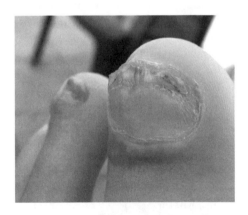

Toenail fungus

or yellowish discoloration. The nail may become brittle and give the appearance of debris under the nail. As the fungus progresses, the nail thickens, which can cause pressure inside footwear. Toenail fungus more often affects men and the chance of its occurring increases with age—but it can affect anyone regardless of age and gender. In spite of these symptoms, many people live with a nail fungus for years because it seldom causes discomfort.

Athletes are at greater risk of developing toenail fungus because of their exposure to specific risk factors.

- Nail trauma can make the nail bed more susceptible to fungal growth.

- Sweaty socks and tight shoes promote a warm, moist environment that can contribute to the growth of the fungus.

- Because nail fungus is contagious, warm and moist environments such as communal showers and locker rooms are places where the fungus can be contracted.

The following steps can reduce your chances of getting toenail fungus:
- Wash and dry feet daily, especially between the toes.

- Wear moisture-absorbing socks.

- Make sure that shoes are completely dry before putting them on.

- Wear shower shoes or flip-flops when showering in public areas.

- Don't apply nail polish to nails that are suspected of infection.

- Wear shoes that breathe and rotate shoes every day.

- Use an antifungal powder or spray.

- Inspect feet regularly and have a doctor check for nail fungus during office visits.

Treating Toenail Fungus

Because the fungus starts in the nail bed and spreads, it is important to stop the progression when symptoms of infection are first seen. Usually doctors will prescribe a strong medication to destroy the fungus. Prescription medications may include oral antifungal medications or topical medications. If you are prescribed an oral medication, be sure to discuss its side effects with your doctor. Because nails grow slowly, treatment can take at least six months to a year or more. This allows the medication to eliminate every last fungal agent around the affected area while a new nail grows in healthy and strong. Podiatrist Christine Dobrowolski, the author of *Those Aching Feet*, talks about treatments for toenail fungus.

The most aggressive and effective treatments are with oral antifungal medications. The most common oral antifungal medications are Sporanox and Lamisil. The most effective topical medication is Penlac lacquer. Another prescription topical is a urea-based medication called Carmol. To increase the effectiveness of the treatment, I recommend combination therapy. If you choose to take an oral medication, make sure you use a topical antifungal agent as well. Nail removal is also an option. Once the nail is removed, the topicals can reach the nail bed and become more effective. The nail will grow back in over a period of eight to ten months. Permanent nail removal is reserved for those with chronic ingrown nails, ulceration under the nails, or pain from the fungal nails.

A fairly new treatment option is the use of a laser to shine through the nail and destroy the specific pathogens embedded in and under your nail causing the infection. The treatment takes about 30 minutes for all ten toes, without pain and no damage to healthy tissue. In the first clinical study, 88% of the treated patients grew out a normal nail after one treatment. Costs average $1,000 for ten toes. Ask your podiatrist about this treatment or do an online search to find where it is offered.

There are several home remedies that many people try, often successfully. If these do not work for you, do not hesitate to consult a doctor. First, tea tree oil, manuka oil, or eucalyptus oil is often used for nail fungus. For best results, apply a few drops to the affected nail and skin around the nail two to three times daily. Dab it on with a cotton swab or ball. Hold it in place with a bandage or tape. As well as killing the fungi, it helps relieve the associated itching. Test a drop or two on your skin to be sure you are not allergic to the oil. The oils can be found in your local drugstore or pharmacy.

Another nail treatment that has been used with success is Vicks VapoRub. Trim the nail back as far as possible and scrape out as much of the loose nail as possible. Apply a thin coat of VapoRub over the nail and in the space underneath. Cover the nail with a Band-Aid. Repeat every morning and evening, and over a few months the fungus will die out and a new nail will grow in. Soaking your toes twice daily in Listerine and/or Listerine and white vinegar (1:1 solution) has worked for some people. One pedorthist recommends putting a capful of rubbing alcohol on your toenails after showering each day. He says that the icky part of the nail will dry out and flake off, and a new nail will grow in normally.

If you use tea tree oil, manuka oil, eucalyptus oil, or Vicks VapoRub, you must apply it twice daily for at least 90 days (and 180 days is better). Dr. Dobrowolski emphasizes, "With any home remedy or nonprescription topical, you must understand that the effectiveness of the treatment is fairly low, less than 10%. If you do try one of these therapies, make sure to use it every day. File the top of the nail down to roughen up the surface and apply the medication with a cotton swab. We really don't have effective, affordable, safe medications available right now for the treatment of toenail fungus. So, when patients have failed other conventional treatments, I'll recommend trying almost any affordable and safe treatment that has helped others in the past, but I just wouldn't expect much."

John Shannon, MD, wrote, "For about ten years I had problems with toenail fungus. The first few times it was cured with Lamisil. Eventually, I had another infection of my left fourth toenail that would not be cured with Lamisil after two courses of the medicine. The nail looked totally involved, and I could practically take off the top of the nail because it would separate from the nail bed or just above the nail bed. A podiatrist and a dermatologist had both looked at the nail and really didn't help me much, to my disappointment as a fellow physician. I had read online about some people treated with chlorhexidine gluconate, a commonly used antiseptic for surgical hand washing. I got a scrub brush with that chemical on it, took off that top part of the nail, and washed my feet with the scrub brush. In two weeks I had a normal nail growing! I was amazed, to say the least. I think more research should be done for that chemical as a topical treatment for nail fungus. To me, the debridement I did by being able to remove the top part of the nail helped in letting the chemical get to the fungus."

The bottom line, Dr. Dobrowolski adds, is that "treating toenail fungus is very difficult. If you have fungal toenails that cause pressure, pain, or infection, consider talking to your doctor about prescription medications, nail removal, or laser treatments. Make sure you take precautions to prevent re-infection and take multiple approaches to eradicate the problem. If your fungal toenails are only unsightly and don't cause any discomfort, try a weekly application of an over-the-counter topical along with methods to prevent re-infection."

Check your local drugstore for over-the-counter medications such as Miranel. Online searches will also give you additional options. Two of these are Fungi-Nail at **www.funginail.com** and Fungisil at **www.fungisil.com,** treatments aimed at the cuticles and nail beds.

Turf Toe

Turf toe is pain at the base of the big toe where it connects to the ball of the foot—a sprain of the big toe metatarsophalangeal joint. It is usually caused from either jamming the toe or hyperextension (bending back) of the big toe. There may also be an associated stiffness and swelling. This injury is especially common among athletes who play on the hard surface of artificial turf. Football and soccer players are most susceptible to it because of all their running and jumping.

The injury is actually a tear of the capsule that surrounds the joint at the base of the toe. Tearing this joint capsule can be extremely painful. It can lead to instability and even dislocation of the joint at the base of the toe. An X-ray is in order.

Robin Fry, a physician's assistant, remembers that during an ultramarathon in 1993, he was "running away from the fire-tower aid station. Suddenly, a terrible pain shot out from my left foot and a swear word or two shot out from my mouth. I had slammed my left great toe into an unseen remnant of a small shrub or tree, barely protruding from the rough trail surface." Years later in 2001, his podiatrist performed surgery to repair the toe, which by then was very deviated laterally, and was crowding the second toe and pushing it into the third toe. After a period of recovery, Robin reports, "I do get some occasional aching in the repaired toe, but it generally stays at a tolerable level and only hurts after some very long, hard efforts. The long-crowded toes of my left foot are gradually resuming a normal alignment. I rarely take any NSAIDS. I have been taking daily Cosamin DS, a glucosamine and chondroitin-sulfate supplement, since early January. And I am back to my old training ways."

Treating Turf Toe

The common treatment consists of resting the sore toe, icing the area, and elevating the foot. Your doctor may prescribe an anti-inflammatory medication and recommend not bearing weight on the affected foot. Avoid playing your sport for about three weeks to allow the joint capsule to heal. When returning to play, you may have to wear a special toe support to protect the joint capsule. Like many injuries, the condition can recur and the rate of rehabilitation can slow with each occurrence. As Robin found out, surgery may be necessary in extreme cases or when the initial injury heals incorrectly.

> **HAPAD DANCER PADS** fit under the ball of the foot with a cutout encompassing the big toe joint to relieve the pain under the first metatarsal joint. The coiled, springlike wool fibers provide firm and resilient support as they mold and shape to the foot. **www.hapad.com**

26

Forefoot Problems

Four conditions commonly affect the front of the foot (the forefoot): bunions, metatarsalgia, Morton's neuroma, and sesamoiditis. Any of them can be bothersome and painful, but when they happen to an athlete, they can make enjoying your sport more challenging.

Bunions

Bunions, or hallux valgus, are one of the most common deformities of the forefoot. A bunion is a bump caused by enlarged bone and tissue at the outer base of the big toe where the joint angles inward toward the other toes. A displacement of the first metatarsal bone toward the midline (center) of the body and a simultaneous displacement of the big toe away from the midline (and toward the smaller toes) cause this bump to appear. Over time, the big toe can come to rest under, or occasionally over, the second toe. The bony bump is a form of arthritis.

The deformity gives you a wide foot and causes a weakening and sagging of the arch. The motion of the joint and shoe pressure can cause pain. There may be corns on the adjacent sides of the first and second toes. A callus may develop over the bunion, and bursitis can form between the skin and the bunion bone.

A similar bump at the outer base of the fifth (small) toe is called a bunionette. These are formed when the little toe moves inward toward the big toe. Bunionettes are sometimes called tailor's bunions.

Bunions are caused by various factors. An abnormal pronated foot that rolls inward is one of the most common causes. Other causes include a family history of bunions, wearing shoes that are too narrow-toed, and limb length discrepancy. Individuals with flat feet are more prone to bunions, calluses, and hammertoes.

Treating Bunions
Be sure that your shoes are wide and deep enough in the forefoot and toe box. If you overpronate, try an arch support or orthotic to reduce the overpronation. Bunion

discomfort may be relieved with wider shoes, pads between the big and first toes, arch supports, and warm soaks. Wearing shoes or boots that are tapered in the toe area can cause bunions to worsen. Check the foot care section of your local drugstore for a current selection of bunion relief products. If there is an inflammation of the bunion, take an anti-inflammatory medication, elevate the foot, and apply ice three times a day, 15 minutes at a time. For information on cold and heat therapy techniques, see page 336.

A full-service shoe shop or a pedorthist should be able to modify a boot to soften a pressure point or stretch a portion of the leather. This may relieve pressure on bunions, corns, and calluses.

To relieve pressure on the painful area, try one of these lacing techniques. Skipping the first set of eyelets is the easiest method to try. Or use two laces per shoe. Lace one through the bottom half of the eyelets, and tie it loosely. Lace the other through the top half of the eyelets, and tie it more tightly than the bottom lace. A third technique is to lace the first few loops loosely, tie a knot, and then lace the rest of the way up the shoe. Both methods allow a looser fit in the forefoot.

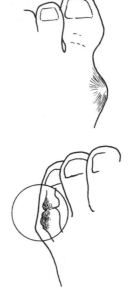

Bunion (top) and
bunionette (bottom)

Two simple big toe stretches can help relieve big toe discomfort associated with bunions.

1. Sit with your foot flat on the floor and then with the heel flat, raise the foot. Gently pull your big toe outward to the side and hold for several seconds. Repeat ten times.

2. While in the same position, raise your foot on its heel, curling your toes tightly downward. Gently push down on your toes. Repeat ten times.

When conservative measures don't provide relief, surgery may be necessary in extreme cases. A bunionectomy removes the bony prominence. In severe cases, an osteotomy procedure realigns the toe joint. In these surgeries, screws, plates, or wires hold the bones in position while they heal. A new procedure, developed by George Holmes, MD, a foot and ankle surgeon with Rush University Medical Center, offers new hope. In this procedure, called the Mini Tightrope, one hole is drilled through the bone leading to the big toe and another through the bone leading to the second toe. A special type of wire, called FiberWire, is fed through the holes, with tiny buttons on each end keeping the wire from slipping out of the bones. The wire is tightened, pulling the outer bone toward the second bone into a better alignment. The surgeon then rebalances the associated ligaments, tendons, and nerves in the toe. Because no bones are cut, healing is faster and with less complications.

BUNION PRODUCTS

Assorted bunion products are available in your local drugstore and pharmacy, among them **DR. SCHOLL'S BUNION CUSHION PADS and HAPAD'S DAYTIME BUNION CUSHION.**

BUNION AID is a flexible splint that realigns the big toe while reducing bunion pain. One size fits all and it can be worn on either foot. While it is meant for 24-hour use, it is too bulky for use during running events. It can be worn in wide shoes or barefoot. **www.bunion-aid.com**

ENGO PATCHES are low-friction patches uniquely applied to areas of footwear and insoles—not skin—for easier, long-lasting bunion protection. Several sizes are available: small ovals for toes or large ovals for the ball of foot. **www. goengo.com**

FOOTSMART carries the Gel Toe Separators and Spreader, Bunion Comforter, and Hydrogel Bunion Guard. **www.footsmart.com**

Metatarsalgia

Metatarsalgia is pain underneath the metatarsal heads of the foot. It typically occurs when one of the metatarsal heads collapses and points downward. Typically the second metatarsal head is affected, but it can also be at the third or fourth metatarsal heads. You may feel as if there is a small stone in your shoe, or you may feel pain, a burning sensation, or swelling at the ball of the foot. By pressing up slightly on each metatarsal head, you can usually identify the painful area. Typically the metatarsal head that is lower than the others is causing the pain and pressure. There will often be a callus at the pressure point. As we age, the fat pads on the bottoms of our feet tend to thin out and our feet become more susceptible to this problem. Metatarsalgia is often associated with Morton's foot.

Shoes that are too narrow in the forefoot or laced too tightly over the forefoot area can cause all of these problems. To see how the pressure in a narrow shoe affects the metatarsals, try this simple test. Grasp your foot around the base of the toes and squeeze gently. See how it forces the metatarsals downward (on the bottom of the foot) and results in increased impact to the area with each step. For proper prevention, start with shoes that fit correctly and use good lacing techniques (for more on these topics, see the chapters "The Magic of Fit," page 43, and "Lacing Options," page 156).

Treating Metatarsalgia

A cushioned metatarsal pad can provide relief from metatarsalgia. If a pad does not help, try cutting a small hole in the insole under the painful metatarsal head. Some metatarsal pads are made in a sleeve that wraps around the foot, and this design may cause problems during sports. To find the right position for a pad, first make a mark at the sore area with a marking pen. Then slide your foot inside your shoe and step down to transfer the ink onto the insole. Stick the pad to the insole with the opening toward the toes.

Wearing shoes with a wide forefoot and high and wide toe box is also recommended. An orthotic may be necessary. If all else fails, ask your podiatrist about a cortisone injection.

METATARSALGIA PRODUCTS

FOOTSMART carries a Silicone Ball-of-Foot Cushion and Metatarsal Pad that redistributes pressure on the metatarsal heads. **www.footsmart.com**

HAPAD makes several pads to relieve metatarsal pain. Metatarsal pads relieve the pain of metatarsalgia and Morton's neuroma. Metatarsal bars relieve pressure on the ball of the foot that causes painful calluses and forefoot irritations. Metatarsal Cookies provide simple metatarsal arch cushioning. The coiled, springlike wool fibers provide firm and resilient support as they mold and shape to the foot. **www.hapad.com**

SPENCO'S METATARSAL ARCH CUSHION is made for the ball of the foot. **www.spenco.com**

VISCOPED INSOLES are made from a noncompressible viscoelastic material with areas of softer density in the raised metatarsal head pad and heel areas. The Viscoped S insole is made with bar of softer silicone in the metatarsal and heel areas. The insoles reduce shock throughout the entire length of the insole, distribute pressure evenly, and are made to relieve pain associated with metatarsalgia and Morton's neuroma. **www.bauerfeindusa.com**

Morton's Neuroma

Morton's neuroma is pain associated with a nerve inflammation usually affecting the third and fourth toes. It will sometimes be felt between the second and third toes. The nerves running between the metatarsal heads and the toes have become inflamed and irritated as they are squeezed at the base of the toes. The painful, swollen nerve is called a neuroma. There is typically tingling or a pins and needles sensation that radiates to the end of the toes—often progressing to a burning sensation with sharp pain. Some people describe the sensation as walking on a pebble. If you press with your thumb at the base of your fourth toe and feel pain, you could have a neuroma. If untreated, scar tissue forms around the nerve and it becomes more painful.

This condition can be caused by a shoe's tight toe box that compresses the forefoot or by the nerves being pressured by the metatarsal heads and the bases of the toes. Sports that place a significant amount of pressure on the forefoot area

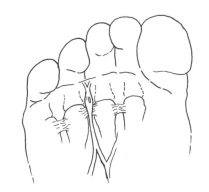

Inflammation of a nerve, indicating Morton's neuroma.

can cause inflammation of the nerves. As we walk or run, we come up onto our toes, and this motion can cause the ligaments supporting the metatarsal bones to compress the nerve between the toes. Limiting your activities for a few days may be enough to allow the inflammation to subside.

Treating Morton's Neuroma

Treatments include applying ice to the pain area, an injection of anti-inflammatory medication, wider shoes, a more cushioned insole, and metatarsal pads that take pressure off the metatarsal heads. The pad reduces forefoot pressure and spreads the toes, which can relieve the pain. To find the right position for a pad, first make a mark at the sore area with a marking pen. Then slide your foot inside your shoe and step down to transfer the ink onto the insole. Stick the pad to the insole with the opening toward the toes. The site **www.footsmart.com** has a number of pads and insoles to help relieve the pain.

Massaging the foot usually helps to relieve the pain. Using icing techniques from the "Cold & Heat Therapy" chapter can help reduce pain and inflammation.

If you overpronate, the metatarsal bones have more movement, which can irritate the nerves running between the metatarsal heads. In this case, wearing firm motion-control shoes may help. Relief may also be gained by inserting a piece of lamb's wool between the toes. The use of an orthotic may be indicated. Bursitis, bunions, or arthritis may also cause metatarsal pain.

When a neuroma has not responded to conservative treatments, cortisone injections can provide relief for months or years. Alternative treatments include alcohol sclerosing injections and surgical excision.

Christine Dobrowolski, a podiatrist and author of *Those Aching Feet*, advises wearing shoes with a low heel to reduce excessive pressure on the ball of the foot, wearing rigid shoes, and using contrasting soaks to reduce inflammation. The soaks start with 5 minutes of heat followed by 5 minutes of ice/cold for 20–30 minutes.

Bob Agazzi's bout with Morton's neuroma over several years led him to study treatment options. He learned of the following treatments, from the least invasive to the most. When he wrote the list, he was down to the last step before surgery.

- Try shoes with a roomy toe box in both height and width, and make sure your socks aren't too tight.

- Try off-the-shelf orthotics.

- Try a metatarsal pad.

- Try deep-tissue massage.

- Try a cortisone injection.

- Try custom orthotics.

- Surgery is the last resort.

TIP: Strengthening Exercises
_____

Toe exercises help to strengthen and tighten the metatarsal arch and stretch the tendons on top of the toes. Practice picking up marbles off a carpeted floor with your toes. Or put a towel on the floor and use your toes to scrunch up the towel and pick it up.

Your podiatrist or orthopedist can help identify the cause of the pain and make recommendations on how to treat the problems. A course of oral anti-inflammatory medication may be suggested. Cortisone injections are sometimes used to control the pain. Serious neuromas may require surgery to release or remove the affected nerve. Try to find a surgeon who goes in from the top of the foot to lessen recovery time and allow you to be more active during recovery.

To relieve pressure on the metatarsal heads and forefoot, try different lacing techniques (see the methods described in the "Bunions" section on page 315). With these methods the metatarsal heads are not squeezed by the pressure of normal lacing. The "Lacing Options" chapter describes other lacing techniques.

MORTON'S NEUROMA PRODUCTS

FOOTSMART offers a Silicone Forefoot Insole, a Forefoot Pad with Metatarsal Dome, and a Plantar Cushion. **www.footsmart.com**

HAPAD makes several pads for neuromas. _See "Metatarsalgia Products," page 318._

SPENCO'S METATARSAL ARCH CUSHION is made for the ball of the foot. **www. spenco.com**

VISCOPED INSOLES may prove helpful. _See "Metatarsalgia Products," page 318._

Sesamoiditis

Sesamoiditis is an inflammation of the two little bones beneath the ball of the foot under the joint that moves the big toe. These two sesamoid bones can become bruised and inflamed, resulting in either sharp, constant pain or pain that occurs with movement of the big toe. The bones can also fracture, resulting in sudden, intense pain and the inability to bear weight on the foot.

Athletes involved in sports that place repetitive and excessive pressure on the forefoot area can experience sesamoid pain. The increasing emphasis on minimalist-style footwear and landing on the ball of the foot might lead to sesamoiditis. Shoes with poor cushioning that offer inadequate protection against rocks can cause trauma to the sesamoid bones.

Rich Schick, a physician's assistant, points out that the sesamoid under the first metatarsal is often composed of several small bones:

If the bones on an X-ray were smooth appearing with no rough or jagged edges, this is likely the situation. Even if it is a fracture, these bones only act as shock absorbers in the first place. One can continue to run with nothing to fear but pain. I high-centered on a sharp rock some years back and fractured mine. On X-ray there were two pieces like half moons with the round side smooth and the straight sides jagged as one would expect if you broke a round object in half. The literature said that these fractures could lead to chronic pain and the fragments could need to be surgically removed. As this worst case didn't seem all that frightening, I opted to train and race as normal. The thing bothered me for about a year, but for the last several years has given me no pain at all.

These two little bones can became a major problem. The ball of Lyal Holmberg's left foot became painful during a short 5-mile run. An X-ray showed the sesamoid bone was broken into three pieces. Lyal reports, "As I continued running, the foot was killing me and caused a tilt toward the right, putting a strain on my left hip." A walking-type boot and an anti-inflammatory was prescribed for two weeks, followed by the use of a small dancer's pad behind the ball of his foot. Lyal says, "If I can walk and run without pain, then the problem is solved. If not, I may need surgery to correct the problem."

Treating Sesamoiditis

The use of soft pads or insoles can help. You can also cut a small hole in your insole under the sesamoid bones. Loosely lacing the forefoot of your shoes, as described in the "Bunions" section on page 315, can help relieve pressure on the sesamoid area. Using icing techniques from the "Cold & Heat Therapy" chapter can help reduce pain and inflammation.

Buddy taping the big toe to the second toe or toes next to it for stabilization will limit movement of the toe. A small piece of gauze, cotton, or tissue between the taped toes will prevent skin breakdown if the tape is on for any great length of time. A firm-soled shoe will help keep the toe in line and the foot-toe joint stable. Nonimpact activities are recommended until the injury has healed.

SESAMOIDITIS PRODUCTS

HAPAD DANCER PADS fit under the ball of the foot with a cutout encompassing the big toe joint to relieve calluses and the painful irritations of sesamoiditis. The coiled, springlike wool fibers provide firm and resilient support as they mold and shape to the foot. **www.hapad.com**

VISCOPED INSOLES may provide relief. See *"Metatarsalgia Products,"* page 318.

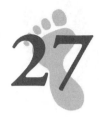

Numb Toes & Feet

Numb feet are usually caused by either transient paresthesia or peripheral neuropathy. Though both are bothersome, the first is usually temporary while the second can be very debilitating. Another form of numbness that is fairly common is Raynaud's syndrome.

If you are diabetic or even prediabetic, pay close attention to any changes in your feet. Neuropathy is a common diabetic foot problem. Likewise, cuts, sores, bruises, and toenail issues can lead to medical problems.

Transient Paresthesia

Transient paresthesia is a temporary nerve compression that can be caused by a gradual buildup of fluids in your feet during extended on-your-feet activity. As the feet swell and blood flow decreases, nerves become compressed. During the compression, the nerves do not receive the oxygen-rich blood they need, resulting in numbness and/or tingling. Tight shoes and/or tightly laced shoes contribute to the problem. Shoes with poor cushioning, coupled with a heavy, pounding gait, can also be a factor.

Numb toes can also be caused by chronic repetitive motions and stresses leading to interdigital neuritis, commonly called Morton's neuroma. Inflammation of the nerves between the metatarsal bones can radiate into the toes.

Ultrarunner and adventure racer Ginny La Forma has battled this numbness in her toes on many occasions. After the Hardrock 100-Mile Run, it lasted a few weeks, but after the Eco Challenge, it lasted over a year. She also suffers from Morton's neuromas.

If the problem continues after your activity has stopped, consider changing to more cushioned shoes and/or wider shoes, and changing insoles and arch supports. There may be some lymph system breakdown in the foot caused by microtrauma. If the problem persists, consult a sports specialist.

Information Resources for Transient Paresthesia and Peripheral Neuropathy

THE FOOT PAIN CENTER, www.footpaincenter.com

THE NEUROPATHY ASSOCIATION, www.neuropathy.org

THE NEUROPATHY TRUST, www.neurocentre.com

NUMB TOES AND ACHING SOLES is a must-read for anyone experiencing peripheral neuropathy. Written by John A. Senneff, who suffers from peripheral neuropathy, the book deals with this disorder from the patient's perspective. Published in 1999 by MedPress.

PERIPHERAL NEUROPATHY: When the Numbness, Weakness, and Pain won't stop, by Norman Latov, published by American Academy of Neurology and Demos Medical Publishing in 2007.

THE NUMB FOOT BOOK, by Drs. Marc Spitz and Alexander McLellan, offered at **www.footpaincenter.com.** Published in 2008 by MedPress.

THE OFFICIAL PATIENT'S SOURCEBOOK ON PERIPHERAL NEUROPATHY, edited by James N. Parker, MD, and Philip M. Parker PhD; published by Icon Health Publications in 2002.

Peripheral Neuropathy

Peripheral neuropathy is a painful nerve condition that can manifest itself as a burning sensation in the feet but that sometimes will appear as a cold sensation. It may start as a mild tingling in the toes and progress to searing pain. It can spread upward in the body, even to the thighs. Other symptoms might include tingling, prickling, or numbness; the sensation of having invisible socks on your feet; a sharp jabbing or electric-type pain; extreme sensitivity to touch; muscle weakness; and a loss of balance or coordination.

The pain results from damage to peripheral nerves that can come from a myriad of causes. A partial list of causes includes poor blood flow to the feet caused by diabetes, kidney, or liver disease; an underactive thyroid; viral and bacterial infections; vitamin deficiencies; and pressure on a single nerve, although often, no cause is identified. It is called neuropathic pain because it occurs in the absence of dangerous stimuli, does not prompt protective reflexes, and does not subside when the danger has passed or the injury healed.

Ken Reed, an ultrarunner who discovered that he had peripheral neuropathy, shares this story. His condition started with a tingling in three of his left foot toes in the summer of 1998 that later turned to numbness. That fall, when the numbness progressed to shooting pains and aches, he sought medical advice. By the spring of 1999 it had progressed to pains in his lower legs, with the numbness also moving upward. Ken reports that when his feet are cold, they constantly ache, buzz, and feel numb. He has resolved to manage the pain and discomfort and hope for a miracle cure.

Treating Peripheral Neuropathy

Treatment often depends on the cause and symptoms of the neuropathy. It can be frustrating to treat, particularly if no reversible cause is identified. Typical treatments include over-the-counter or prescribed pain relievers for mild symptoms, tricyclic antidepressants for burning pain, antiseizure medications for jabbing pain, or other drugs. There is no one mediation or therapy that can reverse the nerve damage.

Self-care treatments include proper care of your feet with loose socks and padded shoes, a semicircular hoop in bed to keep the cover off your feet, cold water soaks and skin moisturizers, massage to improve circulation and stimulate nerves, staying active, and reducing stress levels.

Ask your physician whether Neuragen PN and Neuragen Gel could help your symptoms. These homeopathic topical medications work directly at the site of nerve pain and are available without a prescription. More information can be found at **www.neuragen.com**. Your physician may know of additional medications to try.

Neuro-Reflex Therapy, Bentley Method (NRT) provides a holistic, natural treatment for pain relief and increased circulation for suffers of peripheral neuropathy. Do an online search for Neuro-Reflex Therapy to find a practitioner near you.

Low-level laser treatments (LLLT) are used to treat peripheral neuropathy conditions. Low-intensity light beams penetrate the skin surface and stimulate the damaged cells and tissues, triggering them to function properly and regenerate new, healthy cells. The immune system is stimulated to promote rapid wound healing, reduce the formation of scar tissue, and relieve acute and chronic pain. Studies by the Foot Pain Center (**www.footpaincenter.com**) and **www.chiroweb.com** report significant pain relief from symptoms of chronic neuropathies.

Raynaud's Syndrome

Raynaud's syndrome affects 5–10% of the population. The discomfort is caused by a decreased blood supply to the fingers and toes. Attacks are precipitated by exposure to cold and stress.

Although the severity, duration, and frequency of attacks vary both between individuals and over time, the primary symptoms of Raynaud's syndrome are changes in skin color. The affected areas turn white from the lack of circulation, then blue and cold, and finally numb. When the attack subsides, the affected parts may turn red and may throb, tingle, or swell.

Those affected by Raynaud's Syndrome are more susceptible to cold and wet conditions, which can lead to trench foot. Severe itching and burning—more than normal or that doesn't go away—needs to be checked by your doctor.

Treating Raynaud's Syndrome

Keeping your whole body warm is a good prevention strategy. Wear wind- and water-resistant gloves and socks. Wool or wool-blend socks that retain warmth are good, as arc SealSkinz socks to block moisture. Shoes that block wind and moisture are also recommended. Be sure to allow space in your footwear for thicker socks. Constriction caused by tight socks and footwear can be harmful. Keep fingers and toes dry with talcum powder. If you feel an attack coming on, get inside and warm your hands and feet.

Be careful not to injure the skin in affected areas, and treat injuries without delay. Even minor cuts and scrapes take longer to heal and may be more susceptible to infection when circulation is impaired.

If you suspect you have Raynaud's syndrome, see your physician. Doctors sometimes recommend medications to help combat this condition. The Raynaud's Association (**www.raynauds.org**) can offer help and support for this painful and frustrating condition.

28

Skin Disorders

Five skin disorders commonly affect the feet: athlete's foot, calluses, corns, fissures, and plantar warts. Dealing with these conditions when they first develop will help prevent more serious problems later.

Athlete's Foot

The facts are startling: 70% of people will be affected by athlete's foot in their lifetime, 45% of people with athlete's foot will suffer from it in episodes for more than ten years, and seven out of ten people with athlete's foot are male.

Athlete's foot, technically called tinea pedis, is a skin disease caused by a fungus. The hot weather and foot perspiration that athletes typically encounter can make athlete's foot a common problem. The combination of a warm and humid environment in the shoes or boots, excessive foot perspiration, and changes in the condition of the skin combine to create a setting for the fungi of athlete's foot to begin growing. Athlete's foot usually occurs between the toes or under the arch of the foot. Typical signs and symptoms of athlete's foot include itching, dry and cracking skin, inflammation with a burning sensation, and pain. Blisters and swelling may develop if left untreated. When these blisters break, small, red areas of raw tissue are exposed. As the infection spreads, the burning and itching will increase.

Another type of tinea infection is often called moccasin foot. In this type, a red rash spreads across the lower portion of the foot in the pattern of a moccasin. The skin in this region gradually becomes dense, white, and scaly. The use of a prescription-strength antifungal cream may be required to treat this infection.

Fungus under and around the nails should be treated promptly with antifungal medications. See the "Toenail Fungus" section (page 310) for information on treating fungal infections.

Preventive measures include washing your feet daily with soap and water; drying them thoroughly, especially between the toes; wearing moisture-wicking socks; regularly changing your shoes and socks to control moisture; and using a good, moisture-absorbing foot powder. Because athlete's foot is contagious, if you use a communal shower or bathroom after an event, or use a gym to train, avoid walking barefoot in these areas. Use thongs, shower booties, or even your shoes or boots.

Treating Athlete's Foot

Treatment includes keeping the feet clean and dry, frequent socks changes, anti-fungal medications, and foot powders (see the "Powders" section, page 117, for more information on choosing a foot powder). An antiperspirant may also help those with excessive foot moisture (see the "Antiperspirants for the Feet" section, page 124, for more information about these products). Because wet socks can create an ideal environment for fungal growth, the use of high-quality socks is essential. Moisture-wicking socks can still leave the feet damp. Drymax socks, with their inner fibers that repel moisture, are even better.

Check your local drugstore or pharmacy for a complete line of athlete's foot antifungal ointments, creams, liquids, powders, and sprays. See your doctor if your feet do not respond to treatment with over-the-counter medications. If the fungus returns, alternate medications because the fungus can sometimes build up a resistance to a particular fungicide.

To treat athlete's foot or a case of foot fungi, give tea tree oil, manuka oil, or eucalyptus oil a try. For best results, apply a few drops to the affected areas two to three times daily. Dab it on with a cotton swab or cotton ball. Hold it in place with a bandage or tape. As well as killing the fungi, it helps relieve the associated itching. Test a drop or two on your skin to be sure you are not allergic to the oil. The oils can be found in your local drugstore or pharmacy.

Plain rubbing alcohol works for some people. After showering, rub your toe-nails with an alcohol-soaked cotton ball.

Swabplus's liquid-filled cotton swabs offer an easy way to carry athlete's foot medications. They offer two packs, one with Clotrimazole for athlete's foot and another with Tolnaftate for fungus relief. Bending one end of the swab releases the liquid medication (**www.swabplus.com**).

Other over-the-counter antifungal creams or solutions commonly available in your local drugstore and pharmacy include Dr. Scholl's Fungal Nail Revitalizer and Fungi Solution, Clotrimazole, and Lamisil. Lotrimin, Micatin, Swabplus, Tinactin, and Tolnaftate are all common. Zeasorb-AF is available as a powder and a lotion/powder combination.

If using alcohol or one of the oils, make sure to continue twice a day. Maintain this regimen for at least 90 days. Whether using an over-the-counter or a prescription medication, use according to the directions.

Calluses

Calluses are one of the most controversial foot care subjects. For every athlete who bemoans their calluses, there are two or three others who love them. I have become passionate in telling athletes about the problems that calluses cause when blisters form underneath the hardened skin.

A callus is an abnormal amount of dead, thickened skin caused by recurring pressure and friction, called hyperkeratosis, and is usually on the sole of the foot, most often on the heels, the balls of the feet, or the bottom of the toes. They may be yellowish in color, layered, or even scaly due to excessive dryness. Calluses can form over any bony prominence. Calluses are never normal—they are signs of poor biomechanics or ill-fitting footgear. If it is a footgear problem, this needs to be identified and remedied. Unfortunately most biomechanical problems are things which we need to learn to live with. In many cases, there is nothing wrong or bad about calluses. They can protect against friction and act as a cushioning pad. Calluses become a problem when they become thick enough to interfere with the normal elasticity of the skin or to act like a foreign body on the foot.

A common callus is called intractable plantar keratosis (IPK); this is a localized callus buildup at or near the metatarsal heads on the ball of the foot. An IPK often has a hard central core, which can cause pain when it is in a pressure area. Calluses are caused by a number of factors: poorly aligned metatarsal bones in the forefoot, an abnormal gait, flat or high-arched feet, excessively long metatarsal bones, and a loss of the fat pads on the underside of the foot. Individuals with flat feet are more prone to calluses, bunions, and hammertoes.

Unless the calluses are troublesome, most people tend to forget about them. Your body has made the callus as protection from pressure at those points with little natural fat or padding. To keep painful calluses from returning, you must correct the biomechanical problem that prompted their growth in the first place. Some calluses may have a deep-seated core, called nucleation, which can be painful to pressure. These are often known as corn kernels.

Calluses will continue to grow as they toughen. This can interfere with the fit of your shoes—which in turn can cause a blister—one way or another. Some degree of toughened skin is fine, but be careful of too-callused skin. The time to treat calluses is before an event. Should you develop blisters underneath the tough, hardened surface of a callus, it will usually form deep in the foot, which makes it hard to treat. Once you have experienced a deep blister, you are likely to work hard to rid your feet of their thick calluses. It is hard to drain these blisters. There is fluid underneath the callus, but finding the right depth and location is almost impossible. The section "Deep Blisters" (see page 253) discusses treating these problem blisters.

Am I a stickler about calluses? You bet. I've seen the grimaces on the faces of athletes who have deep blisters that cannot be repaired without a lot of pain. I've seen them hobble off, knowing it won't get any better. When I work at an event patching feet, I encourage athletes to rid their feet of calluses or at least reduce the size and thickness of their calluses. This will leave a smaller and thinner layer of callus, which will still protect the skin but may not cause as many problems if blisters form underneath.

Treating Calluses

Gently grasp some normal skin on your foot and roll it between your thumb and forefinger. Notice how supple it is. Now attempt to roll the callused area in the same manner. If it is too stiff or causes discomfort, the callus is too thick and is likely to cause pain or blisters. You need to thin it down.

Soak your feet weekly in warm water with a bag of tissue-softening chamomile tea to help soften calluses. After soaking, buff with a pumice stone or callus file to remove any dead skin. After the callused skin is dry, apply your choice of cream, lotion, medication, or pads. If your skin is particularly callused, at night after applying the cream, wrap your feet with plastic wrap to hold in the moisturizer. Socks can be worn to bed instead, but they absorb some of the moisturizer off the skin. Over several weeks, simply keep working at it until all areas are as supple as normal skin.

For many athletes, calluses become rough with edges of skin poking up. These edges can catch on socks and lead to the start of a blister. They can also open up into a fissure, a crack in the skin.

The Heel Smoother Pro is the perfect tool for reducing calluses. This two-speed battery-operated pedicure appliance smooths calluses and removes dry skin on heels, toes, or anywhere on your feet. It stops when too much pressure is placed on the skin, preventing overexfoliating, which can damage the skin. The DuraCrystal Power Tips are made with the same crystals used in professional microdermabrasion treatments. This leaves the skin very smooth. It is the only pedicure appliance to receive the American Podiatric Medical Association Seal of Acceptance.

Check your local drugstore for a callus file. These are usually 8–9 inches in length with a rounded, cupped shape to effectively file rounded parts of your feet. Some have a fine file texture on one side and a coarser texture on the other side. If you can't find them locally, check out **www.footsmart.com.** The as-seen-on-TV PedEgg is an inexpensive alternative to files and can be easily found on many websites. The problem with these tools is that the skin is left with a roughened surface.

Ultrarunner Geraldine Wales has a tendency to get tough calluses on her feet that turn into hot spots and eventually blisters. In the evening she uses a file on the calluses and then applies moisturizing cream to keep her feet soft. Never file too deeply into a corn or callus and do not cut into them with sharp objects. A pumice stone will work as well as a file.

A cushioned insole with a good arch support can help equalize the weight load of the foot, while pads around or near the callus can relieve pressure. To relieve heel discomfort from calluses, try a heel cup or heel pad that will distribute body weight evenly across the heel. Orthotics can help relieve pressure in the callused areas of your feet. While there are a variety of callus pads sold, these are only temporary fixes. The regular use of skin moisturizers will help keep the skin soft and eliminate the thick calluses. To relieve pressure on the painful area, try different lacing techniques (see the lacing discussion in the "Bunions" section, page 315). While there are over-the-counter plantar wart removal compounds available that can also be used on corns and calluses, care must be taken in their use. These products contain salicylic acid. Follow the product's directions to avoid damaging good tissue. Do not use these products if you are a diabetic.

Neil Olsen, an MD from Oregon, wrote that he tried Lac-Hydrin: "I've had several cases of really nasty, hyperkeratotic, fissured feet soften up and smooth out with this." Other products are available at your local drugstore and pharmacy.

CALLUS PRODUCTS

The important tip to remember is to use the lotions below daily or according to the package's directions. Using these lotions once or twice a week will not allow them to work their healing magic on your skin.

ANGELFEET PEDICURE FILES are made from surgical stainless steel with a revolutionary smoothing surface that will never wear out. Available in fine, medium, and coarse styles. **www.angelfeetfile.com**

ENGO PATCHES are low-friction patches uniquely applied to footwear, insoles, socks, and athletic equipment—not skin—for easier, longer-lasting protection from calluses. Ultrathin patches leave footwear volume virtually unaltered. Strong, latex-free adhesive prevents migration and movement, even through moisture and sweat. Scientific and field tests show ENGO's slippery blue surface significantly reduces rubbing, providing immediate relief. Several sizes are available: small ovals for toes; large ovals for the ball of foot, arch, and heel areas; rectangles for custom trimming. **www.goengo.com**

FOOTSMART carries a complete line of skin care products made for calluses. These products will help your feet feel softer and smoother while eliminating calluses. Total Foot Recovery Cream comes in three formulas: Original, Tea Tree Oil, and Shea Butter Formula. Callus Treatment Cream with Urethin breaks down painful, hardened skin. The Credo Callus Rasp reduces thick calluses. Callex Callus Ointment and polymer cushions and pads may also prove helpful. **www.footsmart.com**

HAPAD offers several options for callus control. Metatarsal pads and metatarsal bars, Metatarsal Cookies, Dancer Pads with a cutout encompassing the big toe joint, and Horseshoe Heel Cushions all reduce pressure on areas of calluses. The IPK Pad is made for intractable plantar keratosis. The coiled, springlike wool fibers provide firm and resilient support as they mold and shape to the foot. **www.hapad.com**

The **HEEL SMOOTHER PRO BY ARTEMIS WOMAN** is the best tool made for callus control. With two speeds, it stops when too much pressure is put on the skin. The DuraCrystal Power Tips do quick work on heel, toe, and other calluses. Comes with two tips for all shaped areas of the foot. Choose between a battery-operated and rechargeable model.

KATHY'S FAMILY FOOT BALM, FOOT SCRUB, and FOOT BATH are made with 100% natural and organic ingredients. **www.kathys-family.com**

SKINMD NATURAL is a shielding lotion that enhances the skin's own natural protective factor by hydrating the skin. It also forms an invisible, protective barrier that helps prevent blistering and irritation, while keeping natural moisture in. **www.skinmdnatural.com**

ZIM'S CRACK CREAM helps to moisturize, soothe, and soften dry, cracked, painful skin. You can choose between two formulas: a nighttime liquid or daytime cream. The creams are formulated with their unique herbal base of arnica and myrcia oil. Look for Zim's in your drugstore or pharmacy. **www.crackcream.com**

Corns

A corn is a hard, thickened area of skin, generally on the top of, the tip of, or between the toes, usually caused by friction and pressure. A corn is usually like a kernel of corn, round and yellowish in color. Corns on the outer surface of the toes are usually hard, while those between the toes are usually soft. The larger the corn and the more it rubs against your shoe, the more painful it becomes. Typically the corn is an inverted cone shape with a point that can press on a nerve below, causing pain.

Corns can be caused by tight-fitting socks and footwear, deformed toes, or the foot sliding around the shoe. Soft corns, caused by prominent, irregularly shaped bones and bumps, occur between the toes—soft from the perspiration in the forefoot area.

Treating Corns

Weekly warm water and Epsom salt soaks will help soften corns. Following the soak, apply a moisturizing cream and cover them with plastic wrap for 15 minutes. After removing the wrap, gently buff off any dead tissue with a pumice stone.

To relieve the discomfort of corns, start with properly fitting shoes with extra room in the toe box. You can also pad around the corn with corn pads, small pieces of one of the tapes previously mentioned, or Spenco 2nd Skin. There are many types of corn pads and toe sleeves. Lamb's wool can be wrapped around the toe for cushioning.

Check the foot care section of your local drugstore for a current selection of corn relief products. These may include pads and creams to remove the corns. If your corns persist, consult your podiatrist.

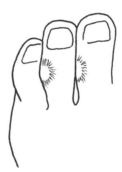

Corns

To control corns, the pressure and friction must be eliminated, usually from improperly fitting shoes. To relieve pressure on the painful area, try the lacing techniques described in the "Bunions" section (page 315). Both methods allow a looser fit in the forefoot.

PRODUCTS FOR CORNS

Assorted corn relief products can be found at your local drugstore and pharmacy. These include Band-Aid Corn Remover, and Dr. Scholl's Corn Cushions, Moisturizing and Corn Remover Kit, and One-Step Corn Remover Pads.

BUNGA OVAL PADS and GEL PADS are made from a medical-grade polymer material. **www.bungapads.com**

HAPAD has Metatarsal Cookies and Pedifix Visco-Gel Corn protectors that provide simple metatarsal arch cushioning. These can relieve the pressure that causes corns and calluses. **www.hapad.com**

Fissures

Fissures often develop in the thickened callused skin on our heels, but they also occur on callused skin on the balls of the feet. These fissures can become infected, may bleed, and can split open into the deeper underlying tissues. Like many foot conditions, fissures can lead to infection if left untreated.

Wearing sandals and going barefoot can contribute to fissures. On vacation one summer, I wore Tevas everyday. My feet were in and out of water all day. After several days of being in the hot, drying sun, I had several deep fissures on one heel. I discovered how painful these cracks can become.

Treating Fissures

Using a moisturizing cream and reducing calluses on your feet will help prevent fissures. If wearing sandals or going barefoot, use the cream morning and evening. The preceding "Calluses" section has information and products that will help in the elimination of fissures. The "Skin Care" section (see page 162) also has a list of products that keep your skin soft and callus free—thus preventing fissures.

Monty Tam, a thru-hiker, has a remedy for deep, dry, cracked heels. At night, rub on lots of petroleum jelly, slip a plastic produce bag over it, slip a sock over the bag, and then elevate your feet and sleep. In the morning your heels will be moist and flexible and won't feel as if you are walking on razor blades.

Rod Dalitz offers a tip on heel cracks or fissures: "Last year I suffered from heel cracks due to wearing sandals in New Zealand in November and December. I fixed them by sanding with some coarse waterproof emery paper glued to a board—more rugged and coarse than what you buy from your local store—and Neutrogena Formula Unscented Hand Cream, which seems a lot more durable than most creams. You don't need much. The sandpaper is so much quicker and more effective than pumice or flimsy commercial boards."

Gail shares how she managed fissures: "The most effective way my husband and I have dealt with these when they occur is by supergluing them together. They heal quickly and the pain is gone immediately. The hardest thing is reaching back to glue them (it's easier to have someone else do it for you). And of course you have to be careful not to glue your fingers to the feet and to let the glue dry completely before stepping down or putting socks on." So if you are bothered by these cracks in the skin, make a note to buy a tube of Gorilla Super Glue, Instant Krazy Glue, or superglue.

Plantar Warts

Plantar warts occasionally rear their ugly heads on the sole of the foot (the *plantar* surface) and cause foot pain. They can appear and then disappear suddenly, without any effort on your part, and may not recur for years. Usually painful from the pressure of standing and walking, plantar warts can become more painful due to sports activities. These warts are typically small, hard, granulated lumps on the skin that can be flesh-colored, white, pink, brown, or gray. They can also feel spongy, thick, and scaly. You may feel as though you have a small stone in your shoe when a wart appears.

Plantar warts are benign tumors caused by common viral infections, usually the human papillomavirus. They generally enter the sole of the foot through cuts and breaks in the skin. The period of time between contact and the wart making its presence known may be several months. There are three types of plantar warts. The first is a single, isolated wart. The second is one wart, often called the mother, surrounded by any number of smaller daughter warts. The third type is a cluster of many warts grouped together, usually on the heels or the balls of the feet. Plantar warts are irregular in shape. While usually small on the skin's surface, they penetrate deep into the foot, where they can cause deep pain.

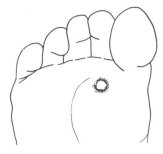

Plantar wart

Moist, cracked skin and open or healing blisters leave one susceptible to the virus. To avoid getting a virus, do not walk barefoot in communal showers or bathrooms. Use flip-flops, shower booties, or even your shoes or boots. Plantar warts thrive in the warm, moist environment found in sports shoes, so be sure to air your feet when able and change into fresh shoes and socks after participating in sports.

Treating Plantar Warts

Most warts disappear without treatment in four to five months. Sometimes, though, when the wart is bothersome or has not gone away on its own, treatment is necessary. While over-the-counter plantar wart removal compounds are available, care must be taken in their use. Many products contain salicylic acid. Follow the product's directions to avoid damaging good tissue. Usually the treatment consists of applying the medication and covering the area with a bandage—repeating daily until the problem is resolved. Check your local drugstore or pharmacy for a complete line of products. These include Compound W Wart Remover Gel, Liquid and Freeze Off, Dr. Scholl's Clear Away Plantar Salicylic Acid Wart Remover System for Feet, DuoFilm Wart Remover, and Wartner Wart Removal System. Do not use these products if you are a diabetic. Some individuals report success simply covering the wart with a piece of duct tape until the wart falls off. You can use moleskin with a hole cut out to relieve painful pressure on the wart. Most drugstores or pharmacies have a selection of pads with cutouts for this purpose.

Kevin Corcoran suffered from plantar warts and used these patches. Each day when he removed the patch, he'd carefully remove the affected layer of skin with a handled razor knife, so that the next patch could further penetrate the skin. He attributes this to greatly reducing the time for the wart to disappear.

Occasionally, it is not a plantar wart but something else. It could be a plugged sweat gland (porokeratotic cyst) or a deep callus with a central core. Check with your doctor if your treatments don't work.

The treatments may put sports activities on hold until after the spot heals, generally in about a week. The common medical treatment by podiatrists for plantar warts involves the use of liquid nitrogen to freeze off the wart. Other treatment options include electrical burning, minor surgery, or laser surgery. Bill Johncock, DPM, recommends trying the simple remedies first, and if those don't work, see a professional. Check with your podiatrist to determine your treatment options.

Duct Tape for Wart Removal?

A study reported in the Archives of Pediatrics & Adolescent Medicine[38] identified duct tape, the all-purpose household fix with hundreds of uses, as an effective wart remover. Researchers say over-the-hardware-counter duct tape is a more effective, less painful alternative to liquid nitrogen, which is used to freeze warts. In the study, patients wore duct tape over their warts for six days. Then they removed the tape, soaked the area in water, and used an emery board or pumice stone to scrape the spot. The tape was reapplied the next morning. The treatment continued for a maximum of two months or until the wart went away. If you have stubborn warts, this duct tape treatment may be worth a try.

The duct tape irritated the warts, and that apparently caused an immune system reaction that attacked the growths, said researcher Dean Richard Focht III, MD, of Cincinnati Children's Hospital Medical Center. He said that researchers did not test other kinds of tape, and so they cannot say whether there is anything special about the gray, heavy-duty, fabric-backed tape.

The study was conducted at the Madigan Army Medical Center near Tacoma, Washington. It began with 61 patients between the ages of 3 and 22, but only 51 patients completed the study. Of the 26 patients treated with duct tape, 85% got rid of their warts compared with 60% of the 25 patients who received the freezing treatment.

Pediatric dermatologist Anthony J. Mancini, MD, of Children's Memorial Hospital in Chicago said he uses a form of duct tape therapy for warts. He combines duct tape with a topical, over-the-counter wart remover for nightly treatments. "The whole point of this is a nonpainful approach," said Dr. Mancini, who was not involved in the study.

Rashes

Capillaritis is a common rash that affects the legs of athletes. Presenting as a funky rash, it simply seems to come out of nowhere and without any related injury. The rash is a harmless skin condition in which reddish-brown patches are caused by leaky capillaries. As the capillaries become inflamed, tiny red dots appear on the skin. The dots form into a flat red patch, which becomes brown and then slowly starts to fade away. Its cause is often unknown, but it tends to develop after exercise. Many times the rash will appear under the socks and gaiters. The rash may be caused by a reaction to Lycra, a common sock fabric, or other fabrics that irritate your skin. It could also be a heat rash from the combination of trapped sweat and hot temperatures. In extreme cases it will present with fluid-filled blisters. It can reoccur and even persist for years.

Delayed pressure urticaria is a form of swelling or hives, edema, or redness of the skin due to some form of pressure upon the skin. It can occur under the elastic of socks or gaiters and can be caused by tight shoes. The rash and pain can last 3–72 hours. Topical applications of Benadryl ointment might help, but usually a more potent corticosteroid is required.

Prickly heat rash is caused by a blockage of sweat glands in areas of heavy sweating, usually beneath clothing. This rash appears as red, itchy, inflamed bumps.

Other possible rashes include poison oak or poison ivy, or rashes that develop because of sensitivity to soap, lotion, or fabrics. These can be ruled out by a physician if they persist.

Treating Rashes

Capillaritis will disappear on its own over a few weeks. The use of a hydrocortisone 1% cream will help control the rash and any related itching. A dermatologist or general physician can be consulted if it does not go away on its own. One useful product is Hand Sense (**www.handsense.com**), a protective cream that enhances the natural lipid system by penetrating the outer layer of skin and bonding with the skin to create a soft shield that prevents irritation of the sensitive living tissue underneath. It works to reduce the incident of rashes on the feet plus it reduces perspiration.

Maddalena Acconci, better known to adventure racers as MA, has a mix of ingredients that she uses for athletes' rashes. She will often mix a batch based on what she sees on feet and ankles. Her basic concoction is triple antibiotic, hydrocortisone, Bag Balm, and either tea tree oil or manuka oil (studies have shown manuka oil is 20–30 times more active than Australian tea tree oil for gram positive bacteria, and 5–10 times more active for fungi). MA says:

> If [the rash] is really bad, I use 1% hydrocortisone and manuka oil. If it's not so very bad, I use 0.5% hydrocortisone and tea tree oil. Sometimes I find people who react badly to antibiotic creams, so I use Burt's Bees Rescue Ointment, which also works great for a whole plethora of race ailments. I don't know if anything I do is unique. I just do what I think will work. For example, I had a racer develop a very mysterious redness on the soles of his feet. None of us could figure out what it was—just red, nothing else. He really wanted to race but his soles were sensitive. I mixed Benadryl cream with Rescue ointment, rubbed it in, cut a layer of Molefoam to shape, and topped it of with a layer of moleskin. I taped it with Leukotape to hold it together. He wore his slightly larger pair of shoes and a thin double-sock combo. It worked, he raced, and the rash went away.

If you are often affected by rashes, try different socks, apply powder under your socks, or wear a thin sock liner made from silk. Prickly heat rash usually lasts for a few days and then disappears on its own, although it may last longer if hot and humid conditions continue.

29

Cold & Heat Therapy

Injuries can be helped through the use of cold and heat therapy. Each has its place in the rehabilitation phase of an injury, as they help healing by reducing swelling, reducing pain, and promoting circulation. The rule of thumb is to start with cold and switch to heat or a cold/heat combination later.

Do not use cold or heat therapy on an area where the skin is broken. First treat the wound. Individuals with known or suspected circulatory problems or cold hypersensitivity, paralysis, areas of impaired sensation, or rheumatoid conditions should consult a physician before using cold compression therapy.

Cold Therapy

Cold therapy, generally referred to as cryotherapy, is an essential part of rehabilitation after an injury, as well as a preventive measure to avoid problems. Icing is usually done in combination with all the other RICE components: rest, compression, and elevation. Remember that all four are important and should be used together for faster recovery from an injury. Cold therapy is effective for sprains and strains, contusions and bruises, muscle pulls, and post-exercise soreness. Those with Raynaud's syndrome or former frostbite sufferers should not use ice on affected body parts.

Icing progresses through four stages—cold, burning, aching, and finally numbness—usually taking about 20 minutes in all. The numbness stage should be reached in order to receive the full benefits of icing; when the area goes numb, stop applying ice. The duration of icing depends on the type and depth of the injury. Body areas with less fat and tissue should be iced for less time than fatty or dense areas (for example, a bony area less than a hamstring). After an injury, soft-tissue damage can cause uncontrolled swelling. This swelling can increase the damage of the initial injury and increase the healing time. The immediate use of ice will reduce the amount of swelling, tissue damage, blood-clot formation, muscle spasms, inflammation, and pain.

Cold therapy works by decreasing the tissue's temperature and constricting the blood vessels in the injured area. This decreases blood flow, venous/lymphatic drainage, and cell metabolism, reducing the chance of hemorrhage and cell death in an acute injury. Once the fourth stage of icing, numbness, is reached, light range of motion can be started. Avoid strenuous exercise during cold therapy.

Cheap Freeze

Homemade ice packs can be made with three parts water and one part rubbing alcohol. Mix in a freezer-grade zip-top bag, and keep one or two in the freezer. The result is a hard slush. If the mix is too hard, let it melt and add a little more alcohol. If it is too liquid, add a little more water. The right consistency will allow the bag to be formed around your foot, ankle, or other body part. Use a towel between the ice bag and your skin. Care must be taken not to get an ice burn from these packs because the alcohol can make them colder than over-the-counter packs.

Do not place ice directly on the skin unless you are using an ice cup or similar delivery system. For these, slide the ice over the area in a slow but steady motion. Ice until the area becomes numb. Otherwise, always use a thin towel, washcloth, or T-shirt between the ice bag and skin. If you have an Ace wrap on the injured part, apply the ice directly over the wrap. Ice cubes in a plastic bag will work, but crushed ice conforms better to the body. When at home, use a bag of frozen peas or corn, which conforms nicely to the curves of the foot or ankle. Use an Ace wrap or other type compression wrap to hold the ice against the injured area. This type of icing is perfect for deeper tissues.

The most effective way to use ice is to ice for 20 minutes, wait 10 minutes, and then reapply the ice for another 20 minutes. Repeat this up to six to eight times a day for three days after an injury

Can you ice too much? As long as you follow the rules of icing, you can ice as many times as you like and as long as it feels helpful. By allowing the skin to warm before re-icing, you can ice over and over—especially for chronic overuse injuries.

TIP: The Ice Masseur Cometh

Ice massage can be done by freezing water in a paper, foam, or plastic cup. When water has frozen, remove part of the cup and rub the ice around the injured area. Because it cools the area faster than normal icing, limit the massage to six to eight minutes at a time, usually three to four times a day. Ice massage is effective when used with range-of-motion exercises and stretching.

Heat Therapy

Heat therapy is used less often than cold therapy. Heat therapy is recommended only after swelling and inflammation have subsided (usually at 48–72 hours after an injury). If the skin is hot and red, swollen, or sensitive to touch, do not use heat. The heat increases blood flow to the injured area, allowing the blood's nutrients to help in the healing process, aid in the removal of waste products from the injured site, and promote healing. Heat can help reduce muscle spasms and pain. Stiffness decreases as tissue elasticity increases. Heat should not be applied for longer than 15–20 minutes at a time and should not be applied to areas of broken skin.

Combination Cold & Heat Therapy

A combination of cold and heat therapy, often called contrast hydrotherapy, can be used 48–72 hours after an injury. This can be easily accomplished by alternating the use of cold and heat packs, ten minutes at a time. An alternative is a contrast bath. Fill two buckets or basins, one with cold water and some ice and the other with tolerable hot water. Alternate your soaking in each for two minutes. With combination therapy, the cold keeps the swelling down while the heat keeps the blood and its nutrients circulating through the injured area.

Avoid contrasting areas that are injured because the heat may aggravate the inflammation more than the cooling phase can control. The heat cycle should be at least one minute and as long as five minutes. Always finish the session with cold. If possible, increase the heat and cold as you work through the contrast cycles.

Dave Barrows, an experienced marathon runner, developed a serious case of bilateral tendinitis. A sports medicine doctor recommended a regimen of contrast baths. Dave had success by following the recommendation:

> Once or twice per day I followed a routine of soaking 5 minutes at a time for 30 minutes per session, first in an ice bath, then immediately into a 105°F hot bath, and back and forth 5 minutes at a time until I had done 15 minutes in each per session. I used a plastic tub for the cold with 10 pounds of crushed ice and water (anything less melts too much before you get to the end of the session). For the hot I filled the bathtub or if at the gym I used the hot tub, which is kept at 104°F. I bought a thermometer for checking the temperature of the hot bath at home. Also, a stopwatch is important to keep you honest about the time. As you might expect, this contrast bath surges blood in and out of the feet with good results. It's time consuming but well worth it. Twice a day for ten days resulted in remarkable improvement for my very serious case.

There are many cold and heat packs available. The list on the opposite page includes options proven to work well for athletes. Along with cold and heat packs are the many topical creams and gels. Products such as Biofreeze (**www.biofreeze. com**), IcyHot (**www.chattem.com**), and Flex-Power Sports Cream (**www.flex power.com**) can be used for localized muscle pain. Check out your local sports store, drugstore, or pharmacy for more options.

COLD & HEAT PRODUCTS

ACTIVEWRAPS provide heat and cold compression therapy to specific areas of the foot and ankle. It is specifically designed and patented for the unique curvatures of these areas. Each ActiveWrap system includes a comfortable plush medical compression wrap and hot/cold (microwave/freezer safe) packs that can be assembled in any position within the wrap. The pack wraps around the foot and stays soft and flexible when cold so they mold comfortably in place. **www.activewrap.com**

CONTOUR PAK makes Cold & Heat Paks, all-purpose cold and heat therapy wraps that contour to the foot and ankle, as well as other parts of the body. This unique wrap uses a nontoxic gel formulation that stays soft and flexible while cold or hot, retaining its therapeutic temperatures for 30–40 minutes. It has a soft, velvety fabric covering that eliminates the need to use a towel between the pack and the skin, and protects against ice or heat burn. Paks are offered in different sizes with Velcro to hold the wrap snugly in place over the injured body part. **www.icewraps.net**

CRYOCUP is a reusable ice massage tool that you fill with water and freeze. **www.cryocup.com**

CRYO-MAX REUSABLE COLD PACKS contain Cryo-Max fluid-filled modules that remain cold for eight hours. The packs can be found in your local drugstores or pharmacies. **www.modularthermaltech.com**

The **MCDAVID ICE BAG WRAP** provides the ability to use ice and compression simultaneously. The ice bag is enclosed in an adjustable neoprene wrap. **www.mcdavidusa.com**

PRO-TEC ICE-UP PORTABLE ICE MASSAGER is a small go-anywhere ice massage device that remains frozen up to ten hours. **www.injurybegone.com**

THERMACARE AIR-ACTIVATED HEATWRAPS are made of comfortable, wearable cloth-like material that conforms to your body's shape to provide therapeutic heat. Each wrap contains small discs made of natural ingredients that heat up when exposed to air, providing at least eight hours of low-level therapeutic heat on the site of pain. Various sizes are available. Look for these wraps in your drugstore or pharmacy. **www.thermacare.com**

TOREX PREMIUM THERMAL MEDICAL DEVICES makes Torex Flat Style Hot/Cold Packs and the Ankle Cold & Compression wrap, which wraps around the foot or ankle to provide maximum pain and swelling relief deep into joints and tissue. **www.torexhealth.com**

30

Foot Care Kits

There are probably few of us who have run, hiked, fast packed, thru-hiked, or adventure raced who have not needed a foot care kit—at least if the outing was for a day or longer. Limping home or back to camp with a blister on your heel that will bother you for days does not make you smarter. The only way to look smarter is to plan for the next time with a foot care kit.

Consider making three types of foot care kits. The first is a basic self-care kit for keeping your feet healthy at home. The second is to carry with you in the field or wherever your sport takes you. The third is an event kit for long-distance or multiday activities. Each is equally important.

The website **www.backpackinglight.com** asked me whether I could put together a 2-ounce foot care kit. I made a small kit that weighed 1.5 ounces and fit in a small plastic bag. It contained a few Spenco Sport Blister Pads, alcohol wipes, compound tincture of benzoin swabs, a pin, a strip of adhesive felt, several feet of tape around a straw, and a small tube of lubricant. Nothing more. Not enough for an expedition-length adventure race but enough for about a week of general use.

You can easily carry a few things just in case you need them. The space and weight is minimal. It could make the difference between being able to continue on foot the next day if you are by yourself. If you are with friends, it could make the difference between holding up the group or continuing on.

Even a minimalist could benefit from carrying a blister patch, an alcohol wipe, a foot of tape, and a pin. A

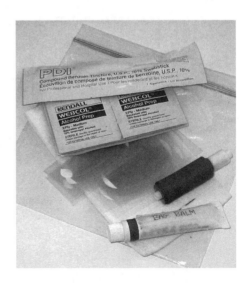

A 2-ounce foot care kit

small 2-by-3-inch bag could easily carry these four items. Too many fail to plan and leave open the door to pain from the unexpected but waiting-to-pounce blister.

You can make your own blister kit or purchase a general first-aid kit or a blister medical kit. Most general first-aid kits contain items for basic first-aid care and can be used for blister care by adding a few more specific items. The kits mentioned in the product section on page 344 are made specifically for blister care. No matter what each kit contains, you should customize the kit to suit your needs and stock it with sufficient equipment for your outing.

Dave told me, "I have carried a small kit in my pack for years. I have not used it on myself but have patched many a runner or hiker met on the trail. I still carry it for that day I'm in need. It's homemade with moleskin patches, and there is a salve made with one-third Vaseline, one-third diaper rash cream (yes, diaper rash cream to keep the area dry), and one-third witch hazel. I stir it using a Popsicle stick and keep the salve in a little travel plastic jar. And there are individual alcohol patches. It's all real 'high tech' and kept inside a zip-top bag."

Spend a bit of time preparing your feet before your trip, and reduce the chances of needing many of the supplies in a kit. Pre-trip preparation includes three steps: reducing calluses with a callus file or creams, getting the skin on your feet in the best possible condition, and trimming your toenails correctly.

If you make a foot care kit, make sure it is stocked with the right materials and you and/or your crew know what's in it and how to use it. Lisa Bliss, an MD who

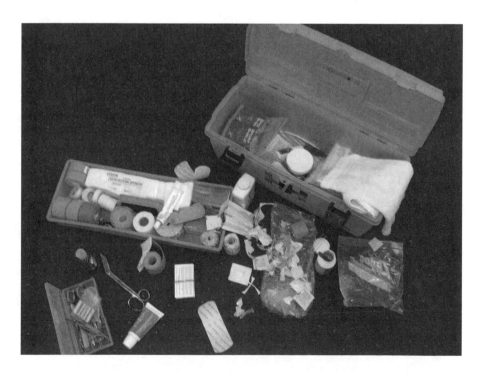

The author's foot care kit for events

helps at Badwater, relates, "Runners have come to the medical HQ with blisters asking for our help in treating them so that they can continue their run. I would ask them what they had in their foot care kit and get blank stares in response: 'Foot care kit?' Then their crews would get a clue and scrounge frantically around through some supplies and pull out—Band-Aids!—even those little circle ones! Just insane!"

Some people have asked about my foot care kit. On the previous page is a picture of the yellow toolbox that carries all my supplies for an event such as Badwater or Western States. I like the removable top tray that holds the stuff I always use. The box is made by Flambeau and is about 20 by 9 by 7.5 inches. It is available through **www.flambeaucases.com** in several sizes. It has a lock tab, which is handy. I have shipped this box to events all over the world. When I do, I wrap the top tray in plastic wrap to hold the contents in place, padding the inside with foot-cleaning cloths.

Basic Self-care Kit for Home Use

A basic self-care kit for good foot treatment does not have to be large. The following items are recommended; add to the kit as necessary for your particular foot conditions.

- Toenail clippers for trimming nails

- File or emery board for smoothing nails after clipping

- Foot powder for absorbing moisture

- Moisturizer cream for softening dry skin, calluses, and corns

- Callus file or pumice stone for removing calluses and dead skin

- Antiseptic ointment for treating cuts and scrapes

Fanny-pack Kit

If you are an athlete who finds yourself continuously bothered by foot problems, or who often covers long distances without crew support, consider making a small foot care kit to carry in a fanny pack. Hikers should carry a kit as part of a larger overall first-aid kit because of their remoteness from assistance. The following items are recommended.

- Compound tincture of benzoin swab sticks or squeeze vials

- Alcohol wipe packets

- A fingernail clipper or pin, and matches for blister puncturing

- Foot powder in a small container

- A small container for your choice of a lubricant

- Your choice of tapes wrapped around a pencil

- A plastic bag with your choice of blister materials and several pieces of toilet paper or tissues

- A small pocketknife with built-in scissors

Depending on your personal needs, you might consider adding a lightweight ankle support; pads for metatarsal, arch, or heel pain; and a heel cup.

Event Kit

If you participate in events in which you or your crew will be providing foot care, a larger kit is necessary. The kit should contain material based on the length and type of event. Do not rely on medical personnel or aid stations to have the materials you need. The following materials form the core of the kit. Add or eliminate materials based on your personal preferences and experience. Look in the tool section of your local hardware stores for a plastic toolbox with trays in which to store the materials.

- Lubricant of choice

- Powder of choice

- Blister patches of choice in various sizes (example: Spenco Sports Blister Pads)

- Spenco 2nd Skin or GlacierGel

- Tapes of choice in a variety of widths

- Compound tincture of benzoin or other tape adherent

- Alcohol pads

- One DuoDerm pad

- Tube of zinc oxide

- 10cc syringe (for zinc oxide)

- 18-gauge needle (for zinc oxide)

- Supply of 25-gauge needles for draining blisters

- Several #11 scalpels for lancing blisters

- Tube of 2% Xylocaine jelly

- Gauze pads (2-by-2-inch and 4-by-4-inch) for draining blisters

- Toenail clippers

- Nail or pedicure file

- Callus file

- Sharp-pointed scissors

- Utility scissors for cutting tape and shoes

- Nail drill

- Tweezers for pulling blister skin to cut a hole in it

- Shoehorn

- Betadine for cleaning dirty wounds/blisters

- Antiseptic ointment

- Extra socks

- Self-adhering wrap

- Ace wrap

- Ankle support

- Pads for metatarsal, arch, or heel pain
- Latex gloves
- Antibacterial hand wipes
- Small basin for soaking feet
- Sponge for cleaning feet
- Hand towel for drying feet
- Plastic bags for garbage

FOOT CARE KIT PRODUCTS

ADVENTURE MEDICAL KITS offers a wide array of kits for any type of activity, any length of event, and any number of people. Their Blister Medic Kit contains adhesive GlacierGel dressings, pre-cut moleskin, alcohol wipes, and antiseptic towelettes. **www.adventuremedicalkits.com**

BRAVE SOLDIER ANTISEPTIC HEALING OINTMENT was made for athletes. Developed by a dermatologist as an effective treatment to keep abrasion wounds moist and protected, Brave Soldier helps heal blisters, road rash, minor cuts, and burns. It's made with tea tree oil as a natural antiseptic, aloe vera gel for its natural healing properties, jojoba oil as a natural moisturizer, vitamin E for rebuilding collagen and skin tissue, shark liver oil for reducing scarring, and comfrey for stimulating skin-cell growth and wound resurfacing. **www.brave soldier.com**

ENGO BLISTER RELIEF KIT contains ENGO Patches, Kinesio Tex tape, benzoin, lancets, folding scissors, instructions, and more in a zippered bag. **www. goengo.com**

SPENCO'S 2ND SKIN BLISTER KIT contains six 2nd Skin 1-inch squares, six sheets of Adhesive Knit, and one sheet of Pressure Pad ovals. The kit comes in a reseal-able pouch. Look for this kit in backpacking or sporting goods stores. **www. spenco.com**

SUPER SALVE is an antioxidant, antibacterial, and antifungal salve that helps soothe and heal dry and cracked skin, abrasions, and skin conditions common to harsh environments. It's made with a combination of herbs, including chaparral leaf, echinacea flower, hops flower, and usnea moss. **www.supersalve.com**

ZOMBIERUNNER offers a Deluxe Foot Kit loaded with blister prevention and patching materials, including folding scissors, tapes, powder, tape adherents, alcohol wipes, 2nd Skin, ENGO Patches, instructions, and more. **www. zombierunner.com**

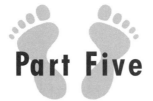

Part Five

Sources & Resources

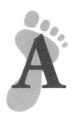

Appendix A:
Product Sources

Rather than use this book as a definitive source for products, use it as a guide to the wide variety of foot care products available. New products are always being developed. Remember, too, that your local stores are an excellent source for what is current in the foot care marketplace.

When products are mentioned in the text, the company name and website (if available) are provided. Generally, your first source for most of these products should be your local stores. Ask at your sporting goods store, running store, backpacking or camping store, pharmacy or drugstore, medical supply store, or orthopedic supply store for the products mentioned. While they may not stock all the products, they may be willing to place a special order. Please be aware that not all companies listed in this book sell retail and therefore their products may have to be ordered through a retailer or medical professional. Please respect their sales policies.

The following companies are sources of many of the products listed in this book:

ZOMBIERUNNER (**www.zombierunner.com/fixingyourfeet**) is a U.S. Web-based company run by ultrarunners that provides equipment and supplies for trail runners, ultrarunners, and other outdoor enthusiasts. They stock hard-to-find items such as tapes, tape adherents, blister patches, lubricants, powders, gaiters, electrolyte caps, and so on. They specialize in materials prepackaged in foot care kits.

FOOTSMART (**www.footsmart.com**) carries a wide assortment of products for flat feet, arch problems, plantar fasciitis, Achilles tendinitis, toenails, bunions, hammertoes, corns, calluses, and skin disorders.

MEDCO SPORTS MEDICINE (**www.medco-athletics.com**) has products including tapes; self-adhering wraps; tape adherents and skin toughening agents; various grades of moleskin; lubricants; powders; antifungal sprays and powders; first-aid equipment; alcohol and compound tincture of benzoin prep pads; hot and cold therapy equipment; physical therapy equipment; ankle supports; Achilles tendon and plantar fasciitis straps; insoles and heel cups; most Cramer, Mueller, and Spenco products; and Johnson & Johnson Band-Aid Blister Relief, Corn Relief, and Callus Relief.

Appendix C lists medical specialists and companies that often offer products related to their services and business. Check it out for additional options for many of the foot problems and disorders in this book.

You may find products similar to those mentioned that are only available in your area. Watching other athletes and their foot care habits will often alert you to new products they have found to be useful. Do not hesitate to ask questions when you see new products.

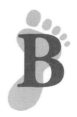

Appendix B:
Shoe & Gear Reviews

The print magazines listed below often offer formal reviews of shoes and foot-related gear and sometimes have additional content on their websites. Check out the magazines and websites to see the extent of their coverage. Many also post their editorial calendars online, allowing you to see which issues cover shoes and boots. The *Fixing Your Feet* blog has reviews and information about new foot care products. You can subscribe at **www.fixingyourfeet.com/blog.**

Backpacker Magazine
www.backpacker.com

Marathon & Beyond Magazine
www.marathonandbeyond.com

Outside Magazine
www.outsidemag.com

Runner's World Magazine
www.runnersworld.com

Running Times Magazine
www.runningtimes.com

Trail Runner Magazine
www.trailrunnermag.com

UltraRunning Magazine
www.ultrarunning.com

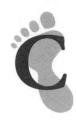

Appendix C:
Medical & Footwear
Specialists

American Academy of Orthopaedic
Surgeons
www.aaos.org

American Academy of Podiatric
Sports Medicine
www.aapsm.org

American Chiropractors Association
www.americhiro.org

American Massage Therapy
Association
www.amtamassage.org

American Orthopaedic Foot and
Ankle Society
www.aofas.org

American Orthotics and Prosthetics
Association
www.aopanet.org

American Physical Therapy Association
www.apta.org

American Podiatric Medical
Association
www.apma.org

International Chiropractic Association
www.chiropractic.org

National Athletic Trainers' Association
www.nata.org

Pedorthic Footwear Association
www.pedorthics.org

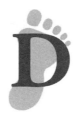

Appendix D:
Feet-related Websites

A free blog about feet, foot-related products, and foot care issues is offered at **www. fixingyourfeet.com.** It also helps athletes learn about new foot care techniques and products between editions of the book.

Websites related to barefoot running and minimalist footwear are listed at the end of the "Barefoot & Minimalist Footwear" chapter.

About Walking
walking.about.com

The Ambulatory Foot Clinic—
Podiatric Pain Management Center
www.footcare4u.com

Dr. Pribut's Running Injuries Page
**www.drpribut.com/sports/sport
frame.html**

Dr. Todd's Relief for the Feet Products
www.drtodds.com

Eneslow Foot Comfort Center
www.eneslow.com

Feet Fixer.com
www.feetfixer.com

Foot and Ankle Link Library
www.footandankle.com/podmed

Footcare Direct—Target In on Your
Foot Care Solutions
www.footcaredirect.com

Foot Express—Footcare Home Health
Products & Treatments
www.footexpress.com

Foot Health Network
www.foot.com

Foot Pain Center
www.footpaincenter.com

Foot Store—Specializing in Foot and
Heel Pain Treatment
www.footstore.com

Foot Web—Footcare Treatment
Information Resource
www.footweb.com

HEALTHYFEETSTORE—
Your online source for footcare
www.healthyfeetstore.com

My Foot Shop—Your Source for
Healthy Feet
www.myfootshop.com

Sports Injury Clinic
www.sportsinjuryclinic.net

Support Your Feet
www.supportyourfeet.com

Notes

1. Roland Mueser, *Long-Distance Hiking: Lessons from the Appalachian Trail* (Camden, ME: Rugged Mountain Press, 1998), 32.

2. J. J. Knapik, K. L. Reynolds, K. L. Duplantis, and B. H. Jones, "Friction Blisters: Pathophysiology, Prevention and Treatment," *Sports Medicine* 20, no. 3 (1995): 140.

3. Karen Berger, *Advanced Backpacking* (New York: W. W. Norton & Company, 1998), 69–70.

4. The usual issues are *Backpacking* (March, the Annual Gear Guide Issue), *Outside* (May Buyer's Guide), *Runner's World* (April and September), *Running Times* (March and September), and *Trail Runner* (spring and fall).

5. J. D. Denton, Dennis Grandy, DPM, and Tom Kennedy, "How to Find the Right Shoe for You," *Running Times* (September 1996): 16; and "How to Find a Shoe That Works," *Running Times* (March 1997): 18.

6. Tom Brunick and Bob Wischnia, "Choosing the Right Shoe" and "Know Your Foot Type," *Runner's World* (April 1997): 52.

7. J. J. Knapik, K. L. Reynolds, K. L. Duplantis, and B. H. Jones, "Friction Blisters: Pathophysiology, Prevention, and Treatment," *Sports Medicine* 20, no. 3 (1995): 142.

8. 12 miles per day times 5,280 feet/mile divided by 2.5 feet/step. For each mile more than 12, add 2,100 steps. For each mile less than 12, subtract 2,100 steps.

9. Ray Jardine, *The Pacific Crest Trail Hiker's Handbook* (LaPine, OR: Adventure Lore Press, 1996), 93.

10. Daniel E. Lieberman, "Biomechanics of Foot Strikes & Applications to Running Barefoot or in Minimal Footwear," **www.barefootrunning.fas.harvard. edu.**

11. William Jungers, "Barefoot Running Strikes Back," *Nature Journal* (January 2010).

12. William A. Rossi, "Why Shoes Make 'Normal Gait' Impossible," *Journal of the American Podiatry Association* (1999).

13. Michael Wharburton, "Barefoot Running," *Sports Science Journal* (Gateway Physiotherapy, Queensland, Australia, 2001).

14. Daniel E. Lieberman, et al, "Foot Strike Patterns and Collision Forces in Habitually Barefoot Versus Shod Runners," *Nature* 463 (January 28, 2010): 531–535.

15. S. D. Perry, A. Radtke, and C. R. Goodwin, "Influence of footwear midsole material hardness on dynamic balance control during unexpected gait termination," *Gait and Posture* 25, no. 1 (January 2007): 94-98.

16. W. Blattler, N. Kreis, B. Lun, J. Winiger, F. Amsler, "Leg Symptoms of Healthy People and Their Treatment with Compression Hosiery," *Phlebology* 23 (2008): 214–221.

17. Tim Noakes, MD, *Lore of Running* (Champaign, IL: Leisure Press, 1991), 460.

18. Robert Boeder, *Beyond the Marathon: The Grand Slam of Trail Ultrarunning* (Vienna, GA: Old Mountain Press, 1996), 22.

19. J. J. Knapik, K. L. Reynolds, K. L. Duplantis, and B. H. Jones, "Friction Blisters: Pathophysiology, Prevention, and Treatment," *Sports Medicine* 20, no. 3 (1995): 139.

20. Andrew Lovy, "New Blister Formula Revealed! Free!" *UltraRunning* (April 1990): 40.

21. Richard Benyo, *The Death Valley 300: Near-Death and Resurrection on the World's Toughest Endurance Course* (Forestville: Specific Publications, 1991), 142.

22. Colin Fletcher, *The Complete Walker III* (New York: Alfred A. Knopf, 1996), 86.

23. Gary Cantrell, "From the South: The Amazing Miracle of Duct Tape," *UltraRunning* (December 1988): 36–37.

24. Donald Baxter, MD; David Porter, MD, PhD; Paul Flahavan, C.Ped; and Charles May, "The Ideal Running Orthosis: A Philosophy of Design," *Biomechanics* (March 1996): 41–44.

25. Tim Noakes, MD, *Lore of Running* (Champaign, IL: Leisure Press, 1991), 459.

26. D. Townes, MD; T. Talbot, MD; I. Wedmore, MD, and R. Billingsly, MD, "Event Medicine: Injury and Illness During an Expedition-Length Adventure Race," *The Journal of Emergency Medicine* 27 (2004): 161-165.

27. J. J. Knapik, K. L. Reynolds, K. L. Duplantis, and B. H. Jones, "Friction Blisters: Pathophysiology, Prevention, and Treatment," *Sports Medicine* 20, no. 3 (1995): 138.

28. Ibid: 140.

29. Ibid: 139.

30. Bryan Bergeron, MD, "A Guide to Blister Management," *The Physician and Sportsmedicine* (February 1995): 40.

31. Ibid: 43.

32. William Trolan, MD, *Blister Fighter Guide* (Seattle: Outdoor Research, 1996).

33. Auleley, Guy-Robert, MD, et al, "Validation of the Ottawa Ankle Rules," *Annals of Emergency Medicine* 32, no. 1 (July 1998): 14–18.

34. "The Conservative Treatment of Plantar Fasciitis: A Prospective Randomized, Multicenter Outcome Study," American Orthopaedic Foot and Ankle Society (October 1996).

35. Robert Nirschl, MD, MS, "Plantar Fasciitis—A New Perspective," *American Medical Joggers Association AMAA Quarterly* (summer 1996).

36. "Heel To Heal: New Stretch Relieves Pain from Plantar Fasciitis Source:" University of Rochester Medical Center (November 13, 2006).

37. Karen Maloney Backstrom, C. Forsyth, B. Walden, Abstract: "Comparison of Two Methods of Stretching the Gastrocnemius and Their Effects on Ankle Range of Motion," University of Colorado Health Services Center (April 1994).

38. Dean R. Focht III, MD; Carole Spicer, RN; and Mary P. Fairchok, MD, "The Efficacy of Duct Tape vs. Cryotherapy in the Treatment of Verruca Vulgaris (the Common Wart)," *Archives of Pediatric & Adolescent Medicine* 156, no. 10 (October 2002).

Glossary

Achilles tendon—the large tendon that runs from the calf to the back of the heel

adventure racing—multisport races over difficult terrain, often done in teams over several days

arch—the curved part of the bottom of the foot

athlete's foot—a fungal infection that causes itchy, red, soggy, flaking, and cracking skin between the toes or fluid-filled bumps on the sides or sole of the foot

biomechanics—the study of the mechanics of a living body, especially of the forces exerted by muscles and gravity on the skeletal structure

blister—a fluid-filled sac between layers of skin that occurs as a result of friction

bone spur—a small, bony growth usually indicating a bone irritation

bruise—an injury in which blood vessels beneath the skin are broken and blood escapes to produce a discolored area

bunion—a bony protrusion at the base of the big toe

bunionette—a bunion on the small toe

bursitis—the formation of an inflamed fluid-filled sac, usually where muscles or tendons glide over bone

calcaneus—the large heel bone

callus—the thickening of skin caused by recurring friction, usually on the sole of the foot, heel, or inner big toe

claw toes—toes that are contracted down at the middle joint but up at the joint at the ball of the foot

contusion—a bruising injury that does not involve a break in the skin

corn—a thickening of the skin, generally on or between the toes, usually caused by friction

dermis—the sensitive connective tissue layer of the skin located below the epidermis, containing nerve endings, sweat and sebaceous glands, and blood and lymph vessels

dislocation—a complete displacement of bone from its normal position at the joint surface

edema—the swelling of body tissues due to excessive fluid

epidermis—the outer, protective, nonvascular layer of the skin covering the dermis

eversion—movement of the foot as it rolls inward at the ankle

fibula—the outer and smaller of the two bones of the lower leg

fissure—crack in the skin, usually found on the toughened, callused skin of the heels

flat foot—a foot that has either a low arch or no arch

forefoot—the ball of the foot and the toes

frostbite—the result of the freezing of skin tissue

Haglund's deformity—a bump in the form of an enlargement of the back of the heel bone (calcaneus) at the area of the insertion of the Achilles tendon

hallux—the great or big toe

hallux valgus—the turning in of the great toe joint that often causes bunions

hammertoes—toes that are contracted at the toe's middle joint, making the toe bend upward at its center and forcing the tip of the toe downward

heel pad—the soft tissue pad on the bottom of the heel

heel-pain syndrome—pain at the heel usually caused by overuse or repetitive stress to the foot's heel

heel spur—a small edge of bone that juts out of the calcaneus

hematoma—a swelling containing blood beneath the skin caused by an injury to a blood vessel

hot spot—a hot and reddened area of skin that has been irritated by friction

hyperhidrosis—excessive moisture

infection—condition in which a part of the body is invaded by a microorganism such as a bacteria or virus

ingrown toenail—when one or both sides of a toenail has grown into the flesh of the toe

inversion—movement of the foot as it rolls outward at the ankle

last—the form over which a shoe or boot is constructed

lateral—the outside of the foot, leg, or body

ligament—the strong, fibrous connective tissue at a joint that connects one bone to another bone

maceration—a breaking down or softening of skin tissue by extended exposure to moisture

mallet toes—toes that are contracted at the end joint only

medial—the inside of the foot, leg, or body

metatarsal—one of the five bones at the ball of the foot

metatarsalgia—pain somewhere underneath the metatarsal heads of the foot

mid-foot—the mid or center part of the foot, containing the arch and five metatarsal bones

Morton's neuroma—pain on the bottom of the foot, usually under the pad of the third or fourth toe

Morton's toe—a foot type where the second toe is longer than the big toe

neuroma—the swelling of a nerve due to an inflammation of the nerve or the tissue surrounding the nerve

NSAIDS—acronym for nonsteroidal anti-inflammatory drugs; used to control pain and swelling after an injury

orthopedist—an orthopedic surgeon specializing in the treatment and surgery of bones and joint injuries, diseases, and problems

orthotic—an insert made from a mold of the bottom of the foot that is then inserted into a shoe or boot to correct a foot abnormality

pedorthist—a specialist trained to work on the fit or modification of shoes and orthotics to alleviate foot problems caused by disease, overuse, or injury

peripheral neuropathy—a painful nerve condition that can manifest itself as a burning sensation in the feet

plantar—the bottom surface of the foot

plantar fascia—the band of fibers along the arch of the foot that connects the heel to the toes

plantar fasciitis—an inflammation of the plantar fascia

plantar warts—small, hard, flesh-colored, white, or pink granulated lumps typically found on the feet and caused by a virus

podiatrist—a doctor of podiatric medicine who specializes in the treatment and surgery of the foot and ankle

pronation—the rolling of the foot toward the inside of the body when weight bearing

Raynaud's syndrome—discomfort caused by a decreased blood supply to the fingers and toes

RICE—acronym for rest, ice, compression, and elevation; describes the typical treatment of sprain and strain injuries

sesamoiditis—an inflammation of the two little bones beneath the ball of the foot and under the joint that moves the big toe

sole—the bottom of the foot

sprain—a joint injury in which ligament damage is sustained

sterilization—the process by which bacteria is removed

strain—muscular injury produced by overuse or abuse of a muscle

stress fracture—typically a small crack in the outer shell of the affected bone caused by sudden or repetitive stress, usually from overuse without proper conditioning

subluxation—an incomplete or partial dislocation

subungual hematoma—a hematoma under the nail plate

supination—the rolling of the foot toward the outside of the body when weight bearing

tendinitis—an inflammation of a tendon or its surrounding sheath

tendon—the elastic tough fibrous tissue that connects muscles to bone

toe box—the front part of a shoe or boot that covers the toes

toenail fungus—nails that are thick and deformed, with a brown, white, or yellowish discoloration

transient paresthesia—a temporary nerve compression that can be caused by a gradual buildup of fluids in your feet during extended on-your-feet activity

trench foot—a serious nonfreezing cold injury that develops when the skin of the feet is exposed to a combination of moisture and cold for extended periods

turf toe—a condition of pain at the base of the big toe at the ball of the foot, usually caused from jamming the toe

ultrarunning—running distances greater than a marathon

virus—a tiny organism that causes disease

wart—a thickened, painful area of skin caused by a virus

Bibliography

Achilles Tendonitis: Prevention & Treatment. London: Peak Performance Publishing, 2002.

Copeland, Glen. *The Foot Book: Relief for Overused, Abused & Ailing Feet*. New York: John Wiley & Sons, 1992.

Davies, Clair, with Amber Davies. *The Trigger Point Therapy Workbook: Your Self-Treatment Guide for Pain Relief*. Oakland, CA: New Harbinger Publications, Inc., 2004.

Dobrowolski, Christine, DPM. *Those Aching Feet: Your Guide to Diagnosis and Treatment of Common Foot Problems (revised edition)*. San Francisco, CA: S.K.I. Publishing Co., 2005.

Ellis, Joe, DPM, with Joe Henderson. *Running Injury-Free*. Emmaus, PA: Rodale Press, 1994.

Egoscue, Pete, with Roger Gittines. *Pain Free: A Revolutionary Method for Stopping Chronic Pain*. New York: Bantam Books, 2000.

Jardine, Ray. *The Pacific Crest Trail Hiker's Handbook*. LaPine, OR: Adventure Lore Press, 1996 (out of print).

Jordan, Ryan, ed. *Lightweight Backpacking & Camping: A Field Guide to Wilderness Equipment, Technique, and Style*. Bozeman, MT: Beartooth Mountain Press, 2005.

Langer, Paul, DPM. *Great Feet for Life: Footcare and Footwear for Healthy Aging*. Minneapolis, MN: Fairview Press, 2007.

Levine, Suzanne M., MD. *My Feet Are Killing Me!* New York: McGraw-Hill Book Company, 1987 (out of print).

Maffetone, Philip, MD. *Fix Your Feet: Build the Best Foundation for Healthy, Pain-Free, Knees, Hips, and Spine*. Guilford, CT: Lyons Press, 2004.

McDougall, Christopher. *Born to Run: A Hidden Tribe, Superathletes, and the Greatest Race the World Has Never Seen*. New York: Alfred A. Knopf, 2009.

McGann, Daniel M., DPM, and L. R. Robinson. *The Doctor's Sore Foot Book*. New York: William Morrow and Company, Inc., 1991 (out of print).

Noakes, Tim, MD. *Lore of Running*, 4th ed. Champaign, IL: Human Kinetics, 2003.

O'Connor, Patrick L., MD, and Thomas M. Schaller, MD. *Footworks II: The Patient's Guide to the Foot and Ankle*. Portage, MI: privately printed, 2001.

Plotkin, Stuart, DPM. *The Hiking Engine: A Hiker's Guide to the Care and Maintenance of Feet and Legs.* Birmingham, AL: Menasha Ridge Press, 2001.

Salmans, Sandra. *Your Feet: Questions You Have . . . Answers You Need.* Allentown, PA: People's Medical Society, 1998 (out of print).

Schneider, Myles J., DPM, and Mark D. Sussman, DPM. *How to Doctor Your Feet Without a Doctor.* Washington, DC: Acropolis Books, Ltd., 1984 (out of print).

Subotnick, Steven I., DPM, MS. *The Running Foot Doctor.* San Francisco: World Publications, 1977 (out of print).

——. *Sports & Exercise Injuries: Conventional, Homeopathic & Alternative Treatments.* Berkeley, CA: North Atlantic Books, 1991.

Taliaferro Blauvelt, Carolyn, and Fred R. T. Nelson. *A Manual of Orthopaedic Terminology,* 6th ed., St. Louis: Mosby, 1998.

Tremain, David M., MD, and Elias M. Awad, PhD. *The Foot & Ankle Sourcebook,* 2nd ed. Lincolnwood, IL: NTC/Contemporary Books Publishing Group, Inc., 1998.

Trolan, William, MD. *Blister Fighter Guide.* Seattle: Outdoor Research, 1996 (out of print).

Weisenfeld, Murry F., MD, with Barbara Burr. *The Runner's Repair Manual.* New York: St. Martin's Press, 1980 (out of print).

About the Author

John Vonhof brings a varied background and extensive experience to *Fixing Your Feet*. This fifth edition, which he wrote and illustrated, is the synthesis of 30 years of experience as a runner and hiker.

His popular website **www.fixing yourfeet.com** is dedicated to providing articles, resources, links, and a blog about foot care, and it serves to inform and educate athletes about all that's new in foot care and to provide foot care advice.

Other medical professionals recognize John's expertise too. In 2009 he was the lead author of a chapter on foot injuries in the textbook *Expedition and Wilderness Medicine* (Cambridge University Press).

A runner since 1982, John discovered trail running and ultras in 1984. He has completed more than 20 ultras: 50Ks, 50-milers, 100-milers, 24-hour runs, and a 72-hour run. He completed the difficult Western States 100-mile

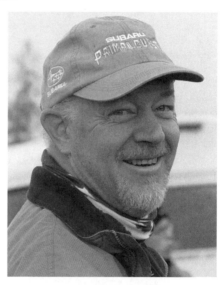

John Vonhof

Endurance Run three times and the Santa Rosa 24-Hour and 12-Hour Track Runs 12 times. In 1987, with fellow runner Will Uher, John fastpacked the 211-mile John Muir Trail in the Sierra Nevada in 8½ days, carrying a 30-pound pack.

As the Ohlone Wilderness 50K Trail Run race director for 15 years, John worked at providing a quality event for runners of all skill levels who participated in this arduous trail ultra.

In 1992 John changed careers, becoming a paramedic, orthopedic technician, and emergency room technician. He now works for an emergency medical services agency in the San Francisco Bay Area as a prehospital care coordinator.

Over the years John has provided volunteer medical aid at numerous sporting events around the world, patching feet, training medical staffs and interested athletes, and providing advice to thousands of athletes. He continues to be sought out for his expertise and experience in providing answers to foot care questions.

Index

A

accommodator orthotics, 290, 296
Achilles Healer, 282
Achilles tendinitis, 278
  exercises, 281
  treating, 279
Achillotrain, 282
aching feet, 195
Acorn Fleece Socks, 103
Activewraps, 339
Adhesive Felt, 241
Adventure Medical Kits, 344
Aetrex Full-Length Anti-Shox
  Sports Orthotics, 148
aging feet, 52
All Terrain's Therapeutic Foot
  Rub, 164
American Academy of
  Orthopaedic Surgeons, 350
American Academy of Podiatric
  Sports Medicine, 350
American Chiropractors
  Association, 350
American Massage Therapy
  Association, 350
American Orthopaedic Foot and
  Ankle Society, 350
American Orthotics and
  Prosthetics Association, 350
American Physical Therapy
  Association, 350
American Podiatric Medical
  Association, 350
Andrew Lovy's formula, 120
Angelfeet Pedicure Files, 330
ankle
  strengthening exercises, 264
  support products, 266
  supports, 262
  tendon injuries, 283
  tendons, 282
  wrapping, 260
Ankle Stabilizing Orthosis
  (ASO), 266

antifungal medications, 311
antiperspirants, 124
Aquaphor Healing Ointment,
  120, 164
Archcrafters CustomComfort
  Insoles, 48
Asics Chafe Free Endurance
  Gel, 120
Asics Chafe Free Powder, 118, 126
ASTYM, 278
athlete's foot, 326
athletic trainers, 22
Avon Silicone Glove, 120

B

Backpacker Magazine, 349
Bag Balm, 120, 335
Balega International Socks, 103
Band-Aid
  Advanced Healing Blister
    Cushions, 246
  Single-Step Liquid Bandage, 246
Ban Roll-On, 126
barefoot running, 76
  avoiding injuries, 83
  books, 92
  function and form, 80
  goals, 90
  precautions, 81
  science on, 79
  tips, 84
  tips to getting started, 90
  websites, 92
barefooted.com, 92
barefooters.org, 93
barefootrunning.com, 92
barefootrunning.fas.harvard.edu, 93
barefootrunninguniversity.com, 92
Baysix Socks, 103
Benadryl Cream, 335
Betadine, 190
big toe problems, 304
Biofreeze, 338
biomechanics, 34

avoiding problems, 37
form and health, 39
gait, 39
birthdayshoes.com, 89, 92
black toenails and electrolytes, 171
Blister Bomber Lubricant, 121
Blister Guard Socks, 98
blisters, 228
 advanced blister patching,
  241, 246
 antiperspirants, 126
 basic blister-care products, 241
 basic repair, 237
 beyond blisters, 254
 blood, 203, 239
 deep blisters, 253
 and dehydration, 160
 draining, 203, 239
 eliminate the problem, 228
 extreme blister patching, 245
 extreme blister prevention, 245
 general care, 236
 hot spots, 229
 patching, 203
 post-event care, 204, 256
 preparation, 11, 202, 218
 preventing infection, 240
 reactive, 225
 taping, 129, 203
 tips on managing, 202
 types of, 235
 under a callus, 253
 understanding, 233
 what changed?, 12
Blistershield Powder, 118
Blist-O-Ban Blister Patches, 246
Bodyglide and Footglide Foot
 Formula, 121
Bodyglide Liquified Powder, 118
Boudreaux's Butt Paste, 178
Brave Soldier Antiseptic Healing
 Ointment, 241, 344
Brave Soldier's Friction Zone, 121
Bridgedale Socks, 103
Bromi-Lotion, 126
Bromi-Talc Powder, 118
Bunga
 Gel Heel Cups, 290, 296
 Oval Pads and Gel Pads, 331

Toe Pads and Toe Caps,
 142, 246
Bunheads Gel Toecaps, 142, 232,
 246, 307
Bunion Aid, 317
bunionette, 315
bunions, 315
bursitis, 284
Burt's Bees
 Coconut Foot Cream, 164
 Rescue Ointment, 335

C
calluses, 327
callus file, 329
capillaritis, 334
Certain Dri Feet, 126
changing your shoes and
 socks, 171
chiropractors, 23
Chi Running, 82
Cho-Pat's
 Achilles Tendon Strap, 282
 Ankle Support, 266
Chris Kock's Secret Formula, 121
claw toes, 305
Coban, 246
cold and wet, 176
cold therapy, 336
cold therapy and heat
 combination, 338
compounds for the feet, 117
compound tincture of benzoin,
 124, 202, 242
conditioning products, 38
Contour Pak, 339
corns, 331
cortisone injections, 275, 286
Count'r-Force Arch Brace, 290
Cramer Heel Cups, 291, 296
Cramer Tuf-Skin, 124
crew support, 197
Crocs, 67
Cropper Medical's Bio Skin, 266
Cryocup, 339
Cryo-Max Reusable Cold
 Packs, 339
custom shoes, 69
CW-X Compression Socks, 103

D

Dahlgren Socks, 103
Darn Tough Vermont Socks, 103
Defeet Socks, 103
dehydration and blisters, 160
dehydration, hydration, and
    sodium, 160
delayed pressure urticaria, 335
Desitin Maximum Strength
    Original Paste, 122, 178
Dirty Girl Gaiters, 154
dislocations, 271
dorsiflexion, 36
Dr. Scholl's
    Blister Treatment, 247
    Ultra Overnight Foot
        Cream, 164
Drymax Socks, 98, 103, 117
Drysol Solution, 126
duct tape, 131, 136
Duenorth All Purpose Traction
    Aid, 184
Duoderm CGF Flexible Sterile
    Dressing, 247

E

Eastern Mountain Sports
    Gaiters, 154
Easy Laces, 160
E-Caps Endurolytes, 170
Elastikon Tape, 131, 136
electrolyte balance, 171
electrolytes and black toenails, 171
endoscopic plantar fasciotomy, 288
Endurafix Tape, 131
Endurasports Tape, 131
Enduro-Sole Insoles, 72
ENGO
    Blister Relief Kit, 344
    Cushion Heel Wrap, 280, 282
    Patches, 142, 235, 242, 247,
        282, 317, 330
Epsom salts, 256
Equinox Gaiters, 154
eucalyptus oil, 312, 327
eversion, 36
Extracorporeal Shock-Wave
    Therapies, 288
extreme conditions, 174
    cold and wet, 176
    frostbite, 181
    heat, 185
    immersion foot, 180
    jungle rot, 189
    maceration, 177
    sand, 187
    snow and ice, 182
    trench foot, 180
EZ Runner Orthotic, 148

F

FabriFoam Anklewrap, 266
feet
    aging, 26
    arch types, 48
    conditioning, 32
    flat-arched, 48
    golden rule for, 6
    high-arched, 48
    know your, 47
    normal-arched, 48
    related websites, 351
Feetures Socks, 103
fissures, 329, 332
fit, 43
    components of a good, 50
    fitting insoles, 44
    tips for a good, 52
fixingyourfeet.com, 351, 361
flaxseed oil, 164
Flexi Care Transparent
    Bandages, 247
Flex-Power Sports Cream, 338
foot care
    are your feet prepared, 9
    for athletes, 201
    basics, 7, 25
    daily ritual, 24
    event kit, 343
    kits, 199, 202, 204, 340
    self-education, 8
    team, 201
Footfix Insoles, 72
Footherapy Natural Mineral Foot
    Bath, 164
Footsmart, 164, 306, 309, 317,
    318, 320, 330, 347
foot solution, 127

footwear
anatomy of, 58
brand loyalty, 57
buying, 45
customizing your, 53
donating, 59
drying your, 178
minimalist, 76
modifying, 193
tossing shoes and boots, 59
forefoot problems, 315
4 Desert Gaiters, 154
Fox River Socks, 103
fractures, 268
treating, 269
types of, 268
Fresh Force, 173
frostbite, 181

G
gait, 39
gaiters, 150, 187
custom-made, 151
making your own, 151
repairing gaiter straps, 152
Gillette Clinical Strength
Antiperspirant, 126
Glaciergel Blister and Burn
Dressings, 247
Gold Bond Powder, 118, 127
Gorilla Glue, 151, 250

H
Haglund's deformity, 296
hammertoes, 305
Hand Sense, 127, 164
Hapad, 142, 147, 306, 318, 320,
330, 331
Arch Pads, 291, 296
Comf-Orthotic Insoles, 72
Dancer Pads, 314, 321
Heel Pads and Cushions,
291, 296
Orthotics, 148
Three-Quarter–Length Heel
Wedges, 282
Toe Caps and Jelly Tips, 307
Tongue Cushions, 160

heat
and cold combination, 338
conditions, 185
rash, 101
therapy, 336
Heel Hugger, 296
heel-pain syndrome, 294
Heel Smoother Pro, 164,
329, 330
heel spurs, 294
hiking boots, 64
buying, 67
hiking socks, 100
Holey Soles, 67
hot spots, 229
howtorunbarefoot.com, 92
hydration
dehydration and sodium, 160
and electrolytes, 170
Hydropel Sports Ointment,
122, 178
Hypafix Tape, 131
hyperkeratosis, 328

I
IcyHot, 338
immersion foot, 180
infection, 240
Injinji Socks, 98, 103
Inov-8, 87, 93
Debri Gaiter, 154
Debrisock, 154
insoles, 72, 145
Dryz Insoles, 127
fitting, 44
Instant Krazy Glue, 249
International Chiropractic
Association, 350
intractable plantar keratosis
(IPK), 328
inversion, 36
invisibleshoe.com, 92

J
Joetrailman Gaiters, 154
Johnson & Johnson's No More
Rash, 165
jungle rot, 189

K

Kahtoola Microspikes, 184
Kallassy Ankle Support, 266
Kastner Tracktion Soles, 184
Kathy's Family Foot Balm,
    165, 330
Keen Footwear, 71
Kerasal Ultra 20 Extra Strength
    Foot Cream, 165
Kinesio Tex Tape, 131, 132,
    135, 242
Kinesys Sport's Soothing Foot
    Spray, 165
Kiwi's Camp Dry, 177
KT Tape, 132

L

lace locks, 160
Lace-Stick, 160
lacing
    methods, 157
    options, 156
    products, 160
    tips, 157
lanolin cream, 122
Leukotape P Tape, 131
Liquicell Blister Bands, 247
Lock-Laces, 160
Lorpen Socks, 103
lubricants, 119
    products, 120
Lynco Biomechanical Orthotic
    System, 149, 291
Lysol, 164, 173

M

maceration, 177
mallet toes, 305
manuka oil, 312, 327, 335
Marathon & Beyond Magazine,
    349
massage
    active release techniques, 168
    deep-tissue muscle, 168
    foot, 167
    products, 169
    self, 168
    therapists, 23
Mastisol, 124

McDavid Ice Bag Wrap, 339
Medco Sports Medicine, 347
medical specialist, 21
    and footwear specialists, 350
Medipore Tape, 132
metatarsalgia, 317
Microfoam Tape, 132
Micropore Tape, 131
minimalist footwear, 76
    choices, 85
    value of, 78
    websites, 92
Mini Tightrope, 316
moccasin foot, 326
moleskin, 237, 241
Montbell Stretch Gaiters, 155
Morton's neuroma, 318
Morton's toe, 308
Mountain Hardwear Gaiters, 155
Mueller Tuffner Clear Spray, 124
multiday
    blister tips, 203
    events, 174, 191, 194

N

National Athletic Trainers'
    Association, 350
needles, 250
neuroma, 318
Neutrogena Foot Cream, 165
New-Skin, 247
    Liquid Bandage, 125
Newton Running, 77, 87, 93
N'Ice Stretch Night Splint
    Suspension System, 283, 291
night splint, 280, 287
NSAIDS, 259
numb toes and feet, 322

O

Odor-Eaters Foot Powder, 118, 127
off with the toes, 193
onychomycosis, 310
OPTP (Orthopedic Physical
    Therapy Products), 38, 267
orthopedists, 21
Orthosole Insoles, 72
orthotics, 143, 287
    custom-made, 145

getting, 145
over-the-counter, 147
patient compliance, 146
using your, 147
orthotripsy, 288
Outdoor Research Gaiters, 155
Outside Magazine, 349
Oxysocks Compression Socks, 103

P

papillomavirus, 333
Patagonia Socks, 104
pedicures, 165
Pedifix Visco-Gel Toe Caps, 247
Pedorthic Footwear
    Association, 350
pedorthists, 22, 53
Peet Dryer, 178
Pepsom salts, 256
Perform 78 Lateral Ankle
    Stabilizer, 267
peripheral neuropathy, 323
peroneal tendons, 282
PF Night Splint, 291
physical therapists, 22
plantar fasciitis, 284, 290
    stretching exercises for, 288
    treating, 285
plantar fibromas, 293
plantar flexion, 36
plantar warts, 332
podiatrists, 21
Point6 Socks, 104
porokeratotic cyst, 333
Pose Running, 82
posterior tibial tendon, 283
powders, 117
PowerSox Socks, 104
PowerStep Insoles, 72, 149,
    291, 297
Pretty Feet & Hands Ultra
    Moisturizing Cream, 165
preventing infection, 240
prevention, 109
    components of, 112
    finding the right combination,
        115
    running injury, 109
prickly heat rash, 335

proactive, 111
proprioception, 262
Prostretch, 283, 292
Pro-Tec
    Ankle Wrap, 267
    Ice-Up Portable Ice Massager,
        339
    Toe Caps, 142, 247
providing foot care for
    athletes, 201
PSC-Pronation/Spring Control
    Strap, 292, 297
pump bump, 297

R

Raceready Trail Gaiters, 155
rashes, 334
Raynaud's syndrome, 324
REI
    Desert Gaiters, 155
    Socks and Rocky Gore-Tex
        Oversocks, 104
    Trail Gaiters, 155
Relaimed Elastic Tape, 132
retrocalcaneal bursitis, 297
RICE treatment, 259
rocker boards, 38, 263, 267
RockTape, 132
rubbing alcohol, 125
runbare.com, 93
Runner's World Magazine, 349
running shoes, 59
    buying, 61
    construction, 60
    last patterns, 60
    socks, 100
Running Times Magazine, 349
RXSorbo Insoles, 73

S

sandals, 70
sand conditions, 187
SealSkinz Socks, 104
Seirus Stormsocks, 104
self care for your feet, 162
sesamoiditis, 320
Shockblockers Insoles, 72
Shock Doctor Footbeds, 73
shoe deodorizer, 173

Shoelace Book, The, 156
shoes vs. minimalist footwear, 77
Sigvaris Athletic Recovery
    Compression Socks, 104
skin
    products, 164
    toughening agents, 121, 124
skin disorders, 326
Skin Lube, 122
SkinMD Natural, 165, 330
Skin-On-Skin, 247
Skins Compression Socks, 104
Slant Board, 283
SmartKnitActive Socks, 104
SmartWool Socks, 104
snow and ice conditions, 182
Soapy Soles, 162
socks, 94
    buying, 99
    compression, 101
    fibers and construction, 96
    going sockless, 105
    high-technology oversocks, 101
    liners, 100
    products, 103
    putting on your, 94
    tossing, 95
sodium, hydration, and
    dehydration, 160
Sof Sole
    Insoles, 73
    Socks, 104
Sole Custom Footbeds, 73, 149
Sorbothane Performance Insoles, 73
Speed Laces, 160
Spenco
    Adhesive Knit, 248
    Arch Supports, 149
    Cushions, 292, 297
    Insoles, 73
    Metatarsal Arch Cushion,
        318, 320
    Pressure Pads, 241
    2nd Skin, 242
    2nd Skin Blister Kit, 344
    2nd Skin Blister Pads, 248
    2nd Skin Dressings, 248
    Sport Blister Pads, 248
SportSlick, 123

sports medicine doctors, 22
SportsShield, 122
sports shoes, 62
Sportwax, 123
sprains, 257
    treating a, 259
Spyroflex, 249
Stabilicer Sports, 184
StaphAseptic, 241
Stick, The, 169
strain, 257
    treating a, 259
Strassburg Sock, 292
stress fractures, 269
Stretch-EZ, 283
Stromgren Ankle Wraps, 267
Stuffitts Shoe Savers, 178
Succeed! Buffer/Electrolyte
    Caps, 170
Superfeet Insoles, 73
Super Glue, 250
Super Salve, 344
sweat gland, 333
syringes, 250

T
tape adherents, 121, 124
taping
    alternative products, 142
    application, 134
    ball of the foot, 138
    between the toe and foot,
        141
    for blisters, 129
    bottom of the foot, 138
    feet, 137
    removing the tape, 135
    sides and bottom of the heel,
        140
    sides of the foot, 139
    skin preparation, 133
    techniques, 135
    toes, 140
    types of tapes, 131
tailor's bunions, 315
teamwork and crew support, 197
tea tree oil, 312, 327, 335
Teko Socks, 104
tendinitis, 273

tendinosis, 273
tendon
    Achilles, 278
    ankle, 282
    how they heal, 276
    injuries, 273
    injuries, treating, 274
    peroneal, 282
    posterior tibial, 283
terraplana.com, 93
Teva Sandals, 71
ThermaCare Air-Activated
    HeatWraps, 339
Thermoskin Plantar FXT, 292
Thermotabs, 170
therunningbarefoot.com, 93
thesockcompany.com, 100
Thorlos Socks, 104
Tineacide Antifungal Shoe
    Spray, 165
tinea pedis, 326
toes
    clenching your, 301
    little toe triangle, 14
    overlapping, 309
    problems, 299
    strengthening, 299
    stubbed, 309
    turf, 314
toenails, 299
    black, 300
    black and electrolytes, 171
    blood blisters under, 301
    fungus, 310
    ingrown, 307
    laser treatments, 312
    treating black, 302
    trimming, 13, 299
Topaz MicroDebrider, 276, 288
Torex Premium Thermal Medical
    Devices, 339
TP Massage Footballer, Baller
    Block, and Massage Balls, 283,
    292, 297
traction products, 184
Trail Runner Magazine, 349
transient paresthesia, 322
Traumeel, 259, 288
trench foot, 180

trigger point therapy, 277
Tripos Labs' Hydrostat, 165
TriSlide, 123
Tuf-Foot, 125
Tuli's, 297
2XU Compression socks, 103

U
Udder Balm, 123
Ultimate Shoelaces, 160
UltraRunning Magazine, 349

V
Vaseline, 123
Vibram FiveFingers, 76, 85
vibramfivefingers.com, 93
Vicks VapoRub, 164, 312
Viscoped Insoles, 292, 297, 318,
    320, 321
Vogel's Homeopathic 7 Herb
    Cream, 165

W
Waldies, 67
waterproof socks, 102
Wigwam Socks, 98, 104
wobble boards, 38, 263, 267
wrapping an ankle, 260
WrightSock, 104

X
Xeroform Petrolatum Gauze
    Dressing, 249
X-Socks, 104

Y
Yaktrax Pro, 184
Yankz Sure Lace System, 160

Z
Zeasorb Powder, 118, 127
Zim's Crack Cream, 165, 330
zinc oxide, 242, 245
zombierunner.com, 131, 344, 347